The Reticuloendothelial System

A COMPREHENSIVE TREATISE

Volume 6
Immunology

The Reticuloendothelial System

A COMPREHENSIVE TREATISE

General Editors:
Herman Friedman, *University of South Florida, Tampa, Florida*
Mario Escobar, *Medical College of Virginia, Richmond, Virginia*
and
Sherwood M. Reichard, *Medical College of Georgia, Augusta, Georgia*

MORPHOLOGY
Edited by Ian Carr and W. T. Daems

BIOCHEMISTRY AND METABOLISM
Edited by Anthony J. Sbarra and Robert R. Strauss

PHYLOGENY AND ONTOGENY
Edited by Nicholas Cohen and M. Michael Sigel

IMMUNOPATHOLOGY
Edited by Noel R. Rose and Benjamin V. Siegel

CANCER
Edited by Ronald B. Herberman and Herman Friedman

IMMUNOLOGY
Edited by Joseph A. Bellanti and Herbert B. Herscowitz

PHYSIOLOGY (In two parts)
Edited by Sherwood M. Reichard and James P. Filkins

PHARMACOLOGY
Edited by John Hadden and Andor Szentivanyi

HYPERSENSITIVITY
Edited by S. Michael Phillips and Peter Abramoff

INFECTION
Edited by John P. Utz and Mario R. Escobar

The Reticuloendothelial System

A COMPREHENSIVE TREATISE

Volume 6
Immunology

Edited by

JOSEPH A. BELLANTI

Georgetown University School of Medicine
Washington, D.C.

and

HERBERT B. HERSCOWITZ

Georgetown University Schools of Medicine and Dentistry
Washington, D.C.

Springer Science+Business Media, LLC

Library of Congress Cataloging in Publication Data

Main entry under title:

The Reticuloendothelial system.

Includes bibliographies and indexes.
CONTENTS: v. 1. Carr, I., Daems, W. T., and Lobo, A. Morphology.—v. 2. Biochemistry and metabolism.—[etc.]—v. 6. Immunology.
1. Reticulo-endothelial system. 2. Macrophages. I. Friedman, Herman, 1931– . II. Escobar, Mario R. III. Reichard, Sherwood M. [DNLM: 1. Reticuloendothelial system. WH650 R437]
QP115.R47 591.2′95 79-25933

ISBN 978-1-4757-6786-5 ISBN 978-1-4757-6784-1 (eBook)
DOI 10.1007/978-1-4757-6784-1

Originally published by Plenum Press, New York in 1984.
Softcover reprint of the hardcover 1st edition 1984

Contributors

STEPHEN W. CHENSUE • Department of Pathology, University of Michigan Medical School, Ann Arbor, Michigan

DIANE E. COLE • Pediatric Branch, National Cancer Institute, Bethesda, Maryland

PETER ERB • Institute for Microbiology and Hygiene, The University of Basel, Basel, Switzerland

JOSEPH C. FANTONE • Department of Pathology, University of Michigan Medical School, Ann Arbor, Michigan

MARC FELDMANN • Imperial Cancer Research Fund, Tumour Immunology Unit, Department of Zoology, University College London, London, England

RAYMOND B. HESTER • Division of Immunology, St. Jude Children's Research Hospital, Memphis, Tennessee

RICHARD HONG • Department of Pediatrics, University of Wisconsin Clinical Science Center, Madison, Wisconsin

ARTHUR G. JOHNSON • Department of Microbiology and Immunology, The University of Minnesota, Duluth, Minnesota

DAVID R. KATZ • Imperial Cancer Research Fund, Tumour Immunology Unit, Department of Zoology, University College London, London, England

STEVEN L. KUNKEL • Department of Pathology, University of Michigan Medical School, Ann Arbor, Michigan

THOMAS R. MALEK • Laboratory of Immunology, National Institute of Allergy and Infectious Diseases, National Institutes of Health, Bethesda, Maryland

MICHAEL E. MILLER • Department of Pediatrics, University of California at Davis School of Medicine, Davis, California

SIMON L. NEWMAN • Division of Rheumatology–Immunology, Department of Medicine, and Department of Microbiology–Immunology, University of North Carolina, Chapel Hill, North Carolina

RICHARD P. PHIPPS • Department of Microbiology and Immunology, Medical College of Virginia, Virginia Commonwealth University, Richmond, Virginia

CARL W. PIERCE • Department of Pathology and Laboratory Medicine, The Jewish Hospital of St. Louis, and Department of Pathology and of Microbiology and Immunology, Washington University School of Medicine, St. Louis, Missouri

DAVID G. POPLACK • Pediatric Branch, National Cancer Institute, Bethesda, Maryland

PETER RALPH • Memorial Sloan–Kettering Cancer Center, Rye, New York

ROSS ROCKLIN • Allergy Division, Department of Medicine, New England Medical Center, Tufts University School of Medicine, Boston, Massachusetts

GORDON D. ROSS • Division of Rheumatology–Immunology, Department of Medicine, and Department of Microbiology–Immunology, University of North Carolina, Chapel Hill, North Carolina

STUART F. SCHLOSSMAN • Division of Tumor Immunology, Dana-Farber Cancer Institute, and Department of Medicine, Harvard Medical School, Boston, Massachusetts

JON R. SCHMIDTKE • Department of Immunology Research, Lilly Research Laboratories, Indianapolis, Indiana

RICHARD M. SCHULTZ • Department of Immunology Research, Lilly Research Laboratories, Indianapolis, Indiana

ETHAN M. SHEVACH • Laboratory of Immunology, National Institute of Allergy and Infectious Diseases, National Institutes of Health, Bethesda, Maryland

USHA SRINIVASAN • Pediatric Branch, National Cancer Institute, Bethesda, Maryland

HENRY C. STEVENSON • Clinical Investigations Section, Biologic Response Modifiers Program, National Cancer Institute, National Institutes of Health, Frederick, Maryland

GEOFFREY H. SUNSHINE • Imperial Cancer Research Fund, Tumour Immunology Unit, Department of Zoology, University College London, London, England

JOHN G. TEW • Department of Microbiology and Immunology, Medical College of Virginia, Virginia Commonwealth University, Richmond, Virginia

ROBERT F. TODD, III • Division of Tumor Immunology, Dana-Farber Cancer Institute, and Department of Medicine, Harvard Medical School, Boston, Massachusetts

WILLIAM S. WALKER • Division of Immunology, St. Jude Children's Research Hospital, Memphis, Tennessee

PETER A. WARD • Department of Pathology, University of Michigan Medical School, Ann Arbor, Michigan

DAVID D. WOOD • Department of Immunology, Ayerst Research Laboratories, Princeton, New Jersey

Foreword

This comprehensive treatise on the reticuloendothelial system is a project jointly shared by individual members of the Reticuloendothelial (RE) Society and biomedical scientists in general who are interested in the intricate system of cells and molecular moieties derived from those cells which constitute the RES. It may now be more fashionable in some quarters to consider these cells as part of what is called the mononuclear phagocytic system or the lymphoreticular system. Nevertheless, because of historical developments and current interest in the subject by investigators from many diverse areas, it seems advantageous to present in one comprehensive treatise current information and knowledge concerning basic aspects of the RES, such as morphology, biochemistry, phylogeny and ontogeny, physiology, and pharmacology as well as clinical areas including immunopathology, cancer, infectious diseases, allergy, and hypersensitivity. It is anticipated that by presenting information concerning these apparently heterogeneous topics under the unifying umbrella of the RES attention will be focused on the similarities as well as interactions among the cell types constituting the RES from the viewpoint of various disciplines. The treatise editors and their editorial board, consisting predominantly of the editors of individual volumes, are extremely grateful for the enthusiastic cooperation and enormous task undertaken by members of the biomedical community in general and especially by members of the American as well as European and Japanese Reticuloendothelial Societies. The assistance, cooperation, and great support from the editorial staff of Plenum Press are also valued greatly. It is hoped that this unique treatise, the first to offer a fully comprehensive treatment of our knowledge concerning the RES, will provide a unified framework for evaluating what is known and what still has to be investigated in this actively growing field. The various volumes of this treatise provide extensive in-depth and integrated information on classical as well as experimental aspects of the RES. It is expected that these volumes will serve as a major reference for day-to-day examination of various subjects dealing with the RES from many different viewpoints.

Herman Friedman
Mario R. Escobar
Sherwood M. Reichard

Preface

This sixth volume of a multivolume treatise on the reticuloendothelial system presents the pivotal role of the mononuclear phagocyte in immunological processes. The volume is poised in a transitional location in the series and builds upon knowledge set forth in previous volumes and directs the reader to discussions of clinical immunology and immunopathology to be found in subsequent volumes.

Throughout each of its chapters, the book maintains a fidelity to the central role of the macrophage as a regulatory cell in immunologic processes. The volume begins with a general overview of the immunobiology of the macrophage and its interactions with lymphoid cells. Included in this chapter is a discussion of disorders of macrophage function which provides a basis for an understanding of host resistance mechanisms. The volume progresses in logical sequence to a discussion of the role of macrophages in nonspecific processes and describes the mechanisms by which macrophages function in host defense. This chapter reviews clinical abnormalities as they reflect upon "nonspecific" functions and also focuses on important studies of phagocytic cell function in the human neonate, underscoring critical roles of the immature phagocytic cell in the predisposition of the neonate to infection. The heterogeneity of macrophages is discussed in the next chapter which describes the functional diversity of macrophages obtained from different tissues as well as individual differences in macrophages obtained from the same tissue. The chapter also poses a provocative question concerning whether heterogeneity represents differences in maturation of a single cell type or whether it is the result of the existence of separate populations of cells. The use of macrophage cell lines is presented in the next chapter which establishes the role of surface antigens in differentiation and function of macrophages, the cytotoxic capacity of macrophage cell lines, the inductive events in pharmacologic regulation, and the importance of macrophage function in variant lines. This chapter will be of particular importance to the investigator interested in studying the macrophage in relatively homogeneous populations. This is followed by a discussion of the function of dendritic cells in immune responses in the next chapter. It reviews the importance of cells with dendritic morphology and their role in such diverse functions as antigen retention in lymphoid tissue, in mixed lymphocyte reactions, and in T-cell-mediated cytotoxicity. Of particular interest in this chapter is a discussion of the Langerhans cell and its specific function in delayed-type reactions of the skin.

The volume next focuses on a relatively new area of immunologic research in which the use of monoclonal antibodies has found application in the characterization of monocyte-macrophage differentiation antigens. Monoclonal antibody technology, extremely useful for the characterization of surface antigens on lymphoid cells, finds application to the characterization of macrophage elements in both circulating monocytes as well as tissue macrophages and allows the identification of antigens which distinguish members of the monocyte-macrophage lineage.

The role of mononuclear phagocytes as accessory cells in lymphocyte responses is discussed in the next chapter. Both cell-bound Ia antigens on membranes of these cells as well as soluble factors produced by mononuclear phagocytes are described. Next, the role of the macrophage in T-helper cell induction is reviewed and the important role of the macrophage in up-regulation of the immune response through its interaction with T-helper cells is described. The importance of antigen-specific factors produced by macrophages in T-helper cell induction as well as factors which act nonspecifically is also reviewed. The next chapter includes a discussion of the role of macrophages in the processing and presentation of protein antigens to T lymphocytes and reviews the evidence for antigen "processing" by macrophages, the role of antiantigen antibody on T-cell antigen recognition, the role of the nature of the protein antigen in T-cell reactivity, and the critical dependence of antigen concentration on the macrophage cell surface. The volume next progresses to a discussion of the requirement for macrophages in primary and secondary humoral responses. This chapter also includes a discussion of the role of Ia molecules in antigen presentation to responding T cells and B cells. The role of critical membrane receptors for complement and IgG molecules is presented in the next chapter which also describes the complex interactions of the complement system, antibody, and macrophages. The generation of extracellular proteases and their effects on the conversion of plasminogen into plasmin is also described. Presented next is a chapter discussing antigen-nonspecific factors elaborated by macrophages which stimulate lymphocytes. Included in this chapter is a critical discussion of interleukin-1. The chapter stresses the molecular heterogeneity of biologically active proteins secreted by the monocyte-macrophage and points out the need for further isolation and characterization of putatively distinct monokines. The chapter ends with a provocative conclusion that monokines and lymphokines may be the hormones of the inflammatory response and, as in classical endocrinology, these new "hormones" may be regulated by complex feedback loops. The next chapter describes the lymphocyte mediators, i.e., lymphokines that modulate the behavior of macrophages, and reviews the nature of these molecules. This chapter again points out the critical importance of these substances which have marked biological effects on a variety of cell types including T and B lymphocytes, macrophages, eosinophils, basophils, and neutrophils. The volume next progresses to the role of prostaglandins in macrophage function and points out the critical elements of macrophage activation, granulomatous inflammatory reaction, and the possibility that prostaglandins, particularly those of the E series, may play an important role in the modulation of macrophage-dependent inflammatory reactions. The suggestion that the prostaglandins may function as suppressors of tissue destruction and regulators of fibrotic reactions is an intriguing possibility and should provide fertile ground for future investigations in this area. This is followed by a chapter which discusses monocyte-mediated antibody-dependent cellular cytotoxicity and reviews the functions of the macrophage not only from the standpoint of their classical role in removal of debris, antigen processing, antimicrobial resistance, antineoplastic activity, mediation of inflammation, control of granulopoiesis in regulation of the immune response, but also their role in cytotoxic activity functions which are believed to be significant in host resistance to infection, tumor rejection, and certain "autoimmune" reactions. This chapter discusses primarily the antibody-dependent cellular cytotoxicity reactions mediated by viable functionally capable monocytes or macrophages as well as the clinical significance of these events in disease processes.

The volume ends with a review of the role of macrophages in immunopotentiation by adjuvants. This chapter describes up-regulation of macrophages by substances commonly referred to as adjuvants, and describes the mechanisms of stimulation of macrophages including intracellular biochemical pathways as well as the release of extracellular products.

The volume thus sets the stage for discussions of models of drug therapy, potential uses in tumor immunotherapy, and the exciting possibilities of altering immunologically mediated diseases such as allergy, autoimmunity, and malignancy through up-regulation or down-regulation of this important cell type.

Joseph A. Bellanti
Herbert B. Herscowitz

Contents

3. The Functional Heterogeneity of Macrophages

William S. Walker and Raymond B. Hester

4. Differentiation and Functional Regulation in Macrophage Cell Lines

Peter Ralph

5. Immune Functions of Dendritic-Type Cells

JOHN G. TEW and RICHARD P. PHIPPS

6. Utilization of Monoclonal Antibodies in the Characterization of Monocyte-Macrophage Differentiation Antigens

ROBERT F. TODD, III, and STUART F. SCHLOSSMAN

10. Requirement for Macrophages in Primary and Secondary Humoral Responses

CARL W. PIERCE

11. Regulation of Macrophage Functions by Complement, Complement Receptors, and IgG-Fc Receptors

GORDON D. ROSS and SIMON L. NEWMAN

12. Antigen-Nonspecific Factors Elaborated by Macrophages Which Stimulate Lymphocytes: Interleukin-1

David D. Wood

13. Lymphocyte Mediators That Modulate the Behavior of Macrophages

Ross Rocklin

14. Role of Prostaglandins in Macrophage Cell Function

Steven L. Kunkel, Stephen W. Chensue, Joseph C. Fantone, and Peter A. Ward

1

Immunobiology of the Macrophage

RICHARD HONG

1. INTRODUCTION

For years relegated to a position of second-class citizenship as a lowly scavenger devoid of the sophisticated recognition and control mechanisms of lymphocytes, the macrophage has now come into its own. The publication of this volume on the immunology of the reticuloendothelial system (RES) represents the acquisition of a long-deserved position of status among the cellular elite. We now appreciate that in immune reactions the macrophage takes advantage of its ability to interact with antigens nonspecifically, but then imposes profound restrictions upon future specific antigen-dependent reactions. Not only does the macrophage play a key role in initiating an immune reaction, but subsequent modulation of the host response is affected by macrophages. Additionally, macrophages form a major bulwark of host defense mechanisms through their ability to affect inflammation, directly kill microbes, and augment cytolytic lymphocytes. The protean manifestations of macrophage functions in the immune responses are considered in this volume. The purpose of this chapter is to provide a brief overview of the macrophage role in immunity. Detailed and exhaustive treatments of specific topics will be found in the other chapters of this volume. The major areas touched upon here are general characteristics of the monocyte-macrophage systems, lymphocyte interactions, macrophage killing, secretion, ontogeny, and human disorders of the macrophages.

2. GENERAL CHARACTERISTICS

Macrophages may be loosely defined as mononuclear phagocytes. They are present in all tissues, but are most prominently located in the bone marrow,

RICHARD HONG • Department of Pediatrics, University of Wisconsin Clinical Science Center, Madison, Wisconsin 53792.

lymph glands, spleen, liver (Kupffer cells), lung, thymus, and skin (Langerhans cells). The appreciation of the Langerhans cell as a monocyte-macrophage has come about only in recent years. The demonstration of Fc receptors, C3 receptors, and Ia antigens on these cells suggested a functional relationship to macrophages which was confirmed by the demonstration that Langerhans cells presented antigen to T cells in an *H-2*-restricted manner (Stingl *et al.*, 1980). The relative lack of inflammatory capability of the Langerhans cells (few lysosomes) may represent an adaptation of these cells to permit influence upon the immune system without an associated major irritative response. The functions of Langerhans cells in the thymus gland may also take advantage of this adaptation (see below). Other cells found in lymphatics or lymph nodes have some, but not all, of the above-mentioned surface markers or behavioral characteristics of the more classic macrophage-monocyte (reviewed in Thorbecke *et al.*, 1980). They may represent moderately adapted closely related cells or different developmental stages of the macrophage system.

In common with B lymphocytes, macrophages carry Fc receptors, C3 receptors, and Ia antigens on their surface. Ia proteins are of major importance in the initiation of the immune response, as will be described later. Fc receptors may permit cytolytic reactions mediated by small amounts of antibody on the target cell, may promote internalization of antigen–antibody complexes, and C3 may enhance B-cell interactions. Macrophage surface markers have been defined with monoclonal antibodies. OKM-1 was defined recently by Schlossman's group (Breard *et al.*, 1980) as an antibody which defined both Ia^+ and Ia^- cells, cells of variable size, adherent and nonadherent cells, attesting to the heterogeneity of the monocyte population. Raff *et al.* (1980) developed a monoclonal antibody reacting with approximately 40% of peripheral blood monocytes detecting a 120,000-dalton moiety, Mac-120. Mac-120^+ cells are most effective in stimulating the autologous mixed leukocyte response; they may represent the most effective antigen-presenting cells. Another epitope defined by a rat monoclonal antibody is shared by both macrophages and mast cells indicating a commonality of origin or function of these cell lines (Katz *et al.*, 1981).

Many macrophage functions involve phagocytosis as an important first step. This may be enhanced by the Fc and C3 receptors which could promote the ingestion of particles coated by immunoglobulins in a more efficient manner. The additional ability to ingest particles nonspecifically, however, is obviously of import in permitting initial antigen processing in naive animals. Reexpression of the antigen on the macrophage surface is a most important step in immunization, as is discussed extensively throughout this volume.

Macrophages arise primarily from the bone marrow, circulate as monocytes, then migrate to the tissues where, under the stimulus of inflammation, they mature. Macrophages are attracted to sites of inflammation by substances such as complement component C5a and lymphocyte activation products. In the peritoneal cavity and the lung, extensive local proliferation to various stimuli can occur (Dannenberg, 1975).

The macrophages can be thought of as an accessory cell line which augments and regulates many phases of host defense mechanisms. They accomplish these many and varied functions by ubiquitous distribution, ability to respond to specific and nonspecific stimuli, display of membrane proteins, phagocytic and secretory processes.

3. EFFECTS ON LYMPHOCYTES

Macrophages, operating in specific and nonspecific ways, enhance or inhibit growth of lymphoid cell lines. In addition, they play major controlling roles in the development of many cell lines as well as in their responses to stimuli.

3.1. T CELLS

Within the thymus, the site of differentiation and maturation of the T cell, interaction with macrophages exerts a profound effect. Immature thymocytes show a natural tendency to associate with macrophages (Siegel, 1970); when thymocytes are cocultured with macrophages, this behavior is lost concomitant with the acquisition of mitogen responsivity. This observation suggests that macrophages can exert a maturation effect upon thymocytes. Of interest, in some experiments, this effect was not genetically restricted (Van den Tweel and Walker, 1977). A striking macrophage effect was shown by Longo and Schwartz (1980). T cells from nonresponder guinea pigs which develop in a responder thymus can thereafter respond to the synthetic polymer GLϕ. In this remarkable transition, a genotypic nonresponder learns to become a phenotypic responder by acquiring the capability to recognize the antigen plus Ia molecules on macrophages. This education is accomplished in the thymus gland apparently by contact with responder macrophages. Beller and Unanue (1977, 1978) cultured immature thymocytes on a layer of adherent thymic macrophages. Within a period of 48 to 72 hr dramatic changes were observed. Concomitant with a loss of TL antiens, surface H-2 increased to adult levels and the ability to respond in mixed leukocyte culture was attained. Thus, maturation was accomplished *in vitro* after exposure to thymic macrophages. An avid binding of the thymocytes to the monolayer was observed. Pure epithelial cell monolayers, devoid of macrophages, were unable to accomplish these results. Macrophage effects on thymocytes are also brought about by humoral factors (Gery *et al.*, 1972; Calderon *et al.*, 1975; Beller and Unanue, 1979).

Mosier (1967) first showed the importance of adherent cells in the *in vitro* generation of antibody to sheep erythrocytes. Seeger and Oppenheim (1970) extended this observation to T-cell proliferative responses to antigens. The role of the macrophage is to present the antigen to T lymphocytes which it does in the context of histocompatibility products controlled by the *I* region in mice and an analogous locus (*DR*, probably) in man (Rosenthal and Shevach, 1973; Shevach and Rosenthal, 1973). The association of the antigen with a self-product imposes a severe restriction upon future immune responses of the responding cells. Thus, the macrophage in its presentation of the antigen for immunization controls the ultimate target of the effector responder cell. Antigen presented in this way is remarkably efficient in generating T-helper cells, of the order of several thousand times more effective than soluble antigen or antigen bound to plastic dishes (Unanue, 1972). Of interest in this regard is the fact that soluble antigen, in contradistinction to the macrophage-processed antigen, induces T-suppressor cells rather than T helpers (Ishizaka and Adachi, 1976).

In a more global way, antigen presentation (or lack thereof) is controlled by the macrophage in the Biozzi high- and low-responder mice. Mice from an outbred Swiss albino stock show high or low antibody responses to virtually any antigen (Biozzi *et al.*, 1968). The most likely explanation for this phenomenon would be that the B cells of the low responders fail to react appropriately to antigen. Howard *et al.* (1974) showed that B cells were normal in the Biozzi mice and capable of normal antibody production to T-independent antigens. Weiner and Bandieri (1974) showed a marked difference in the morphology of macrophages of high (Ab/H) and low (Ab/L) responders after overnight culture. Ab/H macrophages were well spread out and showed many extensions and an irregular cytoplasmic outline, while Ab/L macrophages assumed a spherical configuration. Furthermore, Ab/L macrophages digested antigen more rapidly leaving less membrane bound for presentation.

3.2. B CELLS

Do macrophages act directly to help B cells produce antibody? It is possible that some T-independent stimulation of B cells by polyclonal activators is macrophage-independent, but the extreme difficulty in preparing macrophage-free cell preparations and the fact that as little as 1% contamination of "pure" B-cell preparations is enough to fulfill the macrophage requirements in many systems account for the wide disparity in results obtained to date (reviewed in Unanue, 1981). In many cases, a requirement for macrophages is quite clear and the effects are probably accomplished by means of a secreted product. B-cell proliferation and differentiation are also promoted by Fc fragments of Ig molecules which have been ingested by macrophages (Morgan and Weigle, 1979, 1980). In addition, macrophages, probably as a result of prostaglandin secretion, exert suppressive effects upon pokeweed mitogen stimulation of B-cell differentiation (Goodwin *et al.*, 1977). Macrophage depletion of *in vitro* lymphocyte cultures markedly increases the number of plasma cells and plaque-forming cells (by 100-fold) (Montazeri *et al.*, 1980).

Kurland (1978) showed that macrophages were important in supporting B-cell clonal proliferation, an example of the more generalized trephocytic function of macrophages for many cell lines. Of interest, in these experiments, *H-2*-incompatible macrophages were as effective as *H-2*-identical; macrophages from neonates, however, did not support B-cell proliferation.

4. MACROPHAGE KILLING

One form of macrophage killing is classic for phagocytes. Following ingestion, a phagocytic vacuole is formed which fuses with lysosomal membranes. Thereafter, the lysosomal enzymes are discharged into the vacuole causing death of the microbe, usually by cell membrane dissolution (Hibbs, 1974). Lipases, lysozyme, and phospholipase are among the important cidal agents involved. Another form of macrophage cidal activity involves the transfer of liposomes via cytoplasmic bridges to kill tumor cells (Hibbs, 1974). Macrophages can also pinch off or ingest parts of tumor cells or protozoans (Dannenberg, 1975).

The above-mentioned mechanisms require cell-to-cell contact. Alternatives, effective with minimal cellular interaction, involve secretory products. Some macrophages, after immune activation, secrete toxic fatty acids; some, after activation, secrete a cationic substance. The hydrogen peroxide peroxidase–halide system may also be an integral part of the killing armamentarium (Klebanoff, 1975; Johnston, 1978); however, van Furth *et al.* (1970) find little myeloperoxidase in macrophages.

The process of "activation," brought on by both specific and nonspecific mechanisms, raises the level of function of the macrophages (Blanden *et al.*, 1966). Mineral oil, peptone, polyanions, and other nonspecific irritants produce higher levels of hydrolytic enzymes and more rapid bacterial destruction. Activation brought about via T cells or immunoglobulins reacting with their inducing antigens is referred to as specific (also termed "arming") (Evans *et al.*, 1972). Antigens stimulate sensitized T cells (and probably B cells) to release lymphokines which produce the state of heightened responsivity in macrophages called "activation." The stage of activation is indicated by increased macrophage adherence, spreading, development of ruffled membranes, increased phagocytosis and metabolic activity (David, 1975; Reikvam *et al.*, 1975). Some immune products direct macrophages from the bloodstream to a given area by exerting a chemotactic effect.

Macrophages utilize antibody to lyse targets specifically in two ways. In one, macrophages are "armed" by cytophilic antibody which directs the attack; in the other, antibody coats the target, the macrophage is attracted and lyses, a process termed "antibody-dependent cellular cytotoxicity" (ADCC) (Perlmann and Holm, 1969; Lovchik and Hong, 1977).

Although not directly involved in the cytolytic process, macrophages are important in the regulation of natural killer (NK) cells. NK cells may play an important role in resistance to tumors. The control of NK activity by macrophages appears to be largely mediated by interferon (Djeu *et al.*, 1979).

5. SECRETORY FUNCTIONS

The ability of the macrophage to manipulate and modulate so many important body processes is mediated by a large number of biologically active products. The range of materials extends from low-molecular-weight compounds such as prostaglandins and cyclic nucleotides to proteins such as complement and lysosomal hydrolases. The appropriate and controlled elaboration of these molecules plays a major role in the magnitude and effectiveness of the body response to external assault (reviewed in Gordon, 1980).

One of the most important stimulatory molecules is lymphocyte-activating factor (LAF), now termed interleukin 1 (IL-1), and first clearly demonstrated by Gery *et al.* (1972). IL-1 is secreted by macrophages which have been stimulated by latex ingestion, antigen–antibody complexes, and endotoxin (Calderon *et al.*, 1975). Immune T cells augment the secretion of IL-1 tremendously; this process is *H-2* restricted (*I* region control). Major effects of IL-1 are to stimulate proliferation of T lymphocytes, augment their response to mitogens, and promote secretion of a very potent lymphocyte stimulant, interleukin-2 (IL-2) (Wagner and Rollinghoff, 1978). Thymic macrophages may exert their profound effect upon intrathymic maturation by means of IL-1. IL-1 or related products play similar roles in potentiating the B-cell responses.

The complex interaction of lymphocyte control of macrophages and vice versa is again demonstrated in the modulation of secretory processes by lymphocytes. Lymphocytes stimulated with antigen induce the secretion of the second component of complement (Littman and Ruddy, 1977) and lymphokines can provoke release of lysosomal enzymes (Pantalone and Page, 1975), interferon (Neumann and Sorg, 1977), collagenase (Wahl *et al.*, 1975), and plasminogen activator (Vassalli and Reich, 1977).

Other macrophage secretions such as collagenase and other neutral proteinases, complement components, arachidonic acid oxygenation products, fibrinolytic initiators, and pyrogens obviously have profound effects upon the inflammatory response.

Macrophages can exert suppressive effects by virtue of a number of compounds. Prostaglandins are synthesized in amounts 60-fold in excess of resting levels upon stimulation by zymosan, antigen–antibody complexes, or phorbol myristate acetate. Intermediates of oxygen metabolism (hydrogen peroxide, superoxide anion, hydroxyl radical) are generated during the metabolic processes of phagocytes. Although of importance in bactericidal and possibly tumoricidal capabilities of the macrophage, these intermediaries are toxic to many cells, and therefore suppressive to immune reactions. Hydrogen peroxide is probably the most important of the above, and catalase addition can reverse the inhibition in many cases. A unique behavior of the macrophage is to release thymidine during culture, probably due to the absence of thymidine kinase; the excess thymidine inhibits DNA synthesis. Finally, macrophages act upon lymphocyte products to convert them to active suppressors of immune responses. For example, the known inhibition of immunoglobulin production by myeloma cells was shown to be due to macrophage action upon a product released by the myeloma cells. The result of the B-cell product and the macrophage interaction was a 6000-dalton compound which inhibited antibody formation *in vitro* (Kennard and Zolla-Pazner, 1980).

Macrophages manifest direct microbicidal action by many mechanisms. In addition to the generation of oxygen metabolites as noted above, they secrete lysozyme. It has been proposed that serum lysozyme concentrations may be used to measure the degree of macrophage activation, especially as a guide to the effectiveness of tumor therapy (DiLuzio, 1979).

6. ONTOGENY

The full competence of the immune system is acquired only after appropriate growth and development of several cell lines. Immaturity or insufficiency of cell number accounts for variable degrees of immunocompetence in different species.

Blaese (1975, 1976) showed that Lewis rats demonstrated a clear-cut sequential ability to respond to various antigens. For example, of the series of antigens administered, newborns responded only to *Brucella abortus*. Over a period of 30 days, they gradually acquired the ability to respond to more of the original set employed. This defect was corrected by the administration of adult macrophages along with the antigen. In humans, neonatal macrophages were shown to promote T-cell-mediated suppression of IgG synthesis, correlating with the diminished IgG responses seen in young infants (Ferguson and Cheung, 1981).

Macrophages from the spleens of young mice characteristically show a lack of Ia (Nadler *et al.*, 1980). Although they behave similarly to adult macrophages in their ability to phagocytize, respond to lymphokines, and secrete lymphostimulatory molecules, they are unable to stimulate T cells to proliferate (Lu *et al.*, 1979). Also, macrophages of neonates behave differently from adult cells in their metabolic reactions. Monocytes show a very high glycolytic rate which is not associated with a correspondingly high ATP content, indicating a vulnerability to metabolic stress. This is in part accounted for by low levels of pyruvate kinase. The deficiency is most profound in the neonate (Das *et al.*, 1979).

Thus, a number of observations indicate that the full macrophage contribution to immunocompetence is not manifest until adult life.

7. MACROPHAGE DISORDERS

Macrophages increase in number (> 10%) under a variety of conditions. Monocytosis may represent a reactive proliferative response to such infections as tuberculosis and brucellosis or to intracellular parasitism. During times of vigorous hemolysis, macrophage proliferation is clinically evident as splenomegaly. Accumulation of excessive amounts of phagocytizable organic material as in a number of genetic enzyme deficiencies (e.g., Gaucher's disease) results in large numbers of distended macrophages throughout the RES. Proliferative responses are also seen, but for unknown reasons, in Felty's syndrome, sarcoidosis, and Wegener's granulomatosis (reviewed in Territo and Cline, 1976).

Monocyte malignancies probably cover a wide spectrum of diseases representing uncontrolled proliferation of a cell at a certain stage of differentiation. In this view, monocytic leukemia and undifferentiated reticulum cell sarcomas involve the very young primarily undifferentiated cells, while chronic monocytic leukemia, well-differentiated reticulum cell sarcomas, Letterer–Siwe disease, and histiocytic medullary reticulosis involve moderately differentiated macrophages. The most mature macrophages are seen in Hand–Schuller–Christian disease, eosinophilic granuloma, and localized histiocytoma. The last-named group, however, may not be true malignancies (Cline and Golde, 1973).

Macrophage dysfunction is a concomitant of the general phagocytic failure of chronic granulomatous disease. The basic defect here is an inability to generate hydrogen peroxide and superoxide after phagocytosis (Rodey *et al.*, 1969). Disproportionate macrophage suppression has been reported as a cause of decreased immunoglobulin production in multiple myeloma (Broder *et al.*, 1975), X-linked infantile agammaglobulinemia (Krantman *et al.*, 1981), tuberculosis (Katz *et al.*, 1979), sarcoidosis (Katz and Fauci, 1978), Hodgkin's disease (Sibbitt *et al.*, 1978), and fungal infections (Stobo, 1977). In many of these instances, it is important to remember that the monocyte dysfunction may be only a secondary epiphenomenon, not of major import in the pathogenesis of the disease. It may, however, modify the clinical presentation in a marked manner.

A single report of defective ADCC function in disseminated nontuberculous mycobacterium infection was presented as evidence for a primary macrophage defect. The ADCC values were 46 to 68% of the simultaneously tested normals. IgE values were markedly elevated (to 8186 IU/ml). This interesting study is difficult to evaluate and will require further corroboration and investigation (Herlin *et al.*, 1981). ADCC, although an interesting phenomenon, has not been definitely shown to play a vital role in body defenses.

Although macrophages have tumoricidal capability, they are seldom found in the area of progressively growing lesions. Cianciolo *et al.* (1981) demonstrated an inhibitor of monocyte chemotaxis in the effusions of 17 patients. Cancers of ovarian, lung, and kidney origin were among those tested; the effusions were, for the most part, pleural or ascitic. Of interest, the inhibitor was reactive with a monoclonal antibody directed against a retrovirus structural protein, $P_{15}(E)$. This observation explains in part the demonstrated poor macrophage chemotaxis observed in cancer patients. Decreased chemotaxis is seen also after steroid administration, viral infections, in Wiskott–Aldrich syndrome, chronic mucocutaneous candidiasis, and Chediak–Higashi syndrome (reviewed in Albrecht and Hong, 1976).

8. SUMMARY

This commentary on the macrophage is intended to impart a brief but broad overview of the many and varied roles which the macrophage assumes in our host defense mechanisms. Rather than suffer from the nonspecific aspects of its response, the macrophage capitalizes upon this characteristic and engages in further specific or nonspecific activities depending upon the needs of the host.

Thus, through its amazing versatility, the lowly macrophage has elevated its status from that of a blue-collar scavenger to managerial and highly directive roles in the complex organization of the human defenses.

REFERENCES

Albrecht, R. M., and Hong, R., 1976, Basic and clinical considerations of the monocyte-macrophage system in man, *J. Pediatr.* **88**:751.

Beller, D. I., and Unanue, E. R., 1977, Thymic maturation *in vitro* by a secretory product from macrophages, *J. Immunol.* **118**:1780.

Beller, D. I., and Unanue, E. R., 1978, Thymic macrophages modulate one stage of T cell differentiation *in vitro, J. Immunol.* **121**:1861.

Beller, D. I., and Unanue, E. R., 1979, Evidence that thymocytes require at least two distinct signals to proliferate, *J. Immunol.* **123**:2890.

Biozzi, G., Stiffel, C., Mouton, D., Bouthillier, Y., and Decreusefond, C., 1968, Artificial selection for antibody production in mice, *Ann. Inst. Pasteur* (Paris) **115**:965.

Blaese, R. M., 1975, Macrophages and the development of immunocompetence, in: *The Phagocytic Cell in Host Resistance* (J. A. Bellanti and D. H. Dayton, eds.), pp. 309–320, Raven Press, New York.

Blaese, R. M., 1976, Macrophage function in the development of immunocompetence and in immunodeficiency, *J. Reticuloendothelial Soc.* **20**:67.

Blanden, R. N., Mackaness, G. B., and Collins, F. M., 1966, Mechanisms of acquired resistance in mouse typhoid, *J. Exp. Med.* **124**:585.

Breard, J., Reinherz, E. L., Kung, P. C., Goldstein, G., and Schlossman, S., 1980, A monoclonal antibody reactive with human peripheral blood monocytes, *J. Immunol.* **124**:1943.

Broder, S., Humphrey, R., Durm, M., Blackman, M., Meade, B., Goldman, C., Strober, W., and Waldmann, T., 1975, Impaired synthesis of polyclonal (non-paraprotein) immunoglobulins by circulating lymphocytes from patients with multiple myeloma, *N. Engl. J. Med.* **293**:887.

Calderon, J., Kiely, J. M., Lefko, J. L., and Unanue, E. R., 1975, The modulation of lymphocyte functions by molecules secreted by macrophages. I. Description and partial biochemical analysis, *J. Exp. Med.* **142**:151.

Cianciolo, G., Hunter, J., Silva, J., Haskill, J. S., and Snyderman, R., 1981, Inhibitors of monocyte responses to chemotaxins are present in human cancerous effusions and react with monoclonal antibodies to the $P_{15}(3)$ structural protein of retroviruses, *J. Clin. Invest.* **68**:831.

Cline, M. J., and Golde, D. W., 1973, A review and reevaluation of the histiocytic disorders, *Am. J. Med.* **55**:49.

Dannenberg, A. M., Jr., 1975, Macrophages in inflammation and infection, *N. Engl. J. Med.* **293**:489.

Das, M., Henderson, T., and Feig, S. A., 1979, Neonatal mononuclear cell metabolism: Further evidence for diminished monocyte function in the neonate, *Pediatr. Res.* **13**:632.

David, J., 1975, Macrophage activation by lymphocyte mediators, *Fed. Proc.* **34**:1730.

DiLuzio, N. R., 1979, Lysozyme, glucan-activated macrophages and neoplasia, *J. Reticuloendothelial Soc.* **26**:67.

Djeu, J. Y., Heinbaugh, J. A., Holden, H. T., and Herberman, R. B., 1979, Role of macrophages in the augmentation of mouse natural killer cell activity by poly I:C and interferon, *J. Immunol.* **122**:182.

Evans, R., Grant, C. K., Cox, H., Steele, K., and Alexander, P., 1972, Thymus-derived lymphocytes produce an immunologically specific macrophage arming factor, *J. Exp. Med.* 136:1318.

Ferguson, A. C., and Cheung, S. S. C., 1981, Modulation of immunoglobulin in M and G synthesis by monocytes and T lymphocytes in the newborn infant, *J. Pediatr.* **98**:385.

Gery, I., Gershon, R. K., and Waksman, B. H., 1972, Potentiation of the T-lymphocyte response to mitogens. I. The responding cell, *J. Exp. Med.* **136**:128.

Goodwin, J. S., Bankhurst, A. D., and Messner, R. P., 1977, Suppression of human T-cell mitogenesis by prostaglandin: Existence of a prostaglandin-producing suppressor cell, *J. Exp. Med.* **146**:1719.

Gordon, S., 1980, Lysozyme and plasminogen activator: Constitutive and induced secretory products of mononuclear phagocytes, in: *Mononuclear Phagocytes. Functional Aspects* (R. van Furth, ed.), p. 1273, Nijhoff, The Hague.

Herlin, T., Thelle, T., Kragballe, K., Borregaard, N., and Thestrup-Pedersen, K., 1981, Sustained depression of monocyte cytotoxicity in a boy with disseminated nontuberculous mycobacteriosis, *J. Pediatr.* **99**:264.

Hibbs, J. B., 1974, Heterocytolysis by macrophages activated by bacillus Calmette-Guerin: Lysosome exocytosis into tumor cells, *Science* **184**:468.

Howard, J. G., Courtenay, B. M., and Desaynaud, C., 1974, Equivalent responses to branched polysaccharides and their dinitrophenyl conjugates in Biozzi high and low responder lines of mice, *Eur. J. Immunol.* **4**:453.

Ishizaka, K., and Adachi, T., 1976, Generation of specific helper cells and suppressor cells *in vitro* for the IgE and IgG antibody responses, *J. Immunol.* **117**:40.

Johnston, R. B., Jr., 1978, Oxygen metabolism and the microbicidal activity of macrophages, *Fed. Proc.* **37**:2759.

Katz, H. R., LeBlanc, P. A., and Russell, S. W., 1981, An antigenic determinant shared by mononuclear phagocytes and mast cells, as defined by monoclonal antibody, *J. Reticuloendothelial Soc.* **30**:349.

Katz, P., and Fauci, A. S., 1978, Inhibition of polyclonal B-cell activation by suppressor monocytes in patients with sarcoidosis, *Clin. Exp. Immunol.* **32**:554.

Katz, P., Goldstein, R. A., and Fauci, A. S., 1979, Immunoregulation in infection caused by *Mycobacterium tuberculosis:* The presence of suppressor monocytes and the alteration of subpopulations of T lymphocytes, *J. Infect. Dis.* **140**:12.

Kennard, J., and Zolla-Pazner, S., 1980, Origin and function of suppressor macrophages in myeloma, *J. Immunol.* **124**:268.

Klebanoff, S. J., 1975, Antimicrobial mechanisms in neutrophilic polymorphonuclear leukocytes, *Semin. Hematol.* **12**:117.

Krantman, H. J., Saxon, A., Stevens, R. H., and Stiehm, E. R., 1981, Phenotypic heterogeneity in X-linked infantile agammaglobulinemia with *in vitro* monocyte suppression of immunoglobulin synthesis, *Clin. Immunol. Immunopathol.* **20**:170.

Kurland, J. I., 1978, Regulatory interaction of the macrophage in B lymphocyte proliferation, *J. Reticuloendothelial Soc.* **24**:19.

Littman, B. H., and Ruddy, S., 1977, Production of the second component of complement by human monocytes: Stimulation by antigen-activated lymphocytes or lymphokines, *J. Exp. Med.* **145**:1344.

Longo, D. H., and Schwartz, R. H., 1980, T-cell specificity for H-2 and Ir gene phenotype correlates with the phenotype of thymic antigen-presenting cells, *Nature (London)* **287**:44.

Lovchik, J., and Hong, R., 1977, Antibody-dependent cell-mediated cytolysis (ADCC): Analyses and projections, *Prog. Allergy* **22**:1.

Lu, C. Y., Calarnai, E. G., and Unanue, E. R., 1979, A defect in the antigen-presenting function of macrophages from neonatal mice, *Nature (London)* **282**:327.

Montazeri, G., Chiorazzi, N., Fu, S. M., and Kunkel, H. G., 1980, Regulatory role of circulating monocytes in the differentiative and proliferative responses of human B lymphocytes, *Clin. Immunol. Immunopathol.* **16**:1.

Morgan, E. L., and Weigle, W. O., 1979, The requirement for adherent cells in the Fc fragment-induced proliferative response of murine spleen cells, *J. Exp. Med.* **150**:256.

Morgan, E. L., and Weigle, W. O., 1980, Polyclonal activation of murine B lymphocytes by Fc fragments. I. The requirement for two signals in the generation of the polyclonal antibody response induced by Fc fragments, *J. Immunol.* **124**:1330.

Mosier, D. E., 1967, A requirement for two cell types for antibody formation *in vitro, Science* **158**:1573.

Nadler, P. I., Klingenstein, R. J., and Hodes, R. J., 1980, Ontogeny of murine accessory cells: Ia antigen expression and accessory cell function in *in vitro* primary antibody responses, *J. Immunol.* **125**:914.

Neumann, C., and Sorg, C., 1977, Immune interferon. I. Production by lymphokine-activated murine macrophages, *Eur. J. Immunol.* **7**:719.

Pantalone, R. M., and Page, R. C., 1975, Lymphokine-induced production and release of lysosomal enzymes by macrophages, *Proc. Natl. Acad. Sci. USA* **72**:2091.

Perlmann, P., and Holm, G., 1969, Cytotoxic effects of lymphoid cells *in vitro, Adv. Immunol.* **11**:117.

Raff, H. V., Picker, L. J., and Stobo, J. D., 1980, Macrophage heterogeneity in man: A subpopulation of HLA-Dr-bearing macrophages required for antigen-induced T-cell activation also contains stimulators for autologous-reactive T-cells, *J. Exp. Med.* **152**:581.

Reikvam, A., Grammeltvedt, R., and Hoiby, E., 1975, Activated mouse macrophages: Morphology, lysosomal biochemistry, and microbiocidal properties of *in vivo* and *in vitro* activated cells, *Acta Pathol. Microbiol. Scand.* **83**:129.

Rodey, G. E., Park, B. H., Windhorst, D. B., and Good, R. A., 1969, Defective bactericidal activity of monocytes in fatal granulomatous disease, *Blood* **33**:813.

Rosenthal, A. S., and Shevach, E. M., 1973, Function of macrophages in antigen recognition by guinea pig T lymphocytes. I. Requirement for histocompatible macrophages and lymphocytes, *J. Exp. Med.* **138**:1194.

Seeger, R. C., and Oppenheim, J. J., 1970, Synergistic interaction of macrophages and lymphocytes in antigen-induced transformation of lymphocytes, *J. Exp. Med.* **132**:44.

Shevach, E. M., and Rosenthal, A. S., 1973, Function of macrophages in antigen recognition. II. Role of the macrophage in regulation of genetic control of the immune response. *J. Exp. Med.* **138**:1213.

Sibbitt, W. L., Jr., Bankhurst, A. D., and Williams, R. C., Jr., 1978, Studies of cell subpopulations mediating mitogen hyporesponsiveness in patients with Hodgkin's disease, *J. Clin Invest.* **61**:55.

Siegel, I., 1970, Natural and antibody-induced adherence of guinea pig phagocytic cells to autologous and heterologous thymocytes, *J. Immunol.* **105**:879.

Stingl, G., Tamaki, K., and Katz, S. I., 1980, Origin and function of epidermal Langerhans cells, *Immunol. Rev.* **53**:149.

Stobo, J. D., 1977, Immunosuppression in man: Suppression by macrophages can be mediated by interactions with regulatory T cells, *J. Immunol.* **119**:918.

Territo, M., and Cline, M., 1976, Macrophages and their disorders in man, in: *Immunobiology of the Macrophage* (D. S. Nelson, ed.), p. 594, Academic Press, New York.

Thorbecke, G. J., Silberberg-Sinakin, I., and Flotte, T. J., 1980, Langerhans cells as macrophages in skin and lymphoid organs, *J. Invest. Dermatol.* **75**:32.

Unanue, E. R., 1972, The regulatory role of macrophages in antigenic stimulation, *Adv. Immunol.* **15**:95.

Unanue, E. R., 1981, The regulatory role of macrophages in antigenic stimulation. II. Symbiotic relationship between lymphocytes and macrophages, *Adv. Immunol.* **31**:1.

Van Den Tweel, J. G., and Walker, W. S., 1977, Macrophage-induced thymic lymphocyte maturation, *Immunology* **33**:817.

van Furth, R., Hirsch, J. G., and Fedorko, M. E., 1970, Morphology and peroxidase cytochemistry of mouse promonocytes, monocytes and macrophages, *J. Exp. Med.* **132**:794.

Vassalli, J. D., and Reich, E., 1977, Macrophage plasminogen activator: Induction by products of activated lymphoid cells, *J. Exp. Med.* **145**:429.

Wagner, H., and Rollinghoff, M., 1978, T–T cell interactions during *in vitro* cytotoxic allograft responses. I. Soluble products from activated Ly 1^+ T cells trigger autonomously antigen primed Ly 23^+ T cells to cell proliferation and cytolytic activity, *J. Exp. Med.* **148**: 1523.

Wahl, L. M., Wahl, S. M., Mergenhagen, S. E., and Martin, G. R., 1975, Collagenase production by lymphokine-activated macrophages, *Science* **187**:261.

Weiner, E., and Bandieri, A., 1974, Difference in antigen handling by peritoneal macrophages from the Biozzi high and low responder lines of mice, *Eur. J. Immunol.* **4**:457.

2

The Role of Macrophages in Nonspecific Processes

MICHAEL E. MILLER

1. INTRODUCTION

Interest in the role of macrophages as "nonspecific" mediators of host defense has been heightened in recent years. The importance of macrophages in the inflammatory response is not a new concept, having been first suggested by Metchnikoff (1893) who noted from his observations of tubercle bacilli that "the polynuclear cells engulf the tubercle bacilli readily, but perish after a short time and then with the microbes they contain, are eaten up by various mononuclear phagocytes which may be classed together under the term of macrophages. These latter cells have a much greater power of resistance and in some cases are even capable of destroying the tubercle bacilli."

In 1962, Mackaness's report immensely heightened interest in the role of the macrophage in the immune inflammatory response. He demonstrated that macrophages which had been infected with the intracellular pathogen *Listeria monocytogenes* were able to significantly inhibit the growth and infectivity of other intracellular organisms. Normal macrophages which had not been previously infected with the *Listeria* were, by contrast, unable to do this. Thus was born the concept of the "activated macrophage" (Cohn, 1978; Karnovsky and Lazdins, 1978; North, 1978). Such cells are larger and adhere and spread more on glass than normal macrophages. A number of functional and biochemical activities are enhanced in activated macrophages over those seen in normal macrophages. Phagocytosis of some but not all materials is increased. Glucose utilization through the hexosemonophosphate shunt is increased. Membrane enzymes such as adenylate cyclase and cytoplasmic enzymes such as lactic dehydrogenase show increased activities. Increased numbers of lysosomes and enhanced release of lysosomal enzymes (e.g., collagenase) are also seen.

The functional consequences of these biochemical and morphologic changes remain unclear. The major effects which have been noted in activated mac-

MICHAEL E. MILLER • Department of Pediatrics, University of California at Davis School of Medicine, Davis, California 95616.

rophages are enhanced bactericidal activities and increased tumor inhibition and killing. These two activities do not, however, consistently correlate. In other words, macrophages which have been "activated" in enhanced killing may not always show increased tumoricidal activities and vice versa.

Central to Metchnikoff's thesis was the idea that phagocyte function was of positive benefit to the host. Prior to his work, it was assumed that phagocytes were harmful to the host and contributed to the untoward clinical effects of infectious organisms. Once Metchnikoff demonstrated, however, that "the essential and primary element in typical inflammation consists in a reaction of the phagocyte *against* a harmful agent," it followed that defects in phagocyte function might predispose the host to increased frequency and toxicity of microbial organisms.

Over the past decade, a spectrum of disorders of phagocyte function involving the monocyte-macrophage system has been described. Through these observations, much has been learned of the normal immune-inflammatory functions of these cells. In the development of our discussion, therefore, it is important to draw upon these "experiments of nature" as they have contributed to our understanding of the functions of macrophages. We will first discuss the basic "nonspecific" mechanisms by which macrophages function in host defense and then review clinical abnormalities of these cells as they reflect upon these functions.

The discussion will apply equally to monocytes and macrophages (MNLs) except where differences between the two cell types are noted.

2. BASIC MECHANISMS

2.1. MOVEMENT OF MONONUCLEAR PHAGOCYTES

A central requirement of an effective mononuclear phagocyte response to infection is the ability of these cells to migrate and accumulate at sites of infection. Studies of the movement process of polymorphonuclear leukocytes (PMNs) have demonstrated at least two distinct phases ofagocyte movement (Gallin and Quie, 1978): (1) turning or orientation and (2) actual locomotion.

The term *chemotaxis,* which had formerly been applied to the overall process of movement, designates the turning or orientation phase of the process. The actual increase in rate of locomotion is known as *chemokinesis.* It has been assumed that MNLs, like PMNs, are capable of both chemotaxis and chemokinesis, although data confirming this assumption are limited. Initial studies of MNL movement employed either *in vivo* study as by the "skin window" technique (Rebuck and Crowley, 1955) or *in vitro* measurements by the filter assay.

While the Boyden (filter) assay (1962) has contributed major information to the understanding of overall cell movement, it is not suited to the study of individual components of the migration process. The cells are placed on one side of the filter and eventually reach the other side, but the mechanism(s) by which they migrate is unknown. Recognition of the complexities of the MNL movement process has derived from the introduction of more specific assays involving visual techniques and studies of deformability (Gallin and Quie, 1978). Although gaps remain in the complete understanding of the triggering and maintaining of sustained cell movement, a number of important correlates have been identified. Initially, electrochemical events result in a brief membrane depolarization coincident with calcium and/or sodium influx. This is followed by prolonged hyperpolarization in association with increased potassium permeability (Gallin *et al.*, 1978). A number of metabolic events follow, including increased levels of intracellular cyclic guanosine monophosphate (cGMP) (Hill, 1978); release of lysosomal enzymes (Becker and Showell, 1974); increased glycolysis and hexosemonophosphate shunt activity (Goetzl and Austen, 1974); increased numbers of microtubules (Stossel, 1978); and probable activation of contractile proteins (Boxer *et al.*, 1974).

The cellular mobilization of macrophages can be mediated by a number of humoral substances with chemoattractant activity. Much work is still required to completely define which of these products are specific for PMNs and which for MNLs. It is probable that most of the identified chemoattractant materials are active toward both cell types. Chemoattractants are usually derived following activation of either the complement pathway or the fibrinolytic and kinin-generating systems (Gallin and Wolff, 1976). Such activation can be triggered by antigen–antibody complexes, endotoxin, or even enzymes from macrophages and neutrophils released during the phagocytic process.

Of the complement pathway-derived materials, C3a and C5a manifest substantial chemotactic activity. Plasminogen activator and kallikrein are chemotactic products of the fibrinolytic and kinin-generating systems (Gallin and Kaplan, 1974).

Cell-derived products which are chemotactic for MNLs are also released during the acute inflammatory process from granulocytes and lymphocytes (Ward *et al.*, 1970). Lymphocytes exposed to antigenic stimulation produce chemoattractant lymphokines such as lymphocyte-derived chemotactic factor (LDCF) (Altman *et al.*, 1973) and, perhaps, transfer factor (Lawrence, 1974). Also, compounds produced as a result of bacterial growth *in vitro* possess chemotactic activity for MNLs.

Full control of the mononuclear phagocytes in the inflammatory response also involves substances which inhibit mononuclear cell movement. Presumably this inhibition of mononuclear phagocyte movement is important in maintaining a population of such cells at the inflammatory site once they have been attracted by chemotaxis. It should be emphasized, however, that this functional sequence is hypothetical, with little direct supportive evidence at present. An important mediator of this inhibition may be migration inhibition factor (MIF). This material is a lymphokine released by antigen-stimulated lymphocytes which (at least *in vitro*) inhibits macophage migration (David, 1973).

2.2. INGESTION (ENDOCYTOSIS)

Once they have arrived at the inflammatory site, MNLs are capable of ingesting a wide variety of materials. This internalization of foreign materials (endocytosis) can involve either microscopic fluid droplets (pinocytosis) or the ingestion of larger particulate matter (phagocytosis). These processes are described elsewhere in detail (Cohn, 1968; Gordon and Cohn, 1973) and are mediated by the presence of a number of distinct membrane receptors on the macrophage (Nelson, 1969). Macrophages and monocytes possess surface receptors both for the Fc portion of the IgG molecule and for the third component of complement (C3) (Berken and Benacerraf, 1966; Lay and Nussenzweig, 1968; Rabinovitch, 1970). Fc binding of immunoglobulins may involve either free immunoglobulin or that bound in antigen–antibody complexes. Specific binding of immunoglobulin classes IgG1 and IgG3 is mediated by the macrophage Fc receptor. Those antibodies which bind to macrophages in their free form are known as cytophilic antibodies. Once bound to the macrophage, these antibodies can serve as a receptor in conferring specificity of antigen binding upon the macrophage. The C3 receptor is biochemically and functionally distinct from the Fc receptor (Griffin *et al.*, 1975). The Fc receptor is trypsin resistant and the C3 receptor trypsin sensitive. The Fc and C3 receptors may act synergistically (Griffin *et al.*, 1975) or may apparently function independently in some kinds of phagocytosis (Scornik, 1976). Thus, Griffin *et al.* (1975) demonstrated that ingestion of opsonized pneumococci via the Fc receptor could occur independently of ingestion of particles simultaneously attached to the C3 receptors of the same cell.

Macrophages are also capable of ingesting a wide variety of substances in the apparent absence of antibody. These include glass or plastic beads, modified erythrocytes (as by tannic acid treatment or heating or aging), and various other sorts of foreign debris. It is presumed that receptors are present which are capable of recognizing and binding such nonspecific particles, although their precise characterization and nature are unknown (Rabinovitch, 1967, 1968; Steinman and Cohn, 1972). Macrophage receptors for fibrinogen and fibrin have also been described (Colvin and Dvorak, 1975). Although the precise contribution these receptors play in the inflammatory response has not been determined, it is possible that they increase the efficiency of macrophage ingestion by enabling the cells to bind the foreign particles more firmly.

Finally, macrophages possess receptors of importance in the specific immune response. The nature of these macrophage-lymphocyte receptors is discussed in more detail elsewhere in this book.

Internalization of foreign particles occurs much the same as in PMNs. The ingested particle becomes enclosed within a vesicle formed by the exterior plasma membrane of the cell. Once internalized, these vesicles fuse with lysosomal products forming phagolysosomes in which the bactericidal and digestive processes take place.

2.3. MICROBICIDAL MECHANISMS

Killing of ingested microorganisms is accomplished by a variety of sophisticated biochemical processes. MNL killing of ingested bacteria utilizes many of the processes identified in PMNs (Cline, 1970; T. E. Miller, 1971; Baehner and Johnston, 1972; Klebanoff and Hamon, 1973). The precise differences by which macrophages may accomplish microbicidal activity from PMNs are not well understood. In PMNs, contact of the membrane with a foreign particle is followed by a sequence which results in the liberation of a number of potentially bactericidal metabolic products. These metabolic products—superoxide anion, hydrogen peroxide, hydroxyl radicals, and singlet oxygen—are involved in normal intracellular killing by PMNs. In mononuclear phagocytes, microbicidal activity for some organisms is decreased under conditions of anaerobiosis. This suggests that, as with PMNs, an oxygen-dependent killing system is also important in MNLs. Identification of hydrogen peroxide, myeloperoxidase, and superoxide generating systems within MNLs lends further support to this contention. Myeloperoxidase has been demonstrated in maturing monocytes but not in fully mature macrophages (van Furth and Cohn, 1968).

Also, monocytes from patients with chronic granulomatous disease (CGD) or myeloperoxidase deficiency share the same bactericidal defects as PMNs from afflicted patients (Davis *et al.*, 1968; Nathan *et al.*, 1969). Comparisons of microbicidal efficiency of monocytes and PMNs suggest that while monocytes do not phagocytize as well as PMNs, the cells are equally bactericidal toward ingested microorganisms (Baehner and Johnston, 1972; Steigbigel *et al.*, 1974).

Some differences may occur in microbicidal mechanisms of mononuclear phagocytes depending upon their state of maturation and location in the body (Cline, 1965; Bennett and Cohn, 1966; Cohn, 1968; Nelson, 1969; Karnovsky *et al.*, 1973). Thus, the major energy source for the monocyte appears to be aerobic glycolysis, while mature macrophages derive their energy from both glycolytic and aerobic pathways (Cohn, 1968; Cline and Lehrer, 1968). Depending upon site of origin, macrophages may utilize either the aerobic or the anaerobic process. Pulmonary macrophages demonstrate a high degree of oxygen consumption, utilizing energy gained through oxidative phosphorylation. Macrophages from other sites utilize anaerobic glycolysis as their main energy source.

Mononuclear phagocytes also contain a wide variety of hydrolytic enzymes which may be important secretory products aiding in the killing and digestion of microbes. At least three distinct kinds of hydrolytic enzymes are elaborated (Axline and Cohn, 1970; Solotorovsky and Soderberg, 1972; Davies and Bonney, 1979):

1. Acid hydrolases
2. Lysozyme
3. Neutral proteinases, including collagenase, plasminogen activator, elastase, and a proteoglycan-degrading enzyme

Macrophages also secrete certain arachidonic acid oxygenation products and a number of components of the classical and alternative pathways of complement. The roles which these various products play in microbicidal function of macrophages are presently unknown.

A number of pathogens which are not usually found within granulocytes preferentially parasitize macrophages and replicate within them (Nathan *et al.*,

1980). Once macrophages are activated, these same intracellular pathogens may be inhibited or destroyed. Included among such organisms are *Listeria, Salmonella, Brucella, Mycobacterium, Chlamydia, Rickettsia, Leishmania, Toxoplasma,* and *Trypanosoma. Legionella pneumophilia,* the agent of Legionnaire's disease, has recently also been found to parasitize mononuclear phagocytes. The mechanisms by which macrophages are activated and the relationship of activation to microbicidal activity are still poorly understood. At present, only lymphocyte mediators have been shown to induce full activation of macrophages, but how this is accomplished is unknown.

3. CLINICAL DISORDERS OF PHAGOCYTE FUNCTION

3.1. DISORDERS OF PHAGOCYTE MICROBICIDAL ACTIVITY

As already outlined, importance of the macrophage in host defenses was first suggested by the basic observations of Metchnikoff. Once he established that phagocytes were helpful rather than harmful to the human host, it followed that defects in phagocyte function might predispose the host to increased numbers and toxicity of infections with foreign microorganisms. Indeed, this was predicted by Metchnikoff and clinical recognition of phagocyte disorders has recently proven him correct. The first evidence of an inborn error of phagocyte function was provided by Holmes *et al.* (1966). They studied patients with chronic granulomatous disease (CGD), a disorder characterized by indolent, granulomatous-type infections. The disorder most frequently occurs in an X-linked pattern and usually proves fatal to afflicted males within the first decade of life. Their studies demonstrated that PMNs from the afflicted children were able to ingest bacteria normally, but were unable to kill the ingested organisms *in vitro.* This was in sharp contrast to normal PMNs which effectively killed the same organisms intracellularly. It was also observed that PMNs from the mothers (presumed carriers in an X-linked disorder) were intermediate in their killing capacity.

Subsequent studies demonstrated a primary metabolic abnormality in PMNs from CGD patients. Reduction of a colorless dye—nitrobule tetrazolium (NBT), which turns to blue formazan in the reduced state—was accomplished by normal PMNs stimulated by bacteria, but not by PMNs from the children with CGD (Baehner and Nathan, 1968). This suggested a biochemical lesion under genetic control as the underlying basis for the bactericidal defect. The abnormal mechanisms involved in CGD have been extensively studied in PMNs and a full discussion is beyond the scope of this chapter (see Johnston and Newman, 1977, for review). The basic molecular defect is deficient activity of an enzyme responsible for conversion of oxygen to a bactericidal species. A number of candidates have been proposed for the critical enzyme, including NADH oxidase, NADPH oxidase, and glutathione peroxidase. Although definitive proof for any one is lacking, most investigators currently favor NADPH oxidase.

In the absence of oxidase activation, the normal postphagocytic "respiratory burst" fails to occur. PMNs from patients with CGD fail to show the normal phagocytosis-associated increase in oxygen consumption, generation of superoxide, and hydrogen peroxide. As a consequence, NBT reduction and chemiluminescence responses fail to occur. Decreased bactericidal activity presumably reflects the absence of these potent bactericidal oxidation products of normal PMN respiration.

Monocytes of patients with CGD also manifest abnormalities in bactericidal and fungicidal activity (Davis *et al.*, 1968; Nathan *et al.*, 1969; Rodey *et al.*, 1969; Lehrer, 1975). The defective monocyte killing is presumably due to the same biochemical defect present in their PMNs.

A defect of monocyte microbicidal activity has been described in patients with myeloperoxidase deficiency (Lehrer and Cline, 1969). This enzyme is not involved in microbial killing by mature macrophages but appears to play a role in the microbicidal mechanisms of monocytes (van Furth and Cohn, 1968).

Monocytes from patients with Chediak–Higashi syndrome are also deficient in microbial killing (Root *et al.*, 1972). The defect is similar to that found in PMNs from afflicted patients and presumably reflect a defect of lysosomal degranulation (Blume and Wolff, 1972).

A number of other reports of diminished monocyte bactericidal activity have involved malakoplakia (Abdou *et al.*, 1977), pulmonary alveolar proteinosis (Golde *et al.*, 1976), protein-calorie malnutrition (Douglas and Schopfer, 1974), and perhaps some lymphoid malignancies (Cline, 1973). The role played by the deficient monocyte bactericidal activity in the clinical presentation of these disorders is unknown.

3.2. DISORDERS OF DEFECTIVE PHAGOCYTOSIS

No intrinsic isolated abnormalities of PMN or MNL phagocytosis have been described. The most common clinical situation encountered with decreased mononuclear cell phagocytosis, however, is splenectomy. Absence of the spleen by either congenital or acquired mechanisms is associated with decreased removal of bacteria from the blood by splenic macrophages. The precise relationship of the decreased mononuclear phagocyte clearance to the clinical picture of overwhelming septicemia in many such subjects is unclear, but it is highly probable that it plays a significant role (Stossel, 1977).

3.3. DISORDERS OF PHAGOCYTE MOVEMENT

Disorders of PMN and MNL movement constitute a large and important group of functional phagocyte deficiencies. As reviewed earlier in this chapter, a number of mechanisms are involved in phagocyte movement and are, therefore, potential sites for clinically significant perturbations. Most of the described disorders of phagocyte movement have been defined in PMNs. In those situations in which PMN and monocyte movement have been studied in the same patient, a parallel defect has been found in both cell lines. There is one possible exception to this observation (reviewed in the following section) in comparing monocytes and PMNs from newborn infants.

Several specific conditions have been studied with specific reference to the monocytes, and defects of movement have been observed. These include Wiskott–Aldrich syndrome, chronic mucocutaneour candidiasis, and Chediak–Higashi syndrome.

3.3.1. Wiskott–Aldrich Syndrome

The serum of Wiskott–Aldrich patients contains high levels of chemotactic activity which may cause normal monocytes to manifest decreased chemotaxis (Altman *et al.*, 1974).

3.3.2. Chronic Mucocutaneous Candidiasis

Monocytes of a patient with chronic mucocutaneous candidiasis were studied by Snyderman *et al.* (1973) and found to show defective chemotaxis to both C5a and LDCF. These *in vitro* defects were partially reversed following the administration of transfer factor.

3.3.3. Chediak–Higashi Syndrome

Both monocytes and granulocytes of patients with Chediak–Higashi syndrome show abnormal chemotactic responsiveness to a number of different chemotactic stimuli (Gallin *et al.*, 1975). Again, the relationship of these chemotactic defects to the increased susceptibility to infections of patients with this disorder is unknown.

Finally, several acquired conditions have been associated with decreased monocyte chemotaxis. Kleinerman *et al.* (1974, 1975) demonstrated peripheral blood monocyte chemotaxis to show diminished *in vitro* movement following *in vitro* infection with herpes simplex or influenza viruses. Monocyte chemotactic defects have also been reported in certain malignancies (Snyderman and Mergenhagen, 1976; Boetcher and Leonard, 1974; Hausman *et al.*, 1975), and an inactivator of chemotactic factor has been observed in Hodgkin's disease (Ward and Berenberg, 1974).

4. PHAGOCYTE FUNCTION IN THE HUMAN NEONATE

Closely related to the clinical disorders of MNL function is the developmental immaturity of these cells in the human neonate. In discussing this area, it is important to compare results obtained with neonatal MNLs to those of neonatal PMNs, since it appears that a functional dichotomy may exist between these two cell lines. If so, full understanding of the relative roles of mononuclear and polymorphonuclear phagocytes in the newborn infant should contribute in a significant way to full understanding of the roles of these cells throughout life.

4.1. MOVEMENT OF NEONATAL PMNs AND MNLs

Movement of neonatal PMNs has been studied by a number of investigators and a variety of techniques with highly consistent results. M. E. Miller (1971) compared movement of neonatal PMNs with that of adult PMNs utilizing a modified Boyden (filter) assay. Neonatal PMNs showed significantly less chemotactic activity than adult PMNs toward any of the chemotactic stimuli employed. In a similar study, Pahwa *et al.* (1977) compared movement of cord blood PMNs with PMNs from healthy adults toward two simuli—LDCF and endotoxin-activated normal serum. In each case, cord blood PMNs were significantly less effective in movement. A similar result was obtained by Klein *et al.* (1977) using the agarose technique.

Studies of movement of neonatal monocytes have yielded less consistent results than with neonatal PMNs. Thus, Klein *et al.* (1977) and Weston *et al.* (1976) found deficient movement of neonatal monocytes as has been reviewed for neonatal PMNs. By contrast, however, Raghunathan *et al.* (1979) and Pahwa *et al.* (1977) found mononuclear cell chemotaxis from cord blood from healthy term infants to be normal in comparison with that of healthy adult subjects.

In an intriguing study, Kretschmer *et al.* (1976) utilized LDCF as the chemoattractant and compared movement of cord blood monocytes with that of adult monocytes. When LDCF which was generated from adult lymphocytes was used as the chemoattractant, cord blood monocytes moved as well as adult monocytes. When the LDCF was generated from cord blood lymphocytes, however, cord blood monocytes responded less well than adult monocytes. Adult monocytes responded normally to LDCF from cord or adult lymphocytes. In attempting to explain their results, the authors hypothesized that the poor response of cord blood monocytes to cord blood LDCF might be the result of an inhibitor of mononuclear cell movement elaborated by neonatal lymphocytes and for which only neonatal monocytes have the receptors. The findings of this study await confirmation.

Further suggestion of a dichotomy between neonatal monocytes and neonatal PMNs is found in studies of deformability of cord blood monocytes and cord blood PMNs. Miller and Myers (1975) adapted the assay of cell elastimetry to the study of neonatal PMNs. Neonatal PMNs showed markedly decreased deformability in comparison to adult PMNs. In other words, significantly greater negative pressures were required to aspirate neonatal PMNs than adult PMNs into micropipets. It was suggested that this increased rigidity of the neonatal PMN might play a significant role in explaining the impaired movement of these cells. Raghunathan *et al.* (1979) compared deformability of human cord blood monocytes with adult monocytes. Unlike neonatal PMNs, cord blood monocytes showed no significant differences from adult monocytes in deformability.

4.2. PHAGOCYTOSIS OF NEONATAL PMNs AND MNLs

Phagocytosis by neonatal PMNs has been studied under two major conditions. In the first group of studies, experiments have been carried out in the presence of normal or near-normal concentrations of plasma or serum (reviewed in Miller, 1978). Under such conditions, neonatal PMNs have shown normal phagocytic activity by comparison with adult PMNs. The second group of studies has been carried out under limiting *in vitro* conditions with serum concentrations less than 10% of normal *in vivo* concentrations. Under such conditions, Matoth (1952) and Miller (1969) have demonstrated decreased efficiency of cord blood PMNs in phagocytic activity when compared with adult PMNs. The clinical significance of these findings may be questioned, since normal PMNs presumably circulate in plasma concentrations well in excess of 2.5%. On the other hand, *in vitro* systems inevitably contain a number of alterations from true *in vivo* conditions. As such, concentrations of test groups may not be comparable to actual body concentrations even though the comparison they measure reflects a clinically significant difference. In studies of PMN phagocytosis comparing cells from normal and sick neonates, Forman and Stiehm (1969) found that PMNs from a high percentage of the sick infants showed deficient phagocytosis relative to PMNs from healthy infants. These studies were carried out in serum concentrations in excess of 10%.

In summary of these studies, it may thus be that under stress or limiting conditions, phagocytosis by PMNs from normal neonates is relatively deficient and plays a role in the compromised host defenses common to this period of life.

Monocyte and macrophage phagocytosis has not been well studied in human neonates. Presumably, these functions are developed at birth as macrophages capable of phagocytosis have been identified in mouse embryos (Cline and Moore, 1972). Phagocytosis by neonatal alveolar macrophages has been studied and was found to be entirely normal by comparison with adult cells in alveolar macrophages from 1-day-old animals (Bellanti *et al.*, 1979). This was true both in percentage of alveolar macrophages with associated bacteria and in average number of bacteria ingested per macrophage. *S. aureus* and *E. coli* were the organisms employed.

4.3. BACTERICIDAL ACTIVITIES OF NEONATAL PMNs AND MNLs

For neonatal PMNs, data on bactericidal activity are much the same as those obtained in studies of phagocytosis. In other words, under relatively normal conditions, bactericidal mechanisms are equivalent to those seen in adult PMNs. Under limiting conditions, however, such as high bacteria : phagocyte ratio or when studied *in vivo* from sick neonates, bactericidal functions of neonatal PMNs are relatively deficient. This decreased bactericidal activity may correlate with impaired metabolic responsiveness. Mills *et al.* (1979) studied chemiluminescence and bactericidal activities of PMNs from infants, their mothers, and normal adult controls. The studies were carried out through a range of bacteria : PMN ratios. At large bacteria : PMN ratios, newborn PMNs showed decreased bactericidal activity compared to maternal and controll PMNs. Chemiluminescence of newborn PMNs was significantly lower than in maternal or control PMNs. Uptake of radiolabeled bacteria was the same in all three groups suggesting that the reduced chemiluminescence of neonatal PMNs was not simply the result of decreased phagocytosis. The authors concluded that PMNs from normal neonates have decreased oxidative metabolic responsiveness and decreased bactericidal activity.

Wright *et al.* (1975) measured bactericidal activities of PMNs from neonates with a variety of clinical abnormalities including sepsis, respiratory distress syndrome, meconium aspiration, hyperbilirubinemia, or premature rupture of the membranes. PMNs from the clinically afflicted infants showed significant impairment in bactericidal activities when compared with those of normal, clinically well neonates. Studies of bactericidal activity in neonatal mononuclear phagocytes have yielded conflicting results. Kretschmer *et al.* (1976) and Orlowski *et al.* (1976) found no difference in bactericidal activity of neonatal monocytes as compared with that in adult control monocytes. In the study of Orlowski *et al.* (1976), the monocytes of both infants and adults were significantly less active in bactericidal activity than PMNs from the corresponding groups, but the bactericidal capacities did not differ appreciably between newborn and adult cells of either type. By contrast, Bellanti *et al.* (1979) found differences in bactericidal capacity between neonatal alveolar macrophages and adult alveolar macrophages from rabbits. Microbicidal activity of rabbit alveolar macrophages did not develop until after the first week of life postnatally and did not reach full adult levels until the first postnatal month. The reasons for the difference in results among these studies are unclear, but the findings may reflect different cell types and/or species.

Limited data are available on metabolic correlates of neonatal monocytes. Kretschmer *et al.* (1976) found that cord blood monocytes were equal to adult monocytes in NBT dye reduction. Bellanti *et al.* (1979) found low levels of superoxide dismutase in neonatal rabbit alveolar macrophages which increased over the first week postnatally.

REFERENCES

Abdou, N. I., Na Pombejara, C., Sagawa, A., Ragland, C., Stechschulte, D. J., Nilsson, V., Gourley, W., Watanabe, I., Lindsey, N. J., and Allen, M. S., 1977, Malakoplakia: Evidence for monocyte lysosomal abnormality correctable by cholinergic agonist *in vitro* and *in vivo*, *N. Engl. J. Med.* **297:**1413.

Altman, L. C., Snyderman, R., Oppenheim, J. J., and Mergenhagen, S. E., 1973, A human monoculear leukocyte chemotactic factor: Characterization, specificity, and kinetics of production by homologous leukocytes, *J. Immunol.* **110:**801.

Altman, L. C., Snyderman, R., and Blaese, R. M., 1974, Abnormalities of chemotactic lymphokine synthesis and monocyte leukocyte chemotaxis in Wiskott–Aldrich syndrome, *J. Clin. Invest.* **54:**486.

Axline, S. G., and Cohn, Z. A., 1970, *In vitro* induction of lysosomal enzymes by phagocytosis, *J. Exp. Med.* **131:**1239.

Baehner, R. L., and Johnston, R. B., 1972, Monocyte function in children with neutropenia and chronic infection, *Blood* **40:**31.

Baehner, R. L., and Nathan, D. G., 1968, Quantitative nitroblue tetrazolium test in chronic granulomatous disease, *N. Engl. J. Med.* **278:**971.

Becker, E. L., and Showell, H. J., 1974, The ability of chemotactic factors to induce lysosomal enzyme release. II. The mechanism of release, *J. Immunol.* **112**:2055.
Bellanti, J. A., Neruikar, L. S., and Zeligs, B. J., 1979, Host defenses in the fetus and neonate: Studies of the alveolar macrophage during maturation, *Pediatrics* **64**(Suppl.):726.
Bennett, W. E., and Cohn, Z. A., 1966, The isolation and selected properties of blood monocytes, *J. Exp. Med.* **123**:145.
Berken, A., and Benacerraf, B., 1966, Properties of antibodies cytophilic for macrophages, *J. Exp. Med.* **123**:119.
Blume, R. S., and Wolff, S. M., 1972, The Chediak–Higashi syndrome: Studies in four patients and a review of the literature, *Medicine* **51**:247.
Boetcher, D. A., and Leonard, E. J., 1974, Abnormal monocyte chemotactic response in cancer patients, *J. Natl. Cancer Inst.* **52**:1091.
Boxer, L. A., Hedley-Whyte, E. T., and Stossel, T. P., 1974, Neutrophil actin dysfunction and abnormal neutrophil behavior, *N. Engl. J. Med.* **291**:1093.
Boyden, S., 1962, The chemotactic effect of mixtures of antibody and antigen on polymorphonuclear leucocytes, *J. Exp. Med.* **115**:453.
Cline, M. J., 1965, Metabolism of the circulating leukocyte, *Physiol. Rev.* **45**:674.
Cline, M. J., 1970, Bactericidal activity of human macrophages: Analysis of factors influencing the killing of *Listeria monocytogens, Infect. Immun.* **2**:156.
Cline, M. J., 1973, Defective mononuclear phagocyte function in patients with myelomonocytic leukemia and in some patients with lymphoma, *J. Clin. Invest.* **52**:2185.
Cline, M. J., and Lehrer, R. I., 1968, Phagocytosis by human monocytes, *Blood* **32**:423.
Cline, M. J., and Moore, M. A. S., 1972, Embryonic origin of the mouse macrophage, *Blood* **39**:842.
Cohn, Z. A., 1968, The structure and function of monocytes and macrophages, *Adv. Immunol.* **9**:163.
Cohn, Z. A., 1978, The activation of mononuclear phagocytes: Fact, fancy, and future, *J. Immunol.* **121**:813.
Colvin, R. B., and Dvorak, H. F., 1975, Fibrinogen/fibrin on the surface of macrophage: Detection, distribution, binding requirements, and possible role in macrophage adherence phenomena, *J. Exp. Med.* **142**:1377.
David, J. R., 1973, Lymphocyte mediators and cellular hypersensitivity, *N. Engl. J. Med.* **288**:143.
Davies, P., and Bonney, R. J., 1979, Secretory products of monoculear phagocytes: A brief review, *J. Reticuloendothelial Soc.* **26**:37.
Davis, W. C., Huber, H., Douglas, D. S., and Fudenberg, H. H., 1968, A defect in circulating monoculear phagocytes in chronic granulomatous disease of childhood, *J. Immunol.* **101**:1094.
Douglas, S. D., and Schopfer, K., 1974, Phagocytic function in protein-caloric malnutrition, *Clin. Exp. Immunol.* **17**:121.
Forman, M. L., and Stiehm, E. R., 1969, Impaired opsonic activity but normal phagocytosis in low birth-weight infants, *N. Engl. J. Med.* **281**:926.
Gallin, J. I., and Kaplan, A. P., 1974, Mononuclear cell chemotactic activity of kallikrein and plasminogen activator and its inhibition by C1 inhibitor and α_2 macroglobulin, *J. Immunol.* **113**:1928.
Gallin, J. I., and Quie, P. G. (eds.), 1978, *Leukocyte Chemotaxis: Methods, Physiology, and Clinical Implications*, Raven Press, New York.
Gallin, J. I., and Wolff, S. M., 1976, Leucocyte chemotaxis: Physiological considerations and abnormalities, *Clin. Haematol.* **4**:567.
Gallin, J. I., Klimerman, J. A., Padgett, G. A., and Wolff, S. M., 1975, Defective mononuclear chemotaxis in the Chediak–Higashi syndrome of humans, mink and cattle, *Blood* **45**:863.
Gallin, J. I., Gallin, E. K., Malech, H. L., and Cramer, E. B., 1978, Structural and ionic events during leukocyte chemotaxis, in: *Leukocyte Chemotaxis* (J. I. Gallin and P. G. Quie, eds.), pp. 123–141, Raven Press, New York.
Goetzl, E. J., and Austen, K. F., 1974, Stimulation of human neutrophil leukocyte aerobic glucose metabolism by purified chemotactic factors, *J. Clin. Invest.* **53**:591.
Golde, D. W., Territo, M., Finley, T. N., and Cline, M. J., 1976, Defective lung macrophages in pulmonary alveolar proteinosis, *Ann. Intern. Med.* **85**:304.
Gordon, S., and Cohn, S. A., 1973, The macrophage, *Int. Rev. Cytol.* **36**:171.
Griffin, F. M., Bianco, C., and Silverstein, S. C., 1975, Characterization of the macrophage receptor

for complement and demonstration of its functional independence from the receptor for the Fc portion of immunglobulin G, *J. Exp. Med.* **141**:1269.

Hausman, M. S., Brosman, S., Snyderman, R., Mickey, M. R., and Fahey, J., 1975, Defective monocyte function in patients with genitourinary carcinoma, *J. Natl. Cancer Inst.* **55**:1047.

Hill, H. R., 1978, Cyclic nucleotides as modulators of leukocyte chemotaxis, in: *Leukocyte Chemotaxis* (J. I. Gallin and P. G. Quie, eds.), pp. 179–193, Raven Press, New York.

Holmes, B., Quie, P. G., Windhorst, D. B., and Good, R. A., 1966, Fatal granulomatous disease of childhood: An inborn abnormality of phagocytic function, *Lancet* **1**:1225.

Johnston, R. B., and Newman, S. L., 1977, Chronic granulomatous disease, *Pediatr. Clin. North Amer.* **24**:365.

Karnovsky, M. L., and Lazdins, J. K., 1978, Biochemical criteria for activated macrophages, *J. Immunol.* **121**:809.

Karnovsky, M. L., Lasdins, J., and Simmons, S. R., 1973, Metabolism of activated mononuclear phagocytes at rest and during phagocytosis, in: *Mononuclear Phagocytes in Immunity, Infection and Pathology* (R. van Furth, ed.), pp. 423–439, Blackwell, Oxford.

Klebanoff, S. J., and Hamon, C. B., 1973, Antimicrobial systems of mononuclear phagocytes, in: *Mononuclear Phagocytes in Immunity, Infection and Pathology* (R. van Furth, ed.), pp. 507–531, Blackwell, Oxford.

Klein, R. B., Fischer, T. J., Gard, S. E., Biberstein, M., Rich, K. C., and Stiehm, E. R., 1977, Decreased mononuclear and polymorphonuclear chemotaxis in newborns, *Pediatrics* **60**:467.

Kleinerman, E. S., Snyderman, R., and Daniels, C. A., 1974, Depression of human monocyte chemotaxis by herpes simplex and influenza viruses, *J. Immunol.* **113**:1562.

Kleinerman, E. S., Snyderman, R., and Daniels, C. A., 1975, Depressed monocyte chemotaxis during acute influenza infection, *Lancet* **2**:1063.

Kretschmer, R. R., Stewardson, B. B., Papiernialo, C. K., and Gotoff, S. P., 1976, Chemotactic and bactericidal capacities of human newborn monocytes, *J. Immunol.* **117**:1303.

Lawrence, H. S., 1974, Transfer factor in cellular immunity, in: *Harvey Lecture Series*, Academic Press, New York.

Lay, W. H., and Nussenzweig, V., 1968, Receptors for complement on leukocytes, *J. Exp. Med.* **128**:991.

Lehrer, R. I., 1975, The fungicidal mechanisms of human monocytes. I. Evidence for myeloperoxidase-linked and myeloperoxidase-independent candidacidal mechanisms, *J. Clin. Invest.* **55**:338.

Lehrer, R. I., and Cline, M. J., 1969, Leukocyte myeloperoxidase deficiency and disseminated candidiasis: The role of myeloperoxidase in resistance to candida infection, *J. Clin. Invest.* **48**:1478.

Mackaness, G. B., 1962, Cellular resistance to infection, *J. Exp. Med.* **116**:381.

Matoth, Y., 1952, Phagocytic and ameboid activities of the leukocytes in the newborn infant, *Pediatrics* **9**:748.

Metchnikoff, E., 1893, *Lectures on the Comparative Pathology of Inflammation*, Kegan, Paul, Trench, Trubner & Co., London.

Miller, M. E., 1969, Phagocytosis in the newborn infant: Humoral and cellular factors, *J. Pediatr.* **74**:255.

Miller, M. E., 1971, Chemotactic function in the human neonate: Humoral and cellular aspects, *Pediatr. Res.* **5**:487.

Miller, M. E., 1978, *Host Defenses in the Human Neonate*, Grune & Stratton, New York.

Miller, M. E., and Myers, K. A., 1975, Cellular deformability of the human peripheral blood polymorphonuclear leukocyte: Method of study, normal variation, and effects of physical and chemical alterations, *J. Reticuloendothelial Soc.* **18**:337.

Miller, T. E., 1971, Metabolic events involved in the bactericidal activity of normal mouse macrophages, *Infect. Immun.* **3**:390.

Mills, E. L., Thompson, T., Björkstén, B., and Quie, P. G., 1979, The chemiluminescence response and bactericidal activity of neutrophils from newborns and their mothers, *Pediatrics* **63**:429.

Nathan, C. F., Murray, H. W., and Cohn, Z. A., 1980, The macrophage as an effector cell, *N. Engl. J. Med.* **303**:622.

Nathan, D. G., Baehner, R. L., and Weaver, D. K., 1969, Failure of nitroblue tetrazolium reduction in the phagocytic vacuoles of leukocytes in chronic granulomatous disease, *J. Clin. Invest.* **48**:1895.

Nelson, D. S., 1969, *Macrophages and Immunity*, North-Holland, Amsterdam.

North, R. J., 1978, The concept of the activated macrophage, *J. Immunol.* **121**:806.

Orlowski, J. P., Sieger, L., and Anthony, B. F., 1976, Bactericidal capacity of monocytes of newborn infants, *J. Pediatr.* **89**:797.

Pahwa, S., Pahwa, R., Grimes, E., and Smithwick, E. M., 1977, Cellular and humoral components of monocyte and neutrophil chemotaxis in cord blood, *Pediatr. Res.* **11**:677.

Rabinovitch, M., 1967, Attachment of modified erythrocytes to phagocyte cells in the absence of serum, *Proc. Soc. Exp. Biol. Med.* **124**:396.

Rabinovitch, M., 1968, Phagocytosis: The engulfment stage, *Semin. Haematol.* **5**:134.

Rabinovitch, M., 1970, Phagocytic recognition, in: *Mononuclear Phagocytes* (R. van Furth, ed.), pp. 299–315, Blackwell, Oxford.

Raghunathan, R., Leake, R. D., and Miller, M. E., 1979, Cord blood monocyte movement: An assessment by chemotaxis and cell elastimetry, *Clin. Res.* **27**:110A.

Rebuck, J. W., and Crowley, J. H., 1955, A method of studying leukocytic functions *in vivo*, *Ann. N.Y. Acad. Sci.* **59**:757.

Rodey, G. E., Park, B. H., Windhorst, D. B., and Good, R. A., 1969, Defective bactericidal activity of monocytes in fatal granulomatous disease, *Blood* **33**:813.

Root, R. K., Rosenthal, A. L., and Balestra, D. J., 1972, Abnormal bactericidal, metabolic, and lysosomal functions of Chediak–Higashi syndrome leukocytes, *J. Clin. Invest.* **51**:649.

Scornik, J. C., 1976, Complement dependent immunoglobulin G receptor function in lymphoid cells, *Science* **192**:563.

Snyderman, R., and Mergenhagen, S. E., 1976, Chemotaxis of macrophages, in: *Immunobiology of the Macrophage* (D. S. Nelson, ed.), pp. 323–348, Academic Press, New York.

Snyderman, R., Altman, L. C., Frankel, A., and Blaese, R. M., 1973, Defective mononuclear leucocyte chemotaxis: A previously unrecognized immune dysfunction, *Ann. Intern. Med.* **78**:509.

Solotorovsky, M., and Soderberg, L., 1972, Host–parasite interactions with macrophages in culture, in: *Macrophages and Cellular Immunity* (A. I. Laskin and H. Lechavalier, eds.), pp. 77–123, CRC Press, Cleveland.

Steigbigel, R. T., Lambert, L. H., and Remington, J. S., 1974, Phagocytic and bacterial properties of normal human monocytes, *J. Clin. Invest.* **53**:131.

Steinman, R. M., and Cohn, Z. A., 1972, The interaction of particulate horseradish peroxidase (HRP)–anti HRP immune complexes with mouse peritoneal macrophages *in vitro*, *J. Cell Biol.* **55**:616.

Stossel, T. P., 1977, Phagocytosis: Clinical disorders of recognition and ingestion, *Am. J. Pathol.* **88**:741.

Stossel, T. P., 1978, The mechanism of leukocyte locomotion, in: *Leukocyte Chemotaxis* (J. I. Gallin and P. G. Quie, eds.), pp. 143–160, Raven Press, New York.

van Furth, R., and Cohn, Z. A., 1968, The origin and kinetics of mononuclear phagocytes, *J. Exp. Med.* **128**:415.

Ward, P. A., and Berenberg, J. L., 1974, Defective regulation of inflammatory mediators in Hodgkin's disease, *J. Pediatr.* **290**:76.

Ward, P. A., Remold, H. G., and David, J. R., 1970, The production by antigen-stimulated lymphocytes of a leukotactic factor distinct from migratory inhibitory factor, *Cell. Immunol.* **1**:162.

Weston, W. L., Carson, B. S., Barkin, R. M., and Slater, G. E., 1976, Monocyte-macrophage function in the newobrn, *Clin. Res.* **28**:182A.

Wright, W. C., Jr., Ank, B. J., Herbert, J., and Stiehm, E. R., 1975, Decreased bactericidal activity of leukocytes of stressed newborn infants, *Pediatrics* **56**:579.

3

The Functional Heterogeneity of Macrophages

WILLIAM S. WALKER and RAYMOND B. HESTER

1. INTRODUCTION

Macrophages are morphologically and functionally diverse. As a group, they comprise cells that play vital roles in homeostasis (Berlin and Berk, 1975) and in host defense reactions against foreign materials, microbial agents (Nelson, 1969; Nathan *et al.*, 1980), and, possibly, neoplasms (Adams and Snyderman, 1979). These activities, as well as their accessory cell functions in immune responses differ widely from one anatomical site to another and, in many cases, within the same population.

It is the purpose of this chapter to bring together recent examples of macrophage diversity, in particular those reported since the last reviews on this subject (Walker, 1976a; Hopper *et al.*, 1979; Lee, 1980), and to discuss possible reasons for macrophage functional heterogeneity.

2. FUNCTIONAL DIVERSITY OF MACROPHAGES FROM DIFFERENT TISSUES

2.1. ALVEOLAR AND PERITONEAL MACROPHAGES

Macrophages display numerous regional differences in morphology, physiology, and function; such differences between alveolar (AM) and peritoneal (PM) macrophages have long been recognized and extensively studied (Table 1; also see previous reviews by Walker, 1976a, and Hopper *et al.*, 1979; Lee, 1980). One of the more striking differences between AM and PM is the manner by which they derive energy. As might be expected, AM rely almost entirely on oxidative metabolism, whereas PM and other tissue macrophages utilize mainly anaerobic metabolism. This difference in energy metabolism appears to be due

WILLIAM S. WALKER and RAYMOND B. HESTER • Division of Immunology, St. Jude Children's Research Hospital, Memphis, Tennessee 38101.

to local tissue adaptation, since the levels of enzymes involved in O_2 metabolism can be modulated, depending upon whether the macrophages are maintained in an aerobic or anaerobic environment (Simon *et al.*, 1977; Bar-Eli *et al.*, 1980).

Other functional differences have been reported (Table 1), but in many instances they appear to be quantitative rather than qualitative. One wonders if some of the apparent differences are not, in fact, the consequence of deficient cell function due, in part, to the application of inappropriate atmospheric conditions to these cell populations.

2.2. MACROPHAGES FROM OTHER TISSUES

The development of *in vitro* methods for more efficient isolation, purification, and propagation of macrophages from tissue sources, other than the lung or peritoneum, has provided increasingly reliable data on the functional potentials of "fixed"-tissue macrophages.

TABLE 1. SOME DIFFERENCES BETWEEN ALVEOLAR AND PERITONEAL MACROPHAGES

Activity	Characteristics and references
Energy metabolism	AM derive energy from oxidative metabolism; PM from glycolysis (Oren *et al.*, 1963; Cohn, 1968)
Activation *in vivo*	Intravenous infusion of *C. parvum* fails to activate AM to either tumoricidal or microbicidal activity, whereas PM can be rendered cytotoxic toward both (Ryning *et al.*, 1981)
Elastase secretion	Resident PM secrete low levels except when phagocytically active; elicited PM and resident AM secrete high levels constitutively (White *et al.*, 1977)
Accessory cell function	Rat AM inhibit T-cell proliferation, whereas PM function as accessory cells (Holt and Batty, 1980). Two subpopulations of AM cells have been noted (Holt, 1979, 1980; van Oud Alblas *et al.*, 1981; Pennline and Herscowitz, 1981). Guinea pig AM are more efficient accessory cells than PM (Gorenberg and Daniele, 1978), and murine Ia^+ AM present *Listeria* to immune T cells less efficiently than Ia^+ resident PM (Weinberg and Unanue, 1981)
Chemotaxis	Elicited murine PM are more active than resident AM (Dohlman and Goetzl, 1978)
Complement receptors	Both resident or elicited PM bear CR1 and suspensions of resident PM contain a high proportion of $CR3^+$ cells; elicited PM are $CR3^-$ (Bianco *et al.*, 1975; Rabellino *et al.*, 1978; Kaplan, 1977; Hearst *et al.*, 1980; Ross, 1980). Guinea pig, human, and rabbit AM also bear CR1 and suspensions of the latter two populations contain $CR3^+$ cells (Reynolds *et al.*, 1975; Hunninghake and Fauci, 1976). Murine AM have been reported to lack both CR1 and CR3 (Hearst *et al.*, 1980; however, see Table 2)
Antigens	There are numerous reports of antigenic differences between AM and PM (Walker, 1976a). A monoclonal antibody reactive only with rat AM has been reported (Rumpold *et al.*, 1981).
Synthesis of complement components	Populations of PM contain a higher proportion of C2- and C4-secreting cells than populations of AM; the latter cells secrete at a higher rate than the former (Cole *et al.*, 1980)

2.2.1. Bone Marrow Macrophages

Macrophages can be grown from bone marrow progenitors (Goud *et al.*, 1975), and such cells possess a number of properties and functions associated with other tissue macrophages. In the mouse, for instance, these include Fc receptors (Goud *et al.*, 1975; Walker and Yen, 1982), complement receptor (CR) 1 but not CR3 (binding sites for C3b and C3bi, respectively; Walker and Yen, 1982), and a distinct subpopulation of bone marrow-derived macrophages that bear surface Ia antigen (Lee and Wong, 1979; Walker *et al.*, 1981; Mottram *et al.*, 1981). Functionally, these culture-derived cells can induce helper T cells (Stern *et al.*, 1979), process and present antigens in an Ia-dependent manner (Lee and Wong, 1979), elicit delayed-type hypersensitivity reactions (Mottram and Miller, 1980), and produce natural killer activity (Lohmann-Matthes *et al.*, 1979).

2.2.2. Liver Macrophages

The liver contains a higher proportion of fixed macrophages (Kupffer cells) than any organ (Walker, 1976a), and as such is the major phagocytic barrier in the host. Experiments performed a few years ago to test the ability of Kupffer cells to process and present ingested antigen indicated that these cells were unable to interact productively with lymphocytes for immune induction (Inchley and Howard, 1969). This view was strengthened by *in vivo* observations that hepatic uptake of antigen failed to result in immune sensitization, whereas the hepatic bypass of the same antigens led to an immune reactive state (Triger *et al.*, 1972). Rogoff and Lipsky (1980) and Nadler *et al.* (1980) have reexamined this question using a highly purified population of guinea pig and murine Kupffer cells. Their results indicated that the cells presented antigen to lymphocytes in an Ia-dependent manner similar, although somewhat less efficiently than peritoneal macrophages. Whether the cells make up a distinct subpopulation situated in an anatomically strategic location in the liver is unknown. It may be pertinent that very early studies implicated the liver as a major depot of antigen (Garvey and Campbell, 1957).

2.2.3. Splenic Macrophages

Populations of macrophages from different tissues vary in their effectiveness as accessory cells in the induction of acquired immunity. For the most part, splenic macrophages perform accessory functions more effectively than equivalent numbers of macrophages from other tissue sources (Schwartz *et al.*, 1978). Whether this difference is due to a high content of Ia-bearing macrophages or rather to a lower proportion of macrophages with suppressor-cell activity is unknown, and will be difficult to decide without populations of macrophages containing only Ia^+ cells.

Additional heterogeneity among splenic macrophages has been noted by Roubin and co-workers (Roubin and Zolla-Pazner, 1979; Roubin *et al.*, 1981), who described a small subpopulation of macrophages that formed, upon overnight culture, cell clusters or so-called "foci." These cells differed from the majority of macrophages by binding and ingesting unopsonized sheep erythrocytes and by bearing surface receptors for IgM. The origin and functional significance of these "focus-forming" macrophages are unknown.

In addition to playing an important immunoregulatory function, splenic macrophages are also involved in the removal of effete cellular elements, in particular senescent erythrocytes (Berlin and Berk, 1975) by mechanism(s) that may involve antibody and macrophages Fc receptors (Kay, 1981).

3. FUNCTIONAL DIVERSITY AMONG MACROPHAGES FROM THE SAME TISSUE

The diversity of functions assigned to macrophages in the induction of acquired immunity suggested that populations of these cells, like populations of lymphocytes, could be grouped into subpopulations of cells that were functionally distinct (Walker, 1976a,b). Support for this view has come from numerous reports showing that many macrophage-associated activities are restricted to or enriched in distinct subpopulations of cells (Table 2).

3.1. ACCESSORY CELL ACTIVITY

An early indication that populations of macrophages were heterogeneous in accessory cell activity came with the observations of Mosier and Coppleson (1968), who concluded from cell-mixing experiments that only 1 to 10 cells per 10,000 murine splenic macrophages were essential for the induction of an *in vitro* immune response. More direct evidence was provided by Walker (1971); and confirmed by Rice and Fishman (1974), who demonstrated that populations of elicited peritoneal macrophages could be separated into density subpopulations of cells with different capacities to form immunogenic RNA capable of inducing specific antibody formation in cultures of spleen cells.

The separation of suspensions of peritoneal macrophages into large and small cells by velocity sedimentation also disclosed marked differences in accessory cell activity. Gorczynski (1976) and Lee and Berry (1977) found that small- to medium-sized macrophages differed from large macrophages in their ability to reconstitute *in vitro* antibody- and cell-mediated immune responses. Further heterogeneity was noted when a distinct subpopulation of carbohydrate-processing macrophages was detected (Gorczynski *et al.*, 1979).

These findings have been extended by Tzehoval *et al.* (1981), who described two major subpopulations of elicited peritoneal macrophages in mice, only one of which efficiently processed and presented antigen to primed T cells and was enriched for cells bearing Ia antigen.

There are a number of morphologically distinguishable types of splenic macrophages located at distinct anatomical sites (Carr, 1973). Recently, Humphrey and Grennan (1981) found that macrophages of the white pulp marginal zone differed from macrophages in the red pulp in the uptake of selected poly-

TABLE 2. SOME EXAMPLES OF HETEROGENEITY AMONG MACROPHAGES FROM A SINGLE TISSUE

Characteristic	References
Morphology	Nelson (1969), Carr (1973), Pels *et al.* (1980), van Furth (1980), Tzehoval *et al.* (1981), Yasaka *et al.* (1981), Norris *et al.* (1979)
Density, size	Zembala and Asherson (1970), Walker (1971, 1974), Rice and Fishman (1974), Gorczynski (1976), Lee *et al.* (1979), Tzehoval *et al.* (1981), Miller *et al.* (1980), Yasaka *et al.* (1981), Norris *et al.* (1979), Norman and Weiner (1981), Pelus *et al.* (1981)
Phagocytic activity	Walker (1971), Kavet and Brain (1977), Roubin and Zolla-Pazner (1979), Tzehoval *et al.* (1981), Yasaka *et al.* (1981)
Fc receptors	Walker (1974), Rhodes (1975), Kavai *et al.* (1979), Melewicz and Spiegelberg (1980), Roubin *et al.* (1981), Yasaka *et al.* (1981)
Complement receptors	Whitcomb (1978), Roubin *et al.* (1981), Walker and Yen (1982)
Ia antigen	Schwartz *et al.* (1976), Yamashita and Shevach (1977), Cowing *et al.* (1978), Beller and Unanue (1981), Lee *et al.* (1979), Henry *et al.* (1979), Lee *et al.* (1981), Tzehoval *et al.* (1981)
Secretion of factors	Pelus *et al.* (1981), Tice *et al.* (1981), Yasaka *et al.* (1981)
Subcellular distribution of ingested antigen	Walker (1976a)
Accessory cell function	Walker (1971), Werdelin *et al.* (1974), Rice and Fishman (1974), Lee and Wong (1979), Gorczynski *et al.* (1979), Lee *et al.* (1979), Tzehoval *et al.* (1981), Humphrey and Grennan (1981)
Enzyme content	Fishman and Weinberg (1979), Schroff *et al.* (1981)
Tumoricidal activity	Walker (1976b), Weinberg *et al.* (1978), Lee and Berry (1977), Miller *et al.* (1980), Campbell *et al.* (1980), Norman and Weiner (1981)
Formation of immunogenic RNA	Walker (1971), Rice and Fishman (1974)
Progenitors	McCarthy and MacVittie (1978)

saccharides. These populations also differed in their content of Ia^+ macrophages: suspensions of marginal zone cells contained few, if any, Ia-bearing cells, while about one-half of the red pulp macrophages bore detectable Ia. The accessory activities of these two populations were not tested directly; nevertheless, the authors suggest that marginal zone macrophages may play a role in presenting T-independent antigens to B cells, whereas the red pulp Ia^+ macrophages may participate in presenting Ir-restricted antigens to T-helper and T-suppressor cells.

3.2. Ia ANTIGENS

Certain antigen responses require Ia-bearing macrophages. Yamashita and Shevach (1977) reported that between 15 and 25% peritoneal macrophages elicited in guinea pigs bore Ia antigens and that antibody and complement abrogated the accessory function of these cells. Heterogeneity in the expression of Ia antigen has been reported for murine peritoneal macrophages (Schwartz *et al.*, 1976) as well as for splenic macrophages involved in antibody responses *in vitro* (Niederhuber, 1978) and antigen-specific T-cell responses (Germain *et al.*, 1980). The proportion of Ia-bearing macrophages in different populations of cells varies depending upon anatomical site, environmental stimuli, and the method used to detect the Ia antigen. Unanue and Beller (1981), for instance, observed that agents such as thioglycollate medium, used to induce inflammatory exudates, did not influence the proportion of Ia^+ macrophages in the elicited population. By contrast, injection of *Listeria* yielded exudates in which the majority of the cells bore Ia antigen.

The levels of Ia antigen on monocytes or macrophages can vary with culture conditions, and some have concluded that the antigen is lost completely from peritoneal macrophages upon culturing (Beller and Unanue, 1981). There is evidence, however, that murine peritoneal macrophages do not lose Ia antigen, since Ia^+-resident macrophages can be detected after 5 to 7 days in culture by use of a rosetting assay (Table 3). Furthermore, such cells are fully capable of presenting the synthetic antigen GAT to primed lymphocytes (Table 4), whose response to the antigen is under Ir-gene control (Germain *et al.*, 1980). These results indicate that the proportion of Ia-bearing cells depends on the type of assay used.

Whether the Ia^+ and Ia^- subpopulations of macrophages represent separate cell lineages (Walker *et al.*, 1981) or simply a particular stage in the differentiation-maturation of a single lineage of cells (Lee *et al.*, 1981; Mottram *et al.*, 1981) is unknown. Scher *et al.* (1980) have described a T-cell-derived factor that renders some but not all Ia^- macrophages Ia^+, a circumstance favoring the single lineage model.

3.3. ACTIVATION OF TUMORICIDAL AND MICROBICIDAL ACTIVITY

Populations of macrophages obtained from normal animals or from animals previously injected with macrophage-activating agents such as BCG or *C. parvum*, exhibit marked heterogeneity in tumoricidal activity. Walker (1976b) noted cytotoxic differences between density-dependent subpopulations of elicited rat peritoneal macrophages cultured with [^{125}I]–UdR-labeled syngeneic tumor cells in a long-term (20 hr) assay. Lee and Berry (1977), using velocity-sedimentation subpopulations, found that the cytotoxic macrophages were confined to larger cells and that the smaller macrophages, which lacked detectable cytotoxic activity, could function as accessory cells in immune induction *in vitro*. Weinberg *et al.* (1978) tested subpopulations of elicited peritoneal macrophages from normal rats for their ability to inhibit tumor cell growth *in vitro* (cytostasis) and found that such activity was limited to light-density macrophages isolated on density gradients of bovine serum albumin. Campbell *et al.* (1980) also found that elicited

TABLE 3. DETECTION OF Ia ANTIGEN ON MURINE RESIDENT PERITONEAL MACROPHAGES[a]

Time in culture	M percent (± range) rosette-positive cells	
	CBA(*H-2*^{k}, Ia. 2^{+})	BALB/c(*H-2*^{d}, Ia. 2^{-})
2 hr	45 ± 9	5 ± 2
5 days	46 ± 3	20 ± 1

[a]Sheep erythrocytes, coupled with monoclonal anti-Ia.2 from hybridoma 11-5.2.1.9 (Oi *et al.*, 1978), were mixed with suspensions of adherent purified resident peritoneal cells obtained from dishes incubated for the indicated times in culture. After incubation at 4°C, the number of macrophages forming rosettes was determined microscopically.

and activated rat peritoneal macrophages, differing in anti-tumor-cell activity, could be separated into subpopulations on discontinuous gradients of Percoll or by centrifugal elutriation (Miller *et al.*, 1980). In contrast to the findings of Weinberg *et al.* (1978), however, Campbell *et al.* (1980) found tumoricidal activity, as observed by Lee and Berry (1977), associated with the high-density macrophages Of particular interest was the observation that light-density macrophages promoted rather than inhibited tumor cell growth *in vitro* and that this could be confirmed *in vivo* by Winn-type experiments (Morahan and Miller, 1981).

Macrophages activated to tumoricidal activity are not necessarily microbicidal and *vice versa*. Wing *et al.* (1977) have dissociated these two effector functions and suggest that different subpopulations of activated macrophages may express these cytotoxic activities. In addition, Meltzer and associates have shown that activation for rickettsicidal and tumoricidal activity can be dissociated in particular strains of mice (Meltzer *et al.*, 1981; Nacy *et al.*, 1981).

TABLE 4 CULTURED RESIDENT PERITONEAL MACROPHAGES SERVE AS ACCESSORY CELLS IN A T-CELL RESPONSE TO THE ANTIGEN GAT[a]

Culture	Macrophages	[^{3}H]-TdR incorporated (cpm) + medium	+ GAT	+ GAT and anti-Ia.2
GAT-primed T cells	—	500	2,700	ND
	Day 0	2500	27,500	3000
	Day 5	2000	17,500	1000

[a]Macrophage-depleted lymph node cells from GAT-primed CBA mice were added to 0- and 5-day cultures of adherent peritoneal cells followed by the addition of medium, GAT, or GAT and anti-Ia.2. The proliferative response of the T cells was measured by [^{3}H]thymidine incorporation after 3 days of culture. The results presented are mean values from duplicate experiments.

3.4. HUMAN BLOOD MONOCYTES

Application of cell separation techniques to suspensions of human blood monocytes has revealed a marked heterogeneity within this population. Density gradient centrifugation, velocity sedimentation, and centrifugal elutriation have all been used to isolate monocyte subpopulations differing in Fc-receptor activity (Norris *et al.*, 1979; Melewicz and Spiegelberg, 1980; Yasaka *et al.*, 1981), antibody-dependent cellular cytotoxicity (Norris *et al.*, 1979), response to colony-stimulating factors (Yasaka *et al.*, 1981; Tice *et al.*, 1981), chemotactic agents (Yasaka *et al.*, 1981), nonspecific esterase activity (Norris *et al.*, 1979; Yasaka *et al.*, 1981), and the capacity to become cytotoxic toward tumor cells (Norman and Weiner, 1981).

In addition, some heterogeneity in surface antigen phenotype has been noted. Raff *et al.* (1980) described a monoclonal antibody (Mac-120) that detects a 120,000-dalton protein on a subpopulation of HLA-Dr monocytes. These cells were required for T-cell reactivity to certain antigens and stimulated autologous mixed leukocyte reactions. Hogg and Slusarenko (1981) have prepared a monoclonal antibody reagent that reacts with an antigen found on the processes of cultured neural cells and some, but not all, adherent human monocytes.

4. POSSIBLE REASONS FOR MACROPHAGE HETEROGENEITY

Differences in cell phenotype among macrophages are usually attributed to changes in stage of differentiation-maturation (van Furth, 1970, 1980) or to local tissue adaptation (Bar-Eli *et al.*, 1980). It is possible, however, that some phenotypic differences arise from differences in cell lineages or from the self-renewal of local macrophage populations (Volkman, 1976a). Thus, the tissue origin of macrophages bears directly on any explanation of functional diversity.

Most agree that macrophages which accumulate at the sites of inflammation are derived mainly from circulating monocytes originating in the bone marrow (Volkman, 1976b; van Furth, 1980). The origin, under normal or steady-state conditions, of resident tissue macrophages is still controversial. In one view, all macrophages, regardless of tissue location, functional property, or morphology, originated from a common progenitor that resides in the bone marrow. Peripheral macrophage populations are thought to be replenished from the circulating pool of monocytes (van Furth, 1970, 1980). Thus, functional differences between and within populations of macrophages would reflect either a continuum of stages in differentiation–maturation or be the result of local tissue adaptation.

Arguments for the single lineage model rest on (1) experiments with bone marrow-derived macrophages that have repopulated lethally irradiated recipients (Balner, 1963; Pinkett *et al.*, 1966; Virolainen, 1968; Brunstetter *et al.*, 1971; Godleski and Brain, 1972; Thomas *et al.*, 1976; Gale *et al.*, 1978; Johnson *et al.*, 1980); (2) the reduction of *in vivo* labeling indices of tissue macrophages in animals rendered monocytopenic with corticosteroids (Crofton *et al.*, 1978); (3)

the finding that only a small fraction of resident tissue macrophages can be labeled with [^{3}H]thymidine *in vivo* (Takahashi *et al.*, 1973; Shands and Axelrod, 1977; van Furth *et al.*, 1980); and (4) the similarity of acid esterase isozyme patterns of human monocyte and resident peritoneal macrophages (Parwaresch *et al.*, 1981).

Conclusions drawn from the bone marrow repopulation studies have been criticized on two grounds (Volkman, 1976b). First, the bone marrow may contain progenitors for more than one type of macrophage and, second, lethally irradiated recipients may not represent a valid steady-state model, since products of dead or dying recipient cells could influence the tissue distribution of macrophages derived from donor bone marrow. Similarly, the use of corticosteroids to produce monocytopenia (Crofton *et al.*, 1978) may produce effects well beyond blocking the efflux of monocytes from the bone marrow (Seljelid, 1980). Finally, similar isoenzyme patterns in resident peritoneal macrophages and circulating monocytes (Parwaresch *et al.*, 1981) are consistent with but do not prove identical lineages for the two cell types.

The opposing scheme holds that resident propulations are capable of self-renewal withough drawing on the pool of circulating monocytes (Volkman, 1976a). Functional heterogeneity, therefore, could be partly explained by the presence of functionally specialized, autonomous populations of macrophages (Walker, 1976a). Evidence for the lineal independence of resident macrophage populations is found in (1) the parabiotic experiments of Volkman (1976a) and of Collins and Auclair (1980), which have been interpreted as inconsistent with a circulating monocyte origin for normal perioneal macrophages, liver Kupffer cells, or alveolar macrophages; (2) the *in vivo* labeling studies of Takahashi *et al.* (1973) and Shands and Axelrod (1977), indicating that a small population of normal peritoneal macrophages become labeled earlier and more intensely than circulating monocytes in mice infused intravenously with [^{3}H]thymidine; (3) the demonstration that populations of resident tissue macrophages contain macrophage progenitors, as determined by their ability to form macrophage colonies *in vitro* (Stewart, 1980); (4) the recent report by Volkman *et al.* (1983) showing that the numbers of resident peritoneal macrophages were unaffected in mice rendered monocytopenic with the bone-seeking isotope ^{89}Sr; (5) the report of Bursuker and Goldman (1979) demonstrating distinct and phenotypically stable 5′-nucleotidase activities in bone marrow-derived macrophages and cultured resident and elicited peritoneal macrophages; and finally (6) the observations of Daems and co-workers (1973, 1976, 1980) and Widmann, Fahimi, and colleagues (1972, 1975), who interpreted the ultrastructural peroxidase-staining patterns of elicited versus resident macrophages as evidence for a separate origin of the latter. The conclusion drawn from the peroxidase data has been challenged by van der Meer *et al.* (1979) on the basis of their finding a transitional macrophage in peritoneal resident populations with an intermediate peroxidase staining pattern, which they believe confirms the lineal relationship from monocyte, to the elicited and normal resident tissue macrophages (see, however, Daems and Van der Rhee, 1980). The validity of peroxidase-staining patterns as a stable marker for defining macrophage lineages has been questioned (Bainton, 1980).

An additional aspect of macrophage heterogeneity concerns the cell cycle. Populations of macrophages contain different proportions of cells synthesizing DNA (Volkman, 1976a; Shands and Axelrod, 1977; van Furth, 1980), and differences in cell cycle phase could contribute to macrophage heterogeneity (Berlin *et al.*, 1978), in particular in populations of macrophages elicited by inflammatory agents. Recent studies (Gandour and Walker, 1981; Gandour and Walker, 1983), using murine macrophage-like cell lines, have shown that the cells are enhanced in their Fc receptor-mediated phagocytic activity as they approach the G2 phase of the cycle, and are diminished in phagocytic activity during the M phase. The bases for the enhanced phagocytic activity are related to the presence of greater numbers of Fc receptors on cells in G2.

5. CONCLUSIONS

This chapter has drawn attention to phenotypic differences between macrophages from different tissues and among macrophages isolated from the same tissue. The issue now is the basis for this morphological and functional diversity.

Clearly, some functional differences can be attributed solely to local tissue adaptation (Bar-Eli *et al.*, 1980), or in many instances to the stage of differentiation-maturation, and as such can be accommodated within the framework of a single lineage model. For instance, the heterogeneity among alveolar macrophages in Fc receptor activity is readily eliminated by *in vitro* culture (Rhodes, 1975). Other phenotypic differences, however, are not so easily explained. Walker and Yen (1982) noted that cells and colonies derived from murine bone marrow, blood, and the elicited peritoneal macrophage population had a common complement receptor phenotype, $CR1^{+}3^{-}$, whereas colonies from the resident peritoneal population contained either $CR1^{+}3^{-}$ or $CR1^{+}3^{+}$ cells. The distribution of cells, and eventually of colonies containing a high proportion of cells bearing either CR phenotype, did not change during culture, indicating the stability of the phenotype. While alternative explanations do exist, these phenotypic differences suggest the presence of at least two clonally derived types of macrophages in the resident population.

The origins of macrophages subpopulations remain uncertain and until this central issue is resolved, it will not be possible to determine with certainty the basis for macrophage functional heterogeneity, i.e., whether it reflects a continuum of differentiation-maturation of a single lineage of cells or is due to the existence of autonomously derived and, possibly, functionally specialized population of cells.

ACKNOWLEDGMENTS. The authors' work has been supported by research grants from the National Institutes of Health, the American Cancer Society, and by ALSAC. The authors acknowledge the editorial and secretarial assistance of Mr. John Gilbert and Ms. Chris Winston, respectively.

REFERENCES

Adams, D. O., and Snyderman, R., 1979, Do macrophages destroy nascent tumors?, *J. Natl. Cancer Inst.* **62**:1341.

Bainton, D. F., 1980, Changes in peroxidase distribution within organelles of blood monocytes and peritoneal macrophages after surface adherence *in vitro* and *in vivo*, in: *Mononuclear Phagocytes—Functional Aspects, Part I* (R. van Furth, ed.), pp. 61–86, Nijhoff, The Hague.

Balner, H., 1963, Identification of peritoneal macrophages in mouse radiation chimers, *Transplantation* **1**:217.

Bar-Eli, M., Territo, M. C., and Cline, M. S., 1980, The progeny of a single progenitor cell can develop characteristics of either a tissue or an alveolar macrophage, *Blood* **57**:95.

Beller, D. I., and Unanue, E. R., 1981, Regulation of macrophage populations: Synthesis and expression of Ia antigen by peritoneal exudate macrophages is a transient event, *J. Immunol.* **126**:263.

Berlin, N. I., and Berk, P. D., 1975, The biological life of the red cell, in: *The Red Blood Cell* (D. MacSurgenor, ed.), pp. 957–1019, Academic Press, New York.

Berlin, R. D., Oliver, J. M., and Walter, R. J., 1978, Surface functions in mitosis. I. Phagocytosis, pinocytosis and mobility of surface bound Con A, *Cell* **15**:327.

Bianco, C., Griffin, F. M., and Silverstein, S. C., 1975, Studies of the macrophage complement receptor: Alteration of receptor function upon macrophage activation, *J. Exp. Med.* **141**:1278.

Brunstetter, M. A., Hardie, J. A., and Schiff, R., 1971, The origin of pulmonary alveolar macrophages, *Arch. Intern. Med.* **127**:1064.

Bursuker, I., and Goldman, R., 1979, Derivation of resident and inflammatory macrophages from precursor cells differing in 5'-nucleotidase activity, *J. Reticuloendothelial Soc.* **26**:205.

Campbell, M. W., Sholley, M. M., and Miller, G. A., 1980, Macrophage heterogeneity in tumor resistance: Cytostatic and cytotoxic activity of *Corynebacterium parvum*-activated and proteose peptone-elicited rat macrophages against Moloney sarcoma tumor cells, *Cell. Immunol.* **50**:153.

Carr, I., 1973, *The Macrophage*, Academic Press, New York.

Cohn, Z., 1968, The structure and function of monocytes and macrophages, *Adv. Immunol.* **9**:163.

Cole, F. S., Matthews, W. J., Marino, J. T., Gash, D. J., and Colten, H. R., 1980, Control of complement synthesis and secretion in bronchoalveolar and peritoneal macrophages, *J. Immunol.* **125**:1120.

Collins, F. M., and Auclair, L. K., 1980, Mononuclear phagocytes in the lungs of unstimulated parabiotic rats, *J. Reticuloendothelial Soc.* **27**:429.

Cowing, C., Schwartz, B. D., and Dickler, H. B., 1978, Macrophage Ia antigens: Macrophage subpopulations differ in their expression of Ia antigens, *J. Immunol.* **120**:378.

Crofton, R. W., Diesselhoff-den Dulk, M. M. C., and van Furth, R., 1978, The origin, kinetics and characteristics of the Kupffer cells in the normal steady state, *J. Exp. Med.* **148**:1.

Daems, W. T., and Brederoo, P., 1973, Electron microscopical studies on the structure, phagocytic properties and peroxidatic activity of resident and exudate peritoneal macrophages, *Z. Zellforsch. Mikrosk. Anat.* **144**:247.

Daems, W. T., and Van der Rhee, H. J., 1980, Peroxidase and catalase in monocytes, macrophages, epithelioid cells and giant cells of the rat, in: *Mononuclear Phagocytes—Functional Aspects, Part I* (R. van Furth, ed.), pp. 43–60, Nijhoff, The Hague.

Daems, W. Th., Koerten, H. K., and Soranzo, M. R., 1976, On the differences between monocyte-derived and tissue macrophages, *Adv. Exp. Med. Biol.* **73**:PT-A2740.

Dohlman, J. G., and Goetzl, E. J., 1978, Unique determinants of alveolar macrophage spontaneous and chemokinetically stimulated migration, *Cell. Immunol.* **39**:36.

Fishman, M., and Weinberg, D. S., 1979, Functional heterogeneity among peritoneal macrophages: Enzyme content of macrophage subpopulations, *Cell. Immunol.* **45**:437.

Gale, R. P., Sparkes, R. S., and Golde, D. W., 1978, Bone marrow origin of hepatic macrophages (Kupffer cells) in humans, *Science* **201**:937.

Gandour, D. M., and Walker, W. S., 1981, Cell cycle-dependent expression of the IgG2a isotypespecific Fc-receptor and IgG2a antibody-dependent phagocytosis by the P388D1 macrophage cell line, Proc. 18th Annu. Natl. Meet. Reticuloendothelial Soc., Milwaukee, Abstract 96.

Gandour, D. M., and Walker, W. S., 1983, Macrophage cell cycling: Influence on Fc receptors and antibody-dependent phagocytosis, *J. Immunol.* **130:**1108–1112.

Garvey, J. S., and Campbell, D. H., 1957, Studies of the retention and properties of S^{35} labeled antigen in livers of immunized rabbits, *J. Immunol.* **76:**36.

Germain, R. N., Pierres, M., and Benacerraf, B., 1980, The role of macrophages in determining the balance of regulatory T-cells specific for L-glutamic acid^{60}-L-alanine^{30}-L-tyrosine^{10} (GAT), in: *Macrophage Regulation of Immunity* (E. R. Unanue and A. S. Rosenthal, eds.), pp. 15–33, Academic Press, New York.

Godleski, J. J., and Brain, J. D., 1972, The origin of alveolar macrophages in mouse radiation chimers, *J. Exp. Med.* **136:**630.

Gorczynski, R. M., 1976, Control of the immune response: Role of macrophages in regulation of antibody- and cell-mediated immune responses, *Scand. J. Immunol.* **5:**1031.

Gorczynski, R. M., MacRae, S., and Jennings, J. J., 1979, A novel role for macrophage: Antigen discrimination of distinct carbohydrate bonds, *Cell. Immunol.* **45:**276.

Gorenberg, D. J., and Daniele, R. P., 1978, The alveolar macrophages: Its capacity to act as an accessory cell in mitogen-stimulated proliferation of guinea pig lymphocytes, *Cell. Immunol.* **36:**115.

Goud, T. J., Shotte, C., and van Furth, R., 1975, Identification and characterization of the monblast in mononuclear phagocyte colonies grown *in vitro, J. Exp. Med.* **142:**1180.

Hearst, J. E., Warr, G. A., and Jakab, G. J., 1980, Characterization of murine lung and peritoneal macrophages, *J. Reticuloendothelial Soc.* **27:**443.

Henry, C., Goodman, J. R., Chan, E., Kimura, J., Lucas, A., and Wofsy, L., 1979, Macrophage Ia antigens: Electron microscopic visualization and relevance in an *in vitro* anti-hapten response, *J. Reticuloendothelial Soc.* **26:**787.

Hogg, N., and Slusarenko, M., 1981, Monoclonal antibodies to subsets of human blood monocytes, in: *Heterogeneity of Mononuclear Phagocytes* (O. Forster and M. Landy, eds.), pp. 60–65, Academic Press, New York.

Holt, P. G., 1979, Studies on the mechanism of inhibition of T-cell proliferation, *Immunology* **37:**437.

Holt, P. G., 1980, Interspecies differences in activity in proliferating lymphocyte cultures, *Cell. Immunol.* **50:**210.

Holt, P. G., and Batty, J. E., 1980, Comparative studies on the antigen presentation activity of guinea pig and rat alveolar macrophages, *Immunology* **36:**257.

Hopper, K. E., Wood, P. R., and Nelson, D. S., 1979, Macrophage heterogeneity, *Vox Sang.* **36:**257.

Humphrey, J. H., and Grennan, D., 1981, Different macrophage populations distinguished by means of fluorescent polysaccharides: Recognition and properties of marginal-zone macrophages, *Eur. J. Immunol.* **121:**221.

Hunninghake, G. W., and Fauci, A. S., 1976, Immunological reactivity of the lung: A guinea pig model for the study of pulmonary mononuclear cell populations, *Cell. Immunol.* **26:**89.

Inchley, C. J., and Howard, J. G., 1969, The immunogenicity of phagocytosed T4 bacteriophage: Cell replacement studies with splenectomized and irradiated mice, *Clin. Exp. Immunol.* **5:**189.

Johnson, K. J., Ward, P. A., Striker, G., and Kunkel, R., 1980, A study of the origin of pulmonary macrophages using the Chediak–Higashi marker, *Am. J. Pathol.* **101:**365.

Kaplan, G., 1977, Differences in the mode of phagocytosis with Fc and C3 receptors in macrophages, *Scand. J. Immunol.* **6:**797.

Kavai, M., Laczko, J., and Csaba, B., 1979, Functional heterogeneity of macrophages, *Immunology* **36:**729.

Kavet, R. I., and Brain, J. D., 1977, Phagocytosis: Quantification of rates and intracellular heterogeneity, *J. Appl. Physiol.* **42:**432.

Kay, M. M. B., 1981, Isolation of the phagocytosis-inducing IgG-binding antigen on senescent somatic cells, *Nature (London)* **289:**491.

Lee, K.-C., 1980, On the origin and mode of action of functionally distinct macrophage subpopulations, *Mol. Cell. Biochem.* **30:**39.

Lee, K.-C., and Berry, D., 1977, Functional heterogeneity in macrophages activated by *Corynebac-*

terium parvum: Characterization of subpopulations with different activities in promoting immune responses and suppressing tumor cell growth, *J. Immunol.* **118:**1530.

Lee, K.-C., and Wong, M., 1979, Functional heterogeneity of culture-grown bone marrow derived macrophages: Antigen presenting function, *J. Immunol.* **125:**86.

Lee, K.-C., Wilkinson, A., and Wong, M., 1979, Antigen-specific murine T-cell proliferation: Role of macrophage surface Ia and factors, *Cell. Immunol.* **48:**79.

Lee, K.-C., Wong, M., and McIntyre, D., 1981, Characterization of macrophage subpopulations responsive to activation by endotoxin and by lymphokines, *J. Immunol.* **126:**2474.

Lohmann-Matthes, M. L., Domzig, W., and Taskov, H., 1979, Antibody-dependent cellular cytotoxicity against tumor cells: Cultivated bone-marrow-derived macrophage kill tumor cells, *Eur. J. Immunol.* **9:**261.

McCarthy, K. F., and MacVittie, T. J., 1978, Velocity sedimentation studies on monocyte-macrophage colony forming cells from marrow, spleen, blood and peritoneal exudate, *J. Reticuloendothelial Soc.* **24:**263.

Melewicz, F. M., and Spiegelberg, H. L., 1980, Fc-receptors for IgE on a subpopulation of human peripheral blood monocytes, *J. Immunol.* **125:**1026.

Meltzer, M. S., Nacy, C. A., and Leonard, E. J., 1981, Genetic analysis of macrophage effector function: Development of nonspecific tumoricidal and microbicidal activities during leukocyte activation, in: *Heterogeneity of Mononuclear Phagocytes* (O. Forster and M. Landy, eds.), pp. 384–389, Academic Press, New York.

Miller, G. A., Campbell, M. V., and Hudson, J. L., 1980, Separation of rat peritoneal macrophages into functionally distinct subclasses by centrifugal elutriation, *J. Reticuloendothelial Soc.* **27:**167.

Morahan, P. S., and Miller, G. A., 1981, Heterogeneity of *Corynebacterium parvum*-elicited macrophages, in: *Heterogeneity of Mononuclear Phagocytes* (O. Forster and M. Landy, eds.), pp. 161–164, Academic Press, New York.

Mosier, D. E., and Coppleson, E., 1968, A three-cell interaction required for the induction of the primary immune response *in vitro*, *Proc. Natl. Acad. Sci. USA* **61:**542.

Mottram, P. L., and Miller, J. F. A. P., 1980, Delayed-type hypersensitivity induced by antigen-pulsed, bone marrow-derived macrophages, *Eur. J. Immunol.* **10:**165.

Mottram, P. L., Potter, T. A., McKenzie, I. F. C., and Miller, J. F. A. P., 1981, Serological analysis of macrophage surface alloantigens, *Cell. Immunol.* **59:**151.

Nacy, C. A., Leonard, E. J., and Meltzer, M. S., 1981, Macrophages in resistance to rickettsial infections: Characterization of lymphokines that induce rickettsiacidal activity in macrophages, *J. Immunol.* **126:**204.

Nadler, P. I., Klingenstein, R. J., Richman, L. K., and Ahmann, G. B., 1980, The murine Kupffer cell: Accessory cell function in *in vitro* primary antibody responses, mitogen-induced proliferation, and stimulation of mixed lymphocytic responses, *J. Immunol.* **125:**2521.

Nathan, C. F., Murray, H. W., and Cohn, Z. A., 1980, The macrophage is an effector cell, *N. Engl. J. Med.* **303:**622.

Nelson, D. S., 1969, *Macrophages and Immunity*, North-Holland, Amsterdam.

Niederhuber, J. E., 1978, The role of *I*-region gene products in macrophage–T lymphocyte interaction, *Immunol. Rev.* **40:**28.

Norman, S. J., and Weiner, R., 1981, Isolation of two subsets of human peripheral blood monocytes differing in tumor cytotoxicity, in: *Heterogeneity of Mononuclear Phagocytes* (O. Forster and M. Landy, eds.), pp. 496–500, Academic Press, New York.

Norris, D. A., Morris, R. M., Sanderson, R. J., and Kohler, P. F., 1979, Isolation of functional subsets of human peripheral blood monocytes, *J. Immunol.* **123:**166.

Oi, V. T., Jones, P. P., Goding, J. W., Herzenberg, L. A., and Herzenberg, L. A., 1978, Properties of monoclonal antibodies to mouse Ig allotypes, H-2, and Ia antigens, *Curr. Top. Microbiol. Immunol.* **81:**115.

Oren, R. A., Farnham, A. E., Saito, K., Milofsky, E., and Karnovsky, M. L., 1963, Metabolic patterns in three types of phagocytosing cells, *J. Cell Biol.* **17:**487.

Parwaresch, M. R., Radzum, H. J., and Dommes, M., 1981, The homogeneity and monocytic origin of human peritoneal macrophages evidenced by comparison of esterase polymorphism, *Am. J. Pathol* **102:**209.

Pels, E., DeGroot, J. W., Mullink, R., van Unnik, J. A. M., and Den Otter, W., 1980, Identification of two different types of mouse peritoneal exudate cells with ring-shaped nuclei, *J. Reticuloendothelial Soc.* **27**:367.

Pelus, L. M., Broxmeyer, H. E., DeSousa, M., and Moore, M. A. S., 1981, Heterogeneity among resident murine peritoneal macrophages: Separation and functional characterization of monocytoid cells producing granulcoyte–macrophage colony stimulating factor (GM-CSF) and responding to regulation by lactoferrin, *J. Immunol.* **126**:1016.

Pennline, K. J., and Herscowitz, H. B., 1981, Dual role for alveolar macrophages in humoral and cell-mediated immune responses: Evidence for suppressor and enhancing factors, *J. Reticuloendothelial Soc.* **30**:205.

Pinkett, M. O., Cowdrey, C. R., and Nowell, P. C., 1966, Mixed hematopoietic and pulmonary origin of alveolar macrophages as demonstrated by chromosome markers, *Am. J. Pathol.* **48**:859.

Rabellino, E. M., Ross, G. D., and Polley, M. J., 1978, Membrane receptors for mouse leukocytes: Two types of complement receptors for different regions of C3, *J. Immunol.* **120**:879.

Raff, H. V., Picker, L. J., and Stobo, J. D., 1980, Macrophage heterogeneity in man: A subpopulation of HLA-Dr-bearing macrophages required for antigen-induced T-cell activation also contains stimulators for autologous-reactive T-cells, *J. Exp. Med.* **152**:581.

Reynolds, H. Y., Atkinson, J. P., Newball, H. H., and Frank, M. M., 1975, Receptors for immunoglobulins and complement on human alveolar macrophage, *J. Immunol.* **114**:1813.

Rhodes, J., 1975, Macrophage heterogeneity in receptor activity: The activation of macrophage Fc-receptor function *in vivo* and *in vitro*, *J. Immunol.* **114**:976.

Rice, S., and Fishman, M., 1974, Functional and morphological heterogeneity among rabbit peritoneal macrophages, *Cell. Immunol.* **11**:130.

Rogoff, T. M., and Lipsky, P. E., 1980, Antigen presentation by isolated guinea pig Kupffer cells, *J. Immunol.* **124**:1740.

Ross, G., 1980, Analysis of different types of leukocyte membrane complement receptors and their interaction with the complement system, *J. Immunol. Methods* **37**:197.

Roubin, R., and Zolla-Pazner, S., 1979, Markers of macrophage heterogeneity: Studies of macrophages from various organs of normal mice, *Eur. J. Immunol.* **9**:972.

Roubin, R., Kennard, J., Foley, D., and Zolla-Pazner, S., 1981, Markers of macrophage heterogeneity: Altered frequency of macrophage subpopulations after various pathologic stimuli, *J. Reticuloendothelial Soc.* **29**:423.

Rumpold, H., Swetly, P., Boltz, G., and Forster, O., 1981, Monoclonal antibodies against macrophage-associated antigens, in: *Heterogeneity of Mononuclear Phagocytes* (O. Forster and M. Landy, eds.), pp. 47–51, Academic Press, New York.

Ryning, F. W., Krahenbuhl, J. L., and Remington, J. S., 1981, Comparison of cytotoxic and microbicidal function of bronchoalveolar and peritoneal macrophages, *Immunology* **42**:513.

Scher, M. G., Beller, D. I., and Unanue, E. R., 1980, Demonstration of a soluble factor that induces exudates rich in Ia-positive macrophage, *J. Exp. Med.* **152**:1684.

Schroff, G., Newmann, C., and Sorg, C., 1981, Transglutaminase as a marker for subsets of murine macrophages, *Eur. J. Immunol.* **11**:637.

Schwartz, R. H., Dickler, H. B., Sachs, D. H., and Schwartz, B. D., 1976, Studies on Ia antigens on immune peritoneal macrophages, *Scand. J. Immunol.* **5**:731.

Schwartz, R. H., Yano, A., and Paul, W. E., 1978, Interaction between antigen-presenting cells and primed T-lymphocytes, *Immunol. Rev.* **40**:152.

Seljelid, R., 1980, Properties of Kupffer cells, in: *Mononuclear Phagocytes—Functional Aspects, Part I* (R. van Furth, ed.), pp. 157–199, Nijhoff, The Hague.

Shands, J. W., and Axelrod, B. J., 1977, Mouse peritoneal macrophages: Tritiated thymidine labeling and cell kinetics, *J. Reticuloendothelial Soc.* **21**:69.

Simon, L. M., Robin, E. D., Phillips, J. R., Acevedo, J., Axline, S. G., and Theodore, T., 1977, Enzymatic basis of bioenergetic differences of alveolar versus peritoneal macrophages and enzyme regulation by molecular O_2, *J. Clin. Invest.* **59**:443.

Stern, A. C., Erb, P., and Gisler, R. H., 1979, Ia-bearing bone-marrow cultured macrophages induce antigen-specific helper T-cells for antibody synthesis, *J. Immunol.* **123**:612.

Stewart, C. C., 1980, Formation of colonies by mononuclear phagocytes outside the bone marrow, in: *Mononuclear Phagocytes—Functional Aspects, Part I* (R. van Furth, ed.), pp. 377–413, Nijhoff, The Hague.

Takahashi, H., Enzan, H., and Ohkita, T., 1973, Studies on cell kinetics of peritoneal macrophages, *Recent Adv. RES Res.* **11**:85.

Thomas, E. D., Ramberg, R. E., Sale, G. E., Sparkes, R. S., and Golde, D. W., 1976, Direct evidence for a bone marrow origin of the alveolar macrophage in man, *Science* **192**:1016.

Tice, D. G., Golberg, J., and Nelson, D. A., 1981, Functional properties of isopycnic fractions of human peripheral blood monocytes, *J. Reticuloendothelial Soc.* **29**:459.

Triger, D. R., Alp, M. H., and Wright, R., 1972, Bacterial and dietary antibodies in liver disease, *Lancet* **1**:60.

Tzehoval, E., DeBaetselier, P., Feldman, M., and Segal, S., 1981, The peritoneal antigen-presenting macrophage: Control and immunogenic properties of distinct subpopulations, *Eur. J. Immunol.* **11**:323.

Unanue, E. R., and Beller, D. I., 1981, Control of Ia expression by macrophages, in: *Heterogeneity of Mononuclear Phagocytes* (O. Forster and M. Landy, eds.), pp. 214–217, Academic Press, New York.

van der Meer, J. W. M., Beelen, R. H. J., Fluitsma, D. M., and van Furth, R., 1979, Ultrastructure of mononuclear phagocytes developing in liquid bone marrow cultures: A study on peroxidatic activity, *J. Exp. Med.* **149**:17.

van Furth, R. (ed.), 1970, The origin and turnover of promonocytes, monocytes and macrophages in normal mice, in: *Mononuclear Phagocytes*, pp. 151–165, Blackwell, Oxford.

van Furth, R. (ed.), 1980, Cells of the mononuclear phagocyte system—Nomenclature in terms of sites and conditions, in: *Mononuclear Phagocytes—Functional Aspects*, pp. 1–30, Nijhoff, The Hague.

van Furth, R., Diesselhoff-den Dulk, M. M. C., Raeburn, J. A., van Zwet, T. L., Crofton, R., and van Oud Alblas, A. B., 1980, Characteristics, origin and kinetics of human and murine mononuclear phagocytes, in: *Mononuclear Phagocytes—Functional Aspects, Part I* (R. van Furth, ed.), pp. 279–298, Nijhoff, The Hague.

van Oud Alblas, A. B., van der Linden-Schrever, B., and van Furth, R., 1981, Origin and kinetics of pulmonary macrophages during an inflammatory reaction induced by intravenous administration of heat-killed bacillus Calmette-Guerin, *J. Exp. Med.* **154**:235.

Virolainen, M., 1968, Hematopoietic origin of macrophages as studied by chromosome markers in mice, *J. Exp. Med.* **127**:943.

Volkman, A., 1976a, Disparity in origin of mononuclear phagocyte populations, *J. Reticuloendothelial Soc.* **19**:249.

Volkman, A., 1976b, Monocyte kinetics and their changes in infection, in: *Immunobiology of the Macrophage* (D. S. Nelson, ed.), pp. 291–322, Academic Press, New York.

Volkman, A., Chang, N. C., Strausbauch, P. H., and Morahan, P. S., 1981, Differential effects of chronic monocyte depletion on macrophage populations laboratory investigation **49**:291–298.

Walker, W. S., 1971, Macrophage functional heterogeneity in the *in vitro*-induced immune response, *Nature New Biol.* **229**:211.

Walker, W. S., 1974, Functional heterogeneity of macrophages: Subclasses of peritoneal macrophages with different antigen binding activities and immune complex receptors, *Immunology* **26**:1025.

Walker, W. S., 1976a, Macrophage functional heterogeneity, in: *Immunobiology of the Macrophage* (D. S. Nelson, ed.), pp. 91–110, Academic Press, New York.

Walker, W. S., 1976b, Macrophage functional heterogeneity in the induction and expression of acquired immunity, *J. Reticuloendothelial Soc.* **20**:57.

Walker, W. S., and Yen, S.-E., 1982, Complement receptor phenotypes of culture-derived murine macrophages, *J. Cell. Physiol.* **110**:227–284.

Walker, W. S., Hester, R. B., Gandour, D. M., and Stewart, C. C., 1981, Evidence of a distinct progenitor for the Ia-bearing murine bone-marrow-derived mononuclear phagocyte, in: *Heterogeneity of Mononuclear Phagocytes* (O. Forster and M. Landy, eds.), pp. 229–232, Academic Press, New York.

Weinberg, D. S., and Unanue, E. R., 1981, Antigen-presenting function of alveolar macrophages:

Uptake and presentation of *Listeria monocytogenes*, *J. Immunol.* **126**:794.

Weinberg, D. S., Fishman, M., and Veit, B. C., 1978, Functional heterogeneity among peritoneal macrophages: Effector cell activity of macrophages against syngenic and xenogeneic tumor cells, *Cell. Immunol.* **38**:94.

Werdelin, O., Braendstrup, O., and Pederson, E., 1974, Macrophage–lymphocyte clusters in the immune response to soluble protein antigen *in vitro*. I. Roles of lymphocytes and macrophages in cluster formation, *J. Exp. Med.* **140**:1245.

Whitcomb, M. E., 1978, Identification of a receptor for complement on the guinea pig alveolar macrophage membrane, *Am. Rev. Respir. Dis.* **118**:431.

White, R., Lin, H.-S., and Kun, C., 1977, Elastase secretion by peritoneal exudative and alveolar macrophages, *J. Exp. Med.* **146**:802.

Widmann, J. J., and Fahimi, H. D., 1975, Proliferation of mononuclear phagocytes (Kupffer cells) and endothelial cells in regenerating liver, *Am. J. Pathol.* **80**:349.

Widmann, J. J., Cotran, R. S., and Fahimi, H. D., 1972, Mononuclear phagocytes (Kupffer cells) and endothelial cells: Identification of two functional cell types in rat liver sinusoids by endogenous peroxidase activity, *J. Cell Biol.* **52**:159.

Wing, E. J., Gardner, I. D., Ryning, F. W., and Remington, J. S., 1977, Dissociation of effector junctions in populations of activated macrophages, *Nature (London)* **268**:642.

Yamashita, V., and Shevach, E. M., 1977, The expression of Ia antigen on immunocompetent cells in the guinea pig: Ia antigens on macrophages, *J. Immunol.* **119**:1584.

Yasaka, T., Mantich, N. M., Boxer, L. A., and Baehner, R. L., 1981, Functions of human monocyte and lymphocyte subsets obtained by countercurrent centrifugal elutriation: Differing functional capacities of human monocyte subsets, *J. Immunol.* **127**:1515.

Zembala, M., and Asherson, G. L., 1970, The rapid purification of peritoneal exudate macrophages by Ficoll (polysucrose) density gradient centrifugation, *Immunology* **19**:677.

4

Differentiation and Functional Regulation in Macrophage Cell Lines

PETER RALPH

1. INTRODUCTION

1.1. ADVANTAGES OF CELL LINES

Macrophage-related cell lines offer many advantages for the study of macrophage function (Table 1). These advantages range from *convenience* in obtaining large numbers of cells of relatively homogenous nature by growth in culture, to *purity* of the cell population ensuring that experimental results obtained are due only to macrophages. A *variety* of cell lines and variants exist which stably differ in degree of maturation, sensitivity to inducing agents, and extent of mature macrophage characteristics. Since the cell lines are growing rapidly, it is relatively easy to synchronize or select cells at different stages of the *cell cycle* for study of physiological functions throughout the cell division process.

1.2. SPECIES OF MACROPHAGE-RELATED CELL LINES

Most macrophage lines are derived from murine macrophage tumors. However, a number of lines have been obtained from long-term cultures of normal macrophages (Ralph, 1981a). One or a few lines have been described from chicken (Pfeifer *et al.*, 1980), rabbit, hamster, pig, goat, sheep, guinea pig, dog, cat, and human (Ralph, 1980; Tsuchiya *et al.*, 1980; Wardley *et al.*, 1980; Ralph, 1981a; Bradley *et al.*, 1982). Adaptation to culture and routine growth of macrophage lines has been reviewed by Ralph (1981b). A number of murine lines are

PETER RALPH • Memorial Sloan–Kettering Cancer Center, Rye, New York 10580.

TABLE 1. ADVANTAGES OF MACROPHAGE CELL LINES

Property	Examples	References
Convenience	Production of IL-1 or CSF	Farrar *et al.* (1980), Williams *et al.* (1978)
	Screening immunomodulators	Ralph *et al.* (1977)
Homogeneity		
Biochemical	Intracellular signals associated with gene activation	Kikutani *et al.* (1981), Rosen *et al.* (1979)
Immunochemical	Hybridoma antibody to Mϕ subsets	Springer (1980)
Functional	Cytotoxic activity in Mϕ subsets	Ralph and Nakoinz (1981)
	(Receptor) differences in response to modulators	Ralph *et al.* (1978a)
	Megakaryocyte potentiator free of mega-CSF	Williams *et al.* (1981)
Exclusion of other cell types	LPS stimulation of PFC independent of T cells	Hoffmann *et al.* (1979)
	Direct effect of agents on macrophages	Taniyama and Holden (1980), Ralph *et al.* (1977, 1978a,b, 1980a)
	Production of IL-1 free from IL-2	Farrar *et al.* (1980)
Selection of variants	Loss of Fc receptors	Unkeless (1979), Diamond *et al.* (1978)
	Phagocytosis defects	Muschel *et al.* (1977)
	Lack of H_2O_2 and O_2^- production	Damiani *et al.* (1980)
Functions throughout the cell cycle	Cessation of endocytosis at mitosis	Berlin *et al.* (1978)
Rapid growth, transformation	Cell type-specific growth inhibitors	Ralph *et al.* (1977, 1978a)
	Cancer type-specific chemotherapy	Ralph (1980)

available from ATCC and Meloy Laboratories, and human line U937 is available from ATCC.*

1.3. PROBLEMS WITH CELL LINES

Cell line characteristics are generally stable over periods of a year. The cells can be stored frozen as a supply for reproducible experiments. However, the possibility of unknown contamination of a culture with a different cell line, and overgrowth by variant clones, requires continual quality control and occasion-

*American Type Culture Collection, Dr. Anita C. Weinblatt, 12301 Parklawn Avenue, Rockville, Md. 02852. Meloy Laboratories, Dr. Cortesi, 6715 Electronic Drive, Springfield, Va. 22151.

ally recloning to maintain or select the desired macrophage properties. I have discussed these problems elsewhere (Ralph, 1981b).

2. SUMMARY OF MACROPHAGE CHARACTERISTICS MAINTAINED BY CELL LINES

2.1. MATURE MACROPHAGE CELL LINES

Table 2 shows a number of well-characterized murine lines, their mouse strain of origin and etiology, and special properties. All the lines have strong expression of surface receptors for immunoglobulin Fc and complement, produce lysozyme, and are highly active in phagocytosis of latex or zymosan beads (Ralph and Nakoinz, 1977a). Most of these lines also exhibit immune or antibody-dependent phagocytosis of red blood cells (Ralph and Nakoinz, 1977b, 1980) and varying degrees of cytolytic activity toward red blood cells and tumor targets induced by lymphokine, lipopolysaccharide (LPS), phorbol myristic acetate (PMA), antitarget antibody, and other agents (Ralph and Nakoinz, 1981).

WEHI-3 is perhaps the most immature in this group, with lysozyme, production of endogenous pyrogen, interleukin-1 (IL-1), myeloid colony-stimulating activity (CSA), and prostaglandin E, zymosan, and latex bead phagocytosis but little immune phagocytosis or cytotoxicity (Ralph and Nakoinz, 1977a,b, 1981; Lachman and Metzgar, 1980; Kurland *et al.*, 1979) and very low pinocytosis (Jones and Byrne, 1980). Other lines have most of the functions of peritoneal macrophages.

None of the lines is as adherent as their normal counterparts, but adherence can be increased by transferring from suspension culture to glass or plastic tissue culture substrate in assays (Muschel *et al.*, 1977). Cells also adhere when incubated without serum, with activating agents such as LPS, or with prostaglandin E (PGE) or choleratoxin.

Macrophage cell lines are generally lacking in Ia surface antigen involved in regulation of induction of T- and B-cell immunity (Ralph, 1980). However, Ia has been detected on macrophage cell lines (Walker *et al.*, 1982).

2.2. CONSTITUTIVE AND INDUCED PRODUCTION OF ENZYMES AND SECRETED PRODUCTS

Monokines produced by cell lines include colony-stimulating and related factors for megakaryocyte, erythrocyte, mast cell or basophil, neutrophil, and macrophage progenitors and their precursors (Table 3). Factors that stimulate induction of cytotoxic T cells and immunoglobulin secretion by B lymphocytes have been described (reviewed in Ralph, 1980) and are probably the same as IL-1 or LAF. The cell lines require LPS, BCG, PMA, or other stimulation to produce most of these factors. The dose–response for induction is closely associated with

TABLE 2. MATURE MURINE MACROPHAGE CELL LINES[a]

Name	Strain	Etiology[b]	Special properties[d]	References
WEHI-3	BALB/c	S	Requires own growth factor	Broxmeyer and Ralph (1977)
			Many hemopoietic factors	Williams *et al.* (1981)
			Monocyte-like migration	Aksamit *et al.* (1981)
J774	BALB/c	Oil	Supports *Leishmania* growth	Chang (1980)
			Phosphokinase studies	Kikutani *et al.* (1981)
			Phosphokinase studies	Rosen *et al.* (1979)
PU5-1.8	BALB/c	S?	Strongly cytotoxic	Ralph and Nakoinz (1981)
			Tumoricidal factor (TNF)	Männel *et al.* (1980)
Fc-1	BALB/c	Fusion[c]	Migration sensitive to MIF	Newman *et al.* (1979)
SKW2	BALB/c	A-MuLV		Ralph and Nakoinz (1981)
RAW264	BAB/14	A-MuLV	Strongly cytotoxic	Ralph and Nakoinz (1981)
RAW309Cr	CX BALB.B	A-MuLV		Raschke *et al.* (1978)
LS23	CAL-20	A-MuLV		Ralph and Nakoinz (1981)
IC-21	C57BL/6	SV40	Unresponsive to stimulators	Taniyama and Holden (1980)
			Lacks plasminogen activator	Neumann and Sorg (1981)
			Functionally different complement receptors	Walker and Gandour (1980)
P388D1	DBA/2	S?	Purification of calmodulin	Jamieson and Vanaman (1980)
			Megakaryocyte potentiator	Williams *et al.* (1981)
			Processes Fc stimulator of T cells	Thoman *et al.* (1981)
426C	DBA/2	OS virus[c]		Ralph *et al.* (1980a)
SK2.2	CBA/J	S[c]		Ralph *et al.* (1980a)
A	A/J	S[c]		Ralph *et al.* (1983a)
NCTC1469	C3H/He Anf	S	Liver origin	van Loveren *et al.* (1981)
BJ-1	C3H/HeJ	SV40	Pulmonary origin	Cahoon and Mills (1981)
427E	$B_6D_2F_1$	F-MuLV[c]		Testa *et al.* (1980)
Several	NZB×B, NZB×W	SV40		Levy *et al.* (1981)

[a]These cell lines manifest Fc and C receptors, latex bead phagocytosis, and lysozyme production.
[b]Tumors except as noted. S, spontaneous; A-MuLV, Abelson murine leukemia virus; OS, osteosarcoma virus; F-MuLV, Friend murine leukemia virus.
[c]Experimental cell fusion or virus transformation *in vitro* or spontaneous outgrowth in culture.
[d]A number of lines exhibit chemotaxis (Aksamit *et al.*, 1981; Snyderman *et al.*, 1977), receptors for CSF-1 (Guilbert and Stanley, 1980), and cytotoxic capacity (see below).

TABLE 3. ENZYMES AND OTHER SECRETIONS OF MURINE MACROPHAGE LINES

Property	References
Hemopoietic factors	
Separate granulocyte and macrophage CSFs	Williams *et al.* (1978)
Megakaryocyte CSF and potentiation factor	Williams *et al.* (1981)
Platelet-stimulating factor	Krizsa and Dexter (1978)
Pre-CFU-C-stimulating factor[a]	Broxmeyer (unpublished)
Erythroid burst-promoting factor (BPA)	Iscove (unpublished)
Erythroid-potentiating factor	Ascensao *et al.* (1981)
Mast cell CSF	Nagao *et al.* (1981); Yung *et al.* (1981)
Acidic isoferritin inhibitor	Broxmeyer *et al.* (1982)
Lymphocyte regulators	
IL-1	Farrar *et al.* (1980), Lachman and Metzgar (1980)
B-lymphocyte differentiation factor	Hoffmann *et al.* (1979)
Prostaglandin E	Kurland *et al.* (1979)
55K suppressor factor	Arene and Pierce (1980)
H_2O_2 and O_2^-	Damiani *et al.* (1980), Sasada and Johnston (1980)
Tumoricidal factors	Aksamit and Kim (1979), Russell *et al.* (1980)
Interferon	Djeu *et al.* (1979), Neumann and Sorg (1981), Cahoon and Mills (1981)
Endogenous pyrogen	Bodel (1978), Bodel *et al.* (1980)
Lysozyme	Ralph *et al.* (1976)
Neutral proteases	Werb *et al.* (1980), Hamilton and Moore (1980)
Lysosomal enzymes	Kaplan and Mørland (1978), Sündstrom and Nilsson (1977), Greenberger *et al.* (1978), Snyderman *et al.* (1977)
Ectoenzymes	Edelson (1981)
Lipogenic enzymes	Okuma *et al.* (1976)
Peroxidase	Ichikawa *et al.* (1976), Greenberger *et al.* (1978), Sündstrom and Nilsson (1976)
Adenosine deaminase	Snyderman *et al.* (1977)
Thymidine kinase	Stadecker (1981)

[a]Pre-CFU-C, cell that becomes a colony-forming unit in culture.

growth inhibition of the macrophage lines, suggesting induction of terminal maturation or differentiation (Ralph *et al.*, 1978a).

For CSF production by PU5-1.8, induction represents a gene activation, requiring new RNA and protein synthesis (Ralph *et al.*, 1977). Under certain growth conditions, perhaps due to stimulation by fetal calf serum, PGE and CSF are secreted continuously (Kurland *et al.*, 1979). LPS, zymosan, Con A, poly I : C, PPD, and even CSF induce or enhance PGE production.

Oxygen metabolites, peroxide, and superoxide anion are secreted by some macrophage lines upon stimulation with PMA, zymosan, or antigen–antibody complexes (Damiani *et al.*, 1980), although this activity is difficult to maintain (Sasada and Johnston, 1980). Spontaneous release of tumoricidal factors and poly I : C-induced interferon production have been reported as well as a number of enzymes (Table 3).

2.3. IMMATURE CELL LINES

Some cell lines express a plurality of macrophage characteristics only after culture with inducing agents (Table 4). These immature lines can be induced with endogenous mediators like CSF, with activating agents like LPS and PMA, and with unphysiological agents like polar solvents and nucleotide analogs (Sachs, 1978; Ralph *et al.*, 1982c). Even inhibitors of normal macrophage growth or function such as corticosteroids (Ralph *et al.*, 1978b; Werb *et al.*, 1978) and PGE (Williams, 1979; Pellus *et al.*, 1979) can induce some maturation in immature cell lines (Sachs, 1978; Honma *et al.*, 1978).

Macrophage characteristics induced in these cells include receptors for complement and Fc region of IgG; production of CSF, lysozyme, and prostaglandin; mobility in agar; adherence; peroxidase and lysosomal enzymes; and nonspecific phagocytosis. There appears to be a limit to the degree of maturation possible in the immature murine cell lines since induction of antibody-dependent phagocytosis and lysis of RBC and tumor targets have not been detected (Ralph and Nakoinz, 1981). Human line U937 shows greater capacity for differentiation in response to lymphokine, nonlymphoid sources of CSF, and tumor promoter PMA (Ralph *et al.*, 1982c) (Table 4). Two other human monoblast-like lines, RC-2A and THP-1, have weak expression of macrophage characteristics.

TABLE 4. PROPERTIES OF IMMATURE MACROPHAGE-LINEAGE LINES

Name	Strain	Etiology[a]	Macrophage properties	Induced properties	References
M1	SL	S		Enzymes, PGE, CSF, phagocytosis	Sachs (1978)
				Mac-1 and 3 antigens	Ralph *et al.* (1983a)
R453	C57BL/6	R-MuLV		Peroxidase, phagocytosis	Ichikawa *et al.* (1976)
RAW8	BALB/c	A-MuLV	Endogenous pyrogen, (lysozyme)	Fc receptors	Bodel (1978), Ralph *et al.* (1982b)
U937	Human	DHL	Lysozyme	Fc and C receptors	Larrick *et al.* (1980)
			Peroxidase	ADCC[b]	
			Pyrogen	Nonspecific cytotoxicity	Ralph *et al.* (1982c)
				Chemotactic receptor	Pike *et al.* (1980)
				Phagocytosis	Ralph *et al.* (1982c)
RC-2A	Human	AMML	Several[c]		Bradley *et al.* (1982)
THP-1	Human	AMOL	Several[c]		Tsuchiya *et al.* (1980)

[a]S, spontaneous; R-MuLV, Rauscher murine leukemia virus; A-MuLV, Abelson murine leukemia virus; DHL, diffuse histiocytic lymphoma; AMML, acute myelomonocytic leukemia; AMOL, acute monocytic leukemia.
[b]ADCC, antibody-dependent cellular cytotoxicity to red blood cell and tumor targets.
[c]Fc receptors, C receptors, and latex bead phagocytosis weakly expressed.

3. PARASITE–HOST INTERACTIONS

Macrophage cell lines support the growth of a variety of viruses, bacteria, and protozoal parasites (Table 5). Lymphokine and/or LPS stimulate murine macrophage cell line cytotoxicity to *Leishmania tropica* (Murray, 1981), *Toxoplasma gondii*, and *Chlamydia psittaci* (Jones and Byrne, 1980), and human U937 line toxicity to *T. gondii* (Wing *et al.*, 1981).

4. ROLE OF SURFACE ANTIGENS IN DIFFERENTIATION AND FUNCTION OF MACROPHAGES

4.1. PRESENCE OF MACROPHAGE-RESTRICTED ANTIGENS ON MURINE CELL LINES

Differentiation is a process involving the coordinated control of many genes to produce different cell types. Some of the cellular changes occurring during differentiation can be identified by the expression of surface antigens which in some cases are restricted to a particular cell lineage and are specific for the stage of differentiation in that lineage (Boyse and Old, 1969). Springer (1980) has described hybridoma rat anti-mouse cell surface antibodies which recognize antigenic structures on macrophages. Mac-1 antigen of molecular weight 190,000 and 105,000 is present on granulocytes, macrophages, and NK cells; Mac-2 antigen of molecular weight 32,000 and 110,000 Mac-3 antigen have been detected only on mononuclear phagocytes. Differentiation from blood monocyte to thioglycollate-induced peritoneal macrophage is accompanied by a large increase in expression of these three antigens in parallel with a large decrease in expression of a heat-stable antigen found on a number of hematopoietic cell types (Springer, 1980).

For screening purposes, a radiolabel-binding assay was employed to detect

TABLE 5. GROWTH OF MICROBIAL PARASITES IN CELL LINES

Species	References
Flavivirus	Peiris *et al.* (1981)
Bunyavirus	Peiris *et al.* (1981)
Avian leukemia virus	Pfeifer *et al.* (1980)
Yellow fever virus	Schlesinger and Brandriss (1981)
Abelson murine leukemia virus	Raschke *et al.* (1978)
Herpesvirus	C. Lopez (unpublished)
Rickettsia akari	C. Nacy and P. Ralph (unpublished)
Leishmania donovani amastigotes	Berens and Marr (1979)
Leishmania donovani promastigotes	Chang (1980)
Leishmania tropica amastigotes	C. Nacy and P. Ralph (unpublished)
Candida	Sasada and Johnston (1980)
Toxoplasma gondii	Wing *et al.* (1981)
Chlamydia psittaci	Jones and Byrne (1980)

differentiation antigens (Ralph *et al.*, 1983a). Table 6 shows that mature macrophage lines have 1–4 × 10^5 molecules of Mac-1, 2, and 3 antigens per cell. This is true for lines RAW 264 and PU5-1.8, which are highly active, and J774.1, moderately active, in nonspecific and antibody-dependent cellular cytotoxicity (ADCC) to tumor targets (Ralph and Nakoinz, 1981). The highest levels of antigens are found on variant J774.16C3C, which is defective in hydrogen peroxide and superoxide anion production (Damiani *et al.*, 1980), intracellular killing of trypanosome parasites (B. R. Bloom, personal communication) and which has a defect in ADCC but not some mechanisms of nonspecific killing of tumor targets (Ralph, 1980a). Levels of Mac antigens within the range of those found on mature macrophage cell lines are present on the immature WEHI-3 line which maintains Fc and C receptors, lysozyme production, and latex bead phagocytosis of macrophages, but is incapable of cytotoxic activities or immune or antibody-dependent phagocytosis (Ralph and Nakoinz, 1981). Therefore, there is no correlation of these three antigens with cytotoxic capacity or production of oxygen intermediates. Comparison of macrophage lines in production of myeloid colony-stimulating activity, PGE, plasminogen activator (Ralph, 1980), and acidic isoferritin inhibitor of myelopoiesis (Broxmeyer *et al.*, 1982) suggests that Mac antigens are not involved in expression of these activities. Similarly, Mac antigen levels are not altered on cell line variants lacking the ectoenzyme 5′-nucleotidase (Ralph *et al.*, 1983).

The immature or myeloblast lines M1 and RFM and myeloid line C1498 do not express significant amounts of Mac antigens, nor do erythroleukemia or T- or B-lymphocyte lineage leukemia lines (Table 6).

TABLE 6. DETECTION OF MACROPHAGE-RESTRICTED ANTIGENS ON MURINE CELL LINE[a]

Line	Type	Mac-1	Mac-2	Mac-3
PU5-1.8	Macrophage	14	9	11
RAW264.10	Macrophage	22	12	7
J774.1	Macrophage	34	28	27
J774.16C3C	Macrophage	39	32	26
NCTC 1469	Macrophage	14	19	17
A2	Macrophage	14	33	6
WEHI-3	Immature macrophage	10	7	7
M1	Myeloblast	< 1	—	< 1
RFM	Myeloblast	—[b]	—	< 2
GM-86	Erythroleukemia	—	—	—
18-8	Pre-B cell	—	—	—
WEHI-231	B cell	—	—	< 3
X-63	Myeloma	—	—	< 1
EL4	T lymphoma	—	—	—
R1	T lymphoma	—	—	—

[a]Molecules per cell (× 10^4) detected by ^{125}I-labeled antibody binding assay using 10^6 cells under saturation conditions (60 min at 4°C, 70 ng antibody/150,000 cpm) (Ralph *et al.*, 1983a).
[b]Less than 0.6 × 10^4 molecules per cell.

The possibility that Mac-1, 2, and 3 antigens are surface receptors for agents stimulating or binding to macrophages was studied in the J774 cell line. No inhibition of labeled antibody binding was seen using LPS, PMA, CSF, lymphokine, dextran sulfate, mannan (for mannose receptor), or *Ulex* or *Lotus* lectins (for terminal fucose residues) as competitors. Con A and phytohemagglutinin, prebound to J774, substantially inhibited binding of these antibodies, indicating that the corresponding antigens are glycoproteins.

4.2. INDUCTION OF Mac ANTIGENS IN MURINE MYELOBLAST LINE M1

The M1 line has been extensively used as a model for induction of granulocyte/macrophage differentiation (Sachs, 1978). Table 7 shows that incubation of M1 cells with a variety of inducing agents greatly increased expression of Mac-1 and Mac-3 antigens. Mac-2 antigen was never observed on M1 in these experiments. As a control, line GM-86 inducible for erythroid properties was treated with the same agents. Mac-1 and Mac-2 antigens were not detected; Mac-3 expression on GM-86 was stimulated slightly (less than three-fold) but remained low (not shown).

The expression of macrophage antigens on M1 cells was apparent by day 2 of culture with inducing agents and increased up to 6 days of treatment (Table

TABLE 7. INDUCTION OF Mac-1 AND Mac-3 ANTIGENS OF M1 MYELOBLAST LINE[a]

Inducer		Mac-1	Mac-2	Mac-3
0		1.0	—[b]	0.9
L-CM	5%	4.4	—	nd[c]
	20%	18.1	—	nd
	50%	17.0	—	nd
WEHI-3 CM	5%	11.6	—	4.7
	20%	13.5	—	13.8
	50%	15.0	—	11.7
Lymphokine	5%	4.3	—	2.2
	20%	15.9	—	13.0
	50%	17.8	—	10.7
DM	10^{-8} M	2.8	—	1.3
	10^{-7} M	17.2	—	2.6
	10^{-6} M	14.7	—	14.5
	10^{-5} M	18.2	—	16.0
LPS	0.01 μg/ml	6.2	—	nd
	0.1 μg/ml	17.0	—	nd

[a]M1 cells cultured with agents as shown, diluted 1:2 with growth medium at day 3, and on day 6 washed and assayed for binding ^{125}I-labeled antibody as in Table 6. Control cultures increased 6- to 10-fold in cell numbers. Cells recovered in treated cultures were within 20% of control cultures except for 0.1 μg/ml LPS which inhibited growth over 80%. Data shown as antigen molecules (× 10^4) per cell.
[b]Less than 0.3 × 10^4 molecules/cell.
[c]nd, Not done.

8), approaching the levels found on the mature macrophage cell lines. Mac-1 and Mac-3 antigens were attained by the induced cells in parallel with induction of Fc and C receptors and latex bead phagocytosis. The lack of Mac-2 antigen on induced M1 cells suggests that this surface structure is not involved in expression of these macrophage characteristics.

4.3. INHIBITION OF ANTIGEN INDUCTION IN M1 CELLS BY ANTIBODY

Since the three Mac antigens are present on mature phagocytic cells but not in appreciable amounts on immature cells, we tested if the antigens had any role in the process of differentiation of these cell types. M1 cells were incubated with inducing agents in the presence of antibody to Mac-1 or Mac-3. Table 9 shows that the presence of anti-Mac-1 blocked the *induction* by dexamethasone (and lymphokine, not shown) of Mac-3 on antigen on M1 cells by more than 70%. Anit-Mac-1 did not block the *assay* for Mac-3 on already induced M1 cells. In contrast, anti-Mac-3 did not affect the induction of Mac-1 antigen. These results were found with two quite different inducing agents, dexamethasone, which presumably diffuses into the cells and interacts with cytoplasmic receptors, and lymphokine, which probably acts via CSF-like molecules binding to cell surface receptors (Guilbert and Stanley, 1980). Therefore, it is unlikely that anti-Mac-1 interferes with binding of inducers to the cells. In assays of the reverse reaction, neither dexamethasone, lymphokine, nor WEHI-3 CM blocked binding of ^{125}I-labeled antibodies to the three Mac antigens on mature macrophage cells (unpublished). These findings with cell lines suggest that Mac antigens will be found to play a role in proliferation and differentiation of normal bone marrow progenitors of macrophages.

4.4. INDUCTION OF Mac ANTIGENS AND INHIBITION OF DIFFERENTIATION BY ANTIBODY IN HUMAN MONOBLAST LINE U937

Rat monoclonal antibodies to mouse macrophages also react with similar human cell types. Anti-Mac-1 recognizes human macrophages, granulocytes, and NK cells; anti-Mac-3 sees macrophages and anti-Mac-2 is negative with human hemopoietic cells (Springer, 1980; Ault and Springer, 1981). Table 10 shows that Mac-1, 2, and 3 antigens are not detected in appreciable amounts on a variety of human T, B, erythroleukemia, myeloblast, or monoblast cell lines.

U937 cells can be induced by lymphokine (Larrick *et al.*, 1980), PMA (Gidlung *et al.*, 1981; Ralph *et al.*, 1982c), and nonlymphoid cytokines (Ralph *et al.*, 1982c) to express Fc and C receptors, latex bead phagocytosis, nonspecific killing of tumor targets (Ralph *et al.*, 1982c), ADCC to chicken erythrocytes (Gidlung *et al.*, 1981) and tumor targets (Larrick *et al.*, 1980; Ralph *et al.*, 1982c), chemotaxis

TABLE 8. TIME COURSE OF INDUCTION OF ANTIGENS ON M1 CELLS[a]

	Mac-1				Mac-3			
Inducer Day:	1	2	4	6	1	2	4	6
0	0.6	0.8	0.6	1.1	0.7	0.6	0.7	0.8
WEHI-3 CM	0.8	1.9	7.3	1.4	0.8	1.6	6.1	10.0
Lymphokine	1.4	2.0	10.9	17.6	0.9	2.1	6.3	12.6
DM	1.4	2.4	5.2	8.7	1.5	2.1	5.4	6.0

[a]M1 cells assayed for antigen expression (molecules $\times 10^4$ per cell) at various times of incubation with 20% WEHI-3 CM, 20% lymphokine, or 10^{-5} M dexamethasone as in Table 7.

and receptors for chemotactic peptide (Pike *et al.*, 1980). Culture of U937 with these agents induces Mac-1 and Mac-3 expression (Table 11). As seen with the murine M1 line, anti-Mac-1 blocks the induction of Mac-3 on U937 but not its expression.

5. CYTOTOXIC CAPACITY OF MACROPHAGE CELL LINES

5.1. CONSTITUTIVE LEVELS OF CYTOTOXICITY

We have previously reviewed the ability of macrophage lines to kill erythrocyte and tumor targets spontaneously with antibody (ADCC), and nonspecifically with activating agents present during the killing assays (Ralph *et al.*, 1980a; Ralph and Nakoinz, 1981; Ralph, 1981a). Macrophage-related lines generally fall into groups expressing (1) no effector functions, (2) weak activity similar to resident cells, and (3) strong cytotoxicity similar to peritoneal exudate cells.

TABLE 9. INHIBITION OF INDUCTION OF Mac-3 ANTIGEN IN M1 CELLS BY ANTI-Mac-1[a]

	Addition		Antigens/cell, $\times 10^4$	
Inducer	During induction	After induction	Mac-1	Mac-3
0			< 0.1	< 0.3
DM			12.8	13.7
DM	Anti-Mac-1		0.2	4.3
DM	Anti-Mac-3		nd	0.5
DM		Anti-Mac-1	< 0.1	14.2
DM		Anti-Mac-3	12.9	1.0

[a]M1 cells were incubated 6 days with 10^{-5} M dexamethasone (DM) in the presence of 1 μg/ml antibody as shown, washed, and assayed for antigens. In parallel cultures after induction, 1 μg/ml antibody was added during the assay for antigens. Anti-Mac-1 antibody inhibited induction of Mac-3, but not its expression after induction.

TABLE 10. EXPRESSION OF MACROPHAGE-RESTRICTED ANTIGENS ON HUMAN CELL LINES[a]

Line	Type	Antigens/cell, × 10^4 Mac-1	Mac-3
DAUDI	B cell	< 0.3	< 0.3
Peer	T cell	< 0.1	< 0.1
K562	Myelo/erythroid	< 1	< 1
HL-60	Myeloblast	< 0.5	< 0.5
U937	Monoblast	< 1.0	< 0.5

[a]Antigens assayed as in Table 7.

TABLE 11. MONOCLONAL ANTIBODIES INHIBIT INDUCTION OF DIFFERENTIATION ANTIGENS ON HUMAN MONOBLAST LINE U937

a. Induction of macrophage antigens[a]

Inducer	Antigens/cell, × 10^4 Mac-1	Mac-3	Mac-2
None	< 0.3	< 0.3	< 0.3
PMA 3 ng/ml	8.2	4.3	< 0.3
5637-CM 20%	7.9	4.2	< 0.3
LK 20%	9.1	3.3	< 0.3
Negative controls (T- and B-cell lines ± inducers)	< 0.3	< 0.3	< 0.3

b. Inhibition of induction of antigens by monoclonal antibodies[b]

Cell	Addition: During induction	Addition: After induction	Antigens/cell, × 10^4 Mac-1	Mac-3
U937			1.0	0.3
PMA-U937			4.1	3.8
PMA-U937	Rat IgG		4.3	3.8
PMA-U937	Anti-Mac-1		0.4	1.2
PMA-U937		Rat IgG	3.8	4.0
PMA-U937		Anti-Mac-1	< 0.1	3.6
PMA-U937		Anti-Mac-2	4.0	0.2

[a]U937 cells incubated 5–6 days with PMA, human bladder carcinoma line 5637 conditioned media containing myeloid colony-stimulating activity (CSA), or LK (supernatant of PHA-stimulated blood cells), conditions optimal for induction of Fc and complement receptors, phagocytosis, and ADCC (Ralph *et al.*, 1982c). Antigens assayed as in Table 7.

[b]Cells induced 5 days with 3 ng/ml PMA with 1 μg/ml normal rat IgG, anti-Mac-1, or anti-Mac-3 present during induction, followed by washing, or antibody present after induction and during the assay for surface antigens.

5.2. CLASS OF ANTIBODY MEDIATING ADCC

The classes of immunoglobulin mediating ADCC and phagocytosis of SRBC were found to be of all four murine IgG isotypes, but not IgM, using monoclonal antibodies (Ralph *et al.*, 1980b). Similarly, monoclonal IgG1 and IgG2b, but not IgM, antiphosphoryl choline could collaborate with macrophages and related cell lines in handling hapten-coupled RBC (P. Ralph and B. Diamond, unpublished; Ralph, 1981a). Using monoclonal antibodies to leukocyte antigens, we determined, again, that all four murine IgG isotypes, but not IgM, could mediate ADCC to tumor targets (Ralph, 1983; Ralph and Nakoinz, 1983). Recently, Diamond and Yelton (1981) have demonstrated a receptor for murine IgG3 distinct from previously characterized receptors for IgG1 and IgG2.

5.3. INDUCTION OF ADCC IN MURINE MACROPHAGES

Previous studies on activation of macrophage cell line cytotoxicity to tumors (Russell *et al.*, 1980; Taniyama and Holden, 1980; Ralph and Nakoinz, 1981) have used protocols that incorporate the nonspecific activating agent in the killing assay. The concept of the "angry" macrophage often refers to protocols of prior *in vivo* or *in vitro* activation with no known stimulant in the killing assay. Pre-

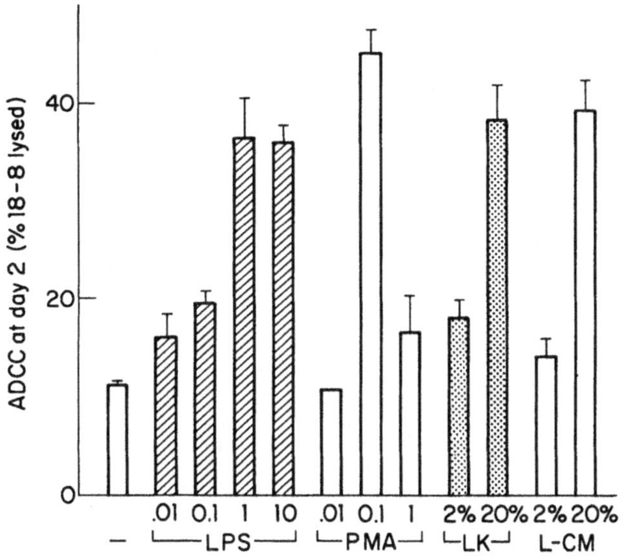

FIGURE 1. Optimal concentrations of agents to stimulate ADCC in murine RAW264 line. RAW264 cells were incubated at 5×10^5/ml for 2 days with 0, 0.01, 0.1, 1 or 10 μg/ml LPS; 0.01, 0.1, or 1 μg/ml PMA; 2 or 20% LK; or 2 or 20% L-CM. Cells were then washed and assayed for lysis of [^{125}I]-UdR-labeled pre-B lymphoma 18-8 at 20 : 1 in a 20-hr incubation (Ralph and Nakoinz, 1981). There was essentially no macrophage toxicity in the absence of antibody.

treatment of cell lines with LPS, PMA, lymphokine, or nonlymphocyte sources of macrophage colony-stimulating factors (CSF) generally did not induce "angry" or nonspecific killing. However, such pretreatment greatly stimulated ADCC (Fig. 1) (Ralph and Nakoinz, 1981). Cell lines (Fig. 2) and resident peritoneal macrophages (Ralph *et al.*, 1982a) require 2 days of pretreatment for optimal ADCC activity. Cell lines lacking effector functions, M1 and WEHI-3, could not be induced for ADCC to either RBC or tumor targets.

Surprisingly, macrophage lines pretreated with any of the agents had strikingly reduced lytic capacity with LPS or PMA added to the assay, in contrast to control LPS or PMA killing (Fig. 3). The inability to maintain an angry, toxic state after removal of an agent may be due to a number of nontrivial reasons. Cell lines, although having most of the properties of peritoneal resident or exudate macrophages, may differ in activation mechanisms for cytotoxicity because of the following:

1. Cell lines grow rapidly. One could propose that passing through a cell cycle erases memory of a previous activation. However, the activating agents actually block cell line growth.
2. Cell lines are transformed, i.e., grow permanently in culture, and this event may alter their regulatory mechanisms.
3. Cell lines are maintained in culture. Recent exposure to the *in vivo* environment may help to maintain the activated state.
4. Cell lines have absolutely no other cell types present. A 1% contamination of peritoneal macrophages by B or T lymphocytes stimulated during prior treatment

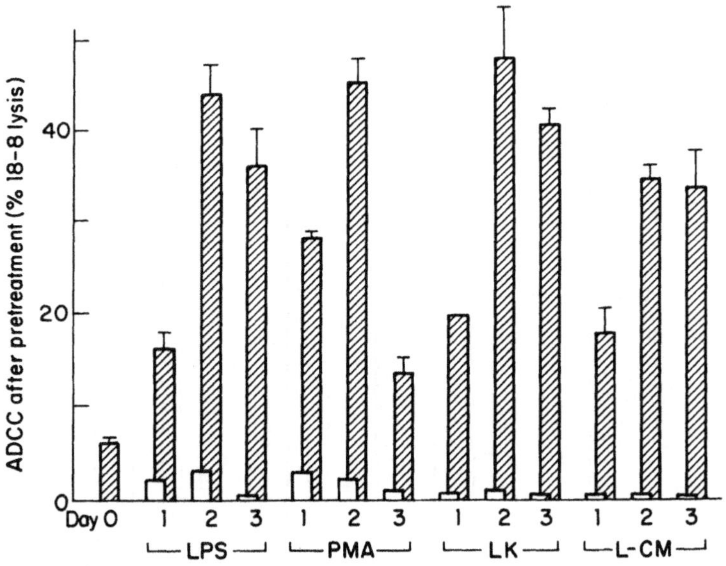

FIGURE 2. Time course for stimulation of RAW264 ADCC. RAW264 cells were incubated 1, 2, or 3 days with 1 μg/ml LPS, 0.1 μg/ml PMA, 10% v/v LK, or 10% v/v L-CM. The cells were then washed and assayed for lysis of 18-8 targets as in Fig. 1. Direct lysis of 18-8 without antibody is shown in open bars. ADCC by control (day 0) and treated RAW264 shown in hatched bars + S.E. Maximal stimulation of ADCC occurred with 2 days' pretreatment.

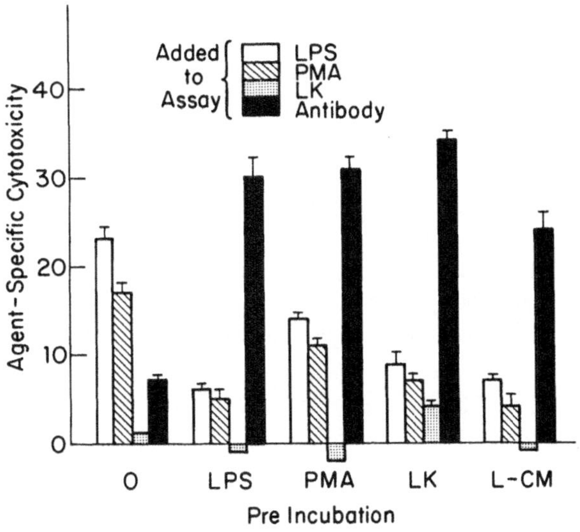

FIGURE 3. Stimulation of ADCC inhibits nonspecific cytotoxicity. RAW264 was incubated 2 days with LPS, PMA, LK, or L-CM and washed as in Fig. 1. The cells were then assayed for killing targets in the presence of 20 μg/ml LPS or 1 μg/ml PMA, concentrations inducing strong cytotoxicity in control RAW264 (Ralph and Nakoinz, 1981), or in the presence of 15% LK or antibody. Spontaneous killing by RAW264 with no agent in the assay varied from 0 to 4% and was subtracted.

may be sufficient to produce antibody or factors enhancing killing during the assay.

Further experiments with animal and culture sources of macrophages are necessary to distinguish among these possibilities, and the results may offer us some surprises.

ADCC to tumor targets could also be induced in cell lines and in resident peritoneal macrophages by pretreatment 2 days with inhibitors of microtubule function. The microtubule-stabilizing drug taxol and depolymerizers, colchicine and cationic anesthetic lidocaine, greatly stimulated ADCC with no activation of nonspecific cytotoxicity to leukemia targets. All agents, used at subtoxic concentrations, had no effect when present during the assay but blocked growth of the macrophage cell line. In contrast, the microfilament-disrupting agent cytochalasin B caused little or no stimulation of ADCC (Ralph and Nakoinz, 1982).

5.4. RELATION OF STIMULATION-OF-ADCC-FACTOR (SAF) TO OTHER ACTIVATING FACTORS

The previous section showed that macrophage activators including crude lymphokine and even nonlymphoid sources (L cell) of CSF could stimulate ADCC against tumor targets. The activity of the protein factor preparations was not due to LPS contaminants because the former were sensitive to heat and resistant to polymyxin B. Since three different sources of CSF contain a factor with ADCC-stimulating activities (stimulation-of-ADCC-factor, SAF) correlating with their CSF content, we must consider the possibility that SAF is CSF. LPS and PMA induce CSF production in macrophage cell lines (Ralph *et al.*, 1977, 1978a), so they may augment ADCC via CSF. This effect, however, would be distinct from direct activation of killing by LPS or PMA.

There is abundant evidence that CSF can increase differentiated functions in mature macrophages, although these cells require more CSF than the bone marrow precursor induced to form colonies (reviewed by Moore *et al.*, 1981). For example, phagocytosis and intracellular killing of *Leishmania tropica* promastigotes (Handman and Burgess, 1979) and *Candida* (Nozawa *et al.*, 1980) microorganisms is stimulated by purified CSF or CSF preparations. CSF in lymphokine and L-cell supernatants is probably the inducer of LAF production (Moore *et al.*, 1980). The J774 line has CSF receptors measured by a radioassay (Guilbert and Stanley, 1980), and purified CSF induces prostaglandin secretion in several macrophage lines (Kurland *et al.*, 1979).

However, several lines of evidence prove that CSF molecules are not SAF.

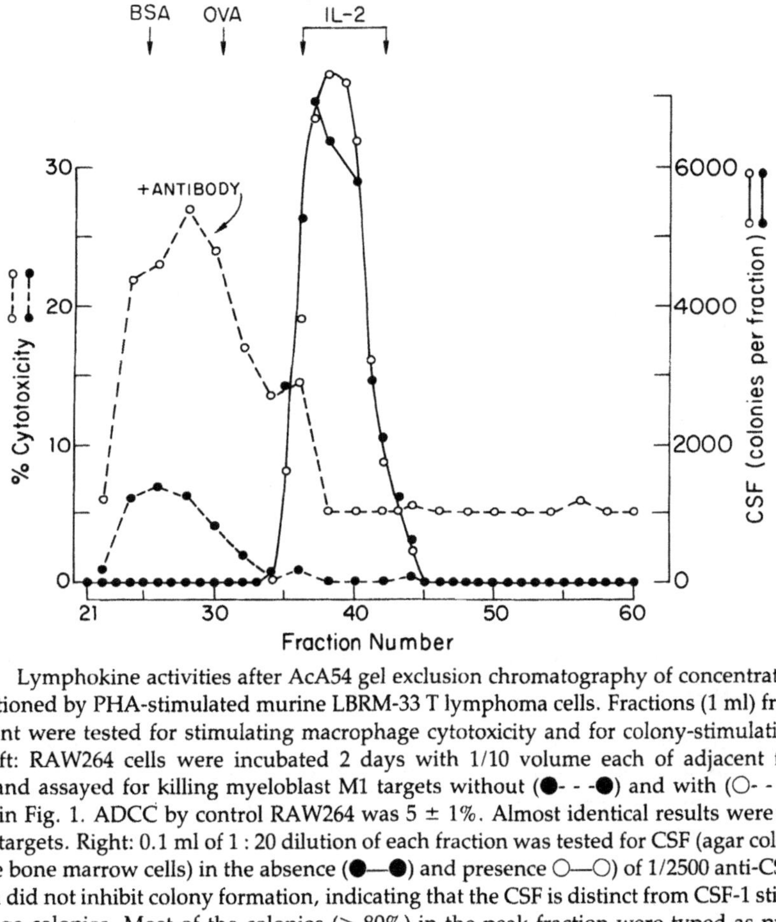

FIGURE 4. Lymphokine activities after AcA54 gel exclusion chromatography of concentrated medium conditioned by PHA-stimulated murine LBRM-33 T lymphoma cells. Fractions (1 ml) from 50 ml supernatant were tested for stimulating macrophage cytotoxicity and for colony-stimulating factor (CSF). Left: RAW264 cells were incubated 2 days with 1/10 volume each of adjacent fractions, washed, and assayed for killing myeloblast M1 targets without (●- - -●) and with (○- - -○) antiserum as in Fig. 1. ADCC by control RAW264 was 5 ± 1%. Almost identical results were obtained with 18-8 targets. Right: 0.1 ml of 1 : 20 dilution of each fraction was tested for CSF (agar colonies per 10^5 mouse bone marrow cells) in the absence (●—●) and presence ○—○) of 1/2500 anti-CSF-1. The antiserum did not inhibit colony formation, indicating that the CSF is distinct from CSF-1 stimulating macrophage colonies. Most of the colonies (> 80%) in the peak fraction were typed as pure granulocytes. Fractions 24–32 were pooled, concentrated 10-fold by ammonium sulfate precipitation, and dialyzed. The activity stimulating ADCC was destroyed by heating (7% of control activity after 10 min at 100°), and was not lost by absorption on sheep erythrocytes which would remove any residual PHA (95% of control activity). (From Ralph *et al.*, 1982a.)

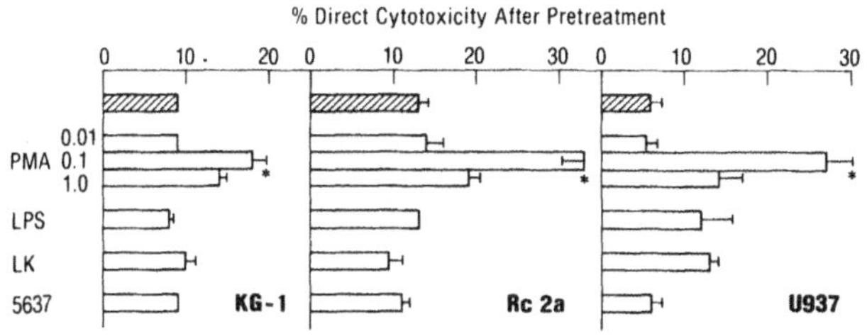

FIGURE 5. Induction of nonspecific tumor cytotoxicity in human monocyte-related lines. U937, Rc-2a, and KG-1 were incubated at 4 × 10^5/ml with 0.1 μg/ml PMA, 20 μg/ml LPS, 20% LK (supernatant of blood mononuclear cells stimulated 2 days with PHA), or 20% supernatant of human urinary bladder carcinoma line 5637. After 5 days, viable cells were counted, washed, and assayed for killing ^{125}I-labeled myeloid leukemia M1 without antitarget serum. Only PMA induced nonspecific cytotoxicity (Ralph *et al.*, 1982c). *Statistically significant, $p < 0.05$.

Purified macrophage-type CSF-1 does not stimulate macrophage ADCC; SAF is present in supernatants of PHA-stimulated T lymphoma LBRM-33 and is of higher molecular weight than the predominantly granulocyte-type CSF produced by these cells (Fig. 4), and SAF in Con A- and antigen-stimulated lymphokine preparations is of a different molecular weight (ca. 60,000) than CSF activities (30,000–50,000) (Ralph *et al.*, 1983b).

SAF is also different from macrophage activation factors for nonspecific lysis of sarcoma targets (45,000–50,000MW) or intracellular *L. tropica* amastigotes (15,000, 80,000, and 120,000) (Ralph *et al.*, 1983b).

5.5. INDUCTION OF ADCC AND NONSPECIFIC CYTOTOXICITY IN HUMAN LINES

Larrick *et al.* (1980) showed induction in U937 cells of ADCC to several targets by preincubation with lymphokine. Gidlung *et al.* (1981) described induc-

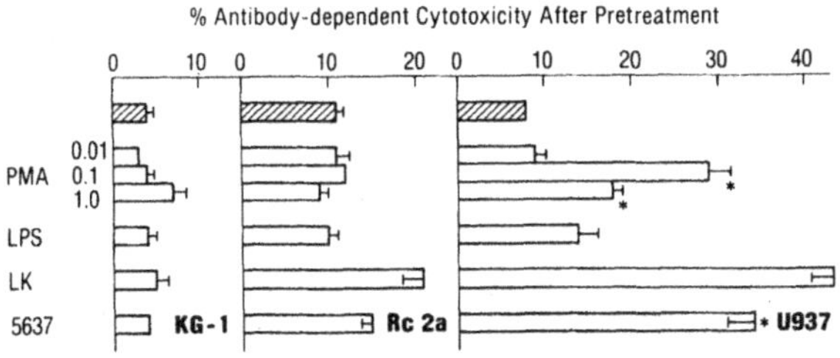

FIGURE 6. Induction of ADCC in human monocyte-related lines. Cells were incubated as in Fig. 5 and assayed for killing M1 targets in the presence of antibody. All agents except LPS induced significant (* = $p < 0.05$) ADCC.

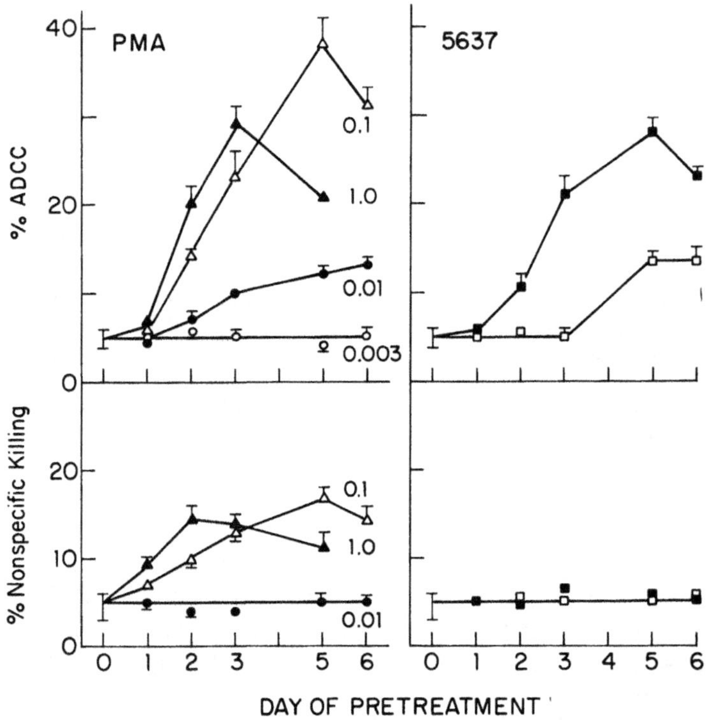

FIGURE 7. Time for stimulation of tumoricidal activity in U937. Cells were incubated with 0.003 (○), 0.01 (●), 0.1 (△), or 1 μg/ml PMA (▲), or with 5% (□) or 20% 5637 supernatant (■) as in Fig. 5. At various times, cells were washed and assayed for tumor killing. The range of control values at each time point for U937 incubated without stimulating agents is shown at day 0. Optimal tumoricidal activity occurred at 5 days' incubation with 0.1 μg/ml PMA or 20% 5637 supernatant; 20% lymphokine gave similar results.

tion of ADCC to chicken RBC using PMA stimulation. We found that PMA induced nonspecific killing of lymphoma targets in two monocyte-related lines, U937 and RC-2A (Fig. 5). Furthermore, PMA, lymphokine, and nonlymphoid sources of CSF, GCT line (GIBCO) and bladder carcinoma line 5637 also induced ADCC in U937 (Fig. 6; Ralph *et al.*, 1982c). The optimum time of pretreatment for induction of ADCC was 3–6 days (Fig. 7).

6. INDUCTIVE EVENTS AND PHARMACOLOGIC REGULATION

Examples of induction or stimulation of macrophage properties have been described in Sections 2.2, 2.3, 3, 4.2, 4.4, 5.3, and 5.5, and have been reviewed previously (Ralph, 1980, 1981a,b). Immunosuppressing corticosteroids are very toxic to the P388D1 line (Werb *et al.*, 1978) in contrast to most macrophage lines (Ralph *et al.*, 1978b), but inhibit plasminogen activator production (Werb *et al.*, 1978; Hamilton and Moore, 1980), induction by LPS and tuberculin PPD of CSF

TABLE 12. VARIANT MACROPHAGE CELL LINES

Parent line	Varient property	Reference
J774	Receptors for immunoglobulin Fc	Unkeless (1979)
FC1	Receptors for immunoglobulin Fc	Diamond and Yelton (1981)
J774	Phagocytosis and pinocytosis	Muschel *et al.* (1977)
FC1	Phagocytosis and pinocytosis	Diamond *et al.* (1978)
J774	Phagocytosis and pinocytosis	Norin (1980)
J774	NBT reduction, O_2^- and H_2O_2 production	Damiani *et al.* (1980)
M1	Macrophage vs. myeloid precursor	Nagata *et al.* (1976)
WEHI-3	Macrophage vs. myeloid precursor	Burgess and Metcalf (1980)

production and ADCC to RBC and tumor targets (Ralph *et al.*, 1978b), and induction by lymphokine of ADCC (Ralph and Nakoinz, 1981) in many of the lines. The corticosteroid dexamethasone is, however, an inducer of differentiation in the M1 line (Table 7; Honma *et al.*, 1978). Corticosteroids abrogate the growth inhibition caused by LPS or PPD in several lines (Ralph *et al.*, 1978b). Werb *et al.* (1978) have analyzed intracellular corticosteroid receptors in P388D1. Regulation of target lysis and phagocytosis by cAMP and insulin (Muschel *et al.*, 1977; Bar *et al.*, 1977) has been studied. It is likely that most regulatory phenomena observed in normal mononuclear phagocytes will be found in cell lines and suitably exploited.

7. VARIANT LINES IN ANALYSIS OF MACROPHAGE FUNCTION

Cell lines which differ in their properties are useful in simplifying scientific study of the bewildering number of reactions in macrophages. A variant line selected for (the absence of) a particular trait is even more valuable since it is likely to be similar to its parent in markers other than those selected. Some variant lines are listed in Table 12.

REFERENCES

Aksamit, R. R., and Kim, K. J., 1979, Macrophage cell lines produce a cytotoxin, *J. Immunol.* **122:**1785.

Aksamit, R. R., Falk, W., and Leonard, E. J., 1981, Chemotaxis by mouse macrophage cell lines, *J. Immunol.* **126:**2194.

Arene, T., and Pierce, C., 1980, Properties of a nonspecific suppressor factor produced by SIRS-treated macrophages, *Fed. Proc.* **39:**1156A.

Ascensao, J. L., Kay, N. E., Earenfight-Engler, T., Koren, H. S., and Zanjani, E. D., 1981, Production of erythroid potentiating factor(s) by a human monocytic cell line, *Blood* **57:**170.

Ault, K. A., and Springer, T. A., 1981, Cross-reaction of a rat-anti-mouse phagocyte-specific monoclonal antibody (anti-Mac-1) with human monocytes and natural killer cells, *J. Immunol.* **126:**359.

Bar, R. S., Kahn, C. R., and Koren, H. S., 1977, Insulin inhibition of antibody-dependent cytotoxicity and insulin receptors in macrophages, *Nature (London)* **265:**632.

Berens, R. L., and Marr, J. J., 1979, Growth of *Leishmania donovani* amastigotes in a continuous macrophage-like cell culture, *J. Protozool.* **26:**453.

Berlin, R. D., Oliver, J. M., and Walter, R. J., 1978. Surface functions during mitosis: Phagocytosis, pinocytosis and mobility of surface-bound Con A, *Cell* **15:**327.

Bodel, P., 1978, Spontaneous pyrogen production by mouse histiocytic and myelomonocytic tumor cell lines *in vitro*, *J. Exp. Med.* **147:**1503.

Bodel, P., Ralph, P., Wenc, K., and Long, J. C., 1980, Endogenous pyrogen production by Hodgkin's disease and human histiocytic lymphoma cell lines *in vitro*, *J. Clin. Invest.* **65:**514.

Boyse, E. A., and Old, L. J., 1969, Some aspects of normal and abnormal cell surface genetics, *Annu. Rev. Genet.* **3:**269.

Bradley, T. R., Pilkington, G., Garson, M., Hodgson, G. S., and Kraft, N., 1982, Cell lines derived from a human myelomonocytic leukaemia, *Br. J. Haematol.* **51:**595.

Broxmeyer, H. E., and Ralph, P., 1977, *In vitro* regulation of a mouse myelomonocytic leukemia line in culture, *Cancer Res.* **37:**3578.

Broxmeyer, H. E., Bognacki, J., Ralph, P., Dorner, M. H., Li, L., and Castro-Malaspina, H., 1982, Monocyte-macrophage derived acidic isoferritins: Normal feedback regulators of granulocyte-macrophage progenitor cells, *Blood* **60:**595.

Burgess, A. W., and Metcalf, D., 1980, Characterization of a serum factor stimulating the differentiation of myelomonocytic leukemic cells, *Int. J. Cancer* **26:**647.

Cahoon, B. E., and Mills, J., 1981, Development and characterization of a continuous line of alveolar macrophages from C3H/HeJ mice, *J. Reticuloendothelial Soc.* **29:**357.

Chang, K.-P., 1980, Human cutaneous *Leishmania* in a mouse macrophage line: Propagation and isolation of intracellular parasites, *Science* **209:**1240.

Damiani, G., Kiyotaki, C., Soeller, W., Sasada, M., Peisach, J., and Bloom, B. R., 1980, Macrophage variants in oxygen metabolism, *J. Exp. Med.* **152:**808.

Diamond, B., and Yelton, D. E., 1981, A new Fc receptor on mouse macrophages binding IgG_3, *J. Exp. Med.* **153:**514.

Diamond, B., Bloom, B. R., and Scharff, M. D., 1978, The Fc receptors of primary and cultured phagocytic cells studied with homogeneous antibodies, *J. Immunol.* **121:**1329.

Djeu, J. Y., Heinbaugh, J. A., Holden, H. T., and Herberman, R. B., 1979, Role of macrophages in the augmentation of mouse natural killer cell activity by poly I : C and interferon, *J. Immunol.* **122:**182.

Edelson, P. J., 1981, Plasma membrane ectoenzymes: Macrophage differentiation antigens, in: *Heterogeneity of Mononuclear Phagocytes* (O. Forster and M. Landy, eds.), pp. 143–149, Academic Press, New York.

Farrar, J. J., Mizel, S. B., Fuller-Farrar, J., Farrar, W. L., and Hilfiker, M. L., 1980, Macrophage-independent activation of helper T cells. I. Production of interleukin 2, *J. Immunol.* **125:**793.

Gidlung, M., Orn, A., Pattengale, P. K., Jannson, M., Wigzell, H., and Nilsson, K., 1981, Natural killer cells kill tumour cells at a given stage of differentiation, *Nature (London)* **292:**848.

Greenberger, J. S., Newberger, P. C., Karpas, A., and Moloney, W. C., 1978, Constitutive and inducible granulocyte–macrophage functions in mouse, rat and human myeloid leukemia-derived culture lines, *Cancer Res.* **38:**3340.

Guilbert, J. L., and Stanley, E. R., 1980, Specific interaction of murine colony-stimulating factor with mononuclear phagocytic cells, *J. Cell Biol.* **85:**153.

Hamilton, J. A., and Moore, M. A. S., 1980, Regulation of the plasminogen activator of macrophage tumor cell lines, *Int. J. Immunopharmacol.* **2:**353.

Handman, E., and Burgess, A. W., 1979, Stimulation by granulocyte–macrophage colony-stimulating factor of *Leishmania tropica* killing by macrophages, *J. Immunol.* **122:**1134.

Hoffmann, M. K., Koenig, S., Mittler, R. S., Oettgen, H. F., Ralph, P., Galanos, C., and Hämmerling, U., 1979, Macrophage factor controlling differentiation of B cells, *J. Immunol.* **122:**497.

Honma, Y., Kasukabe, T., and Hozumi, M., 1978, Production of differentiation-stimulating factor in cultured mouse myeloid leukemia cells treated with glucocorticoids, *Exp. Cell Res.* **111:**261.

Ichikawa, Y., Maeda, M., and Horiuchi, M., 1976, *In vitro* differentiation of Rauscher virus-induced myeloid leukemia cells, *Int. J. Cancer* **17:**789.

Jamieson, G. A., and Vanaman, T. C., 1980, Isolation and characterization of calmodulin from a murine macrophage-like cell line, *J. Immunol.* **125:**1171.

Jones, T. C., and Byrne, G. I., 1980, Interactions of macrophages with intravacuolar bacteria and protozoa, in: *Mononuclear Phagocytes: Functional Aspects* (R. van Furth, ed.), pp. 1611–1629, Nijhoff, The Hague.

Kaplan, G., and Mørland, B., 1978, Properties of a murine monocytic tumor cell line J-774 *in vitro.* I. Morphology and endocytosis, *Exp. Cell Res.* **115:**53.

Kikutani, H., Kishimoto, T., Sakaguchi, N., Nishizawa, Y., Ralph, P., and Yamamura, Y., 1981, Activation of cyclic AMP-dependent protein kinase activity during LPS stimulation of macrophage tumor cell line, J774.1, *Int. J. Immunopharmacol.* **3:**57.

Krizsa, K., and Dexter, T. M., 1978, Cell interactions in long term murine bone marrow culture, *Biomed. Express (Paris)* **29:**162.

Kurland, J. I., Pelus, L., Ralph, P., Bockman, R. S., and Moore, M. A. S., 1979, Synthesis of prostaglandin E by normal and neoplastic macrophages is dependent upon colony-stimulating factors (CSF), *Proc. Natl. Acad. Sci. USA* **76:**2326.

Lachman, L. B., and Metzgar, R. S., 1980, Characterization of high and low ML lymphocyte-activating factor (interleukin I) from P388D1 and J774.1 mouse macrophage cell lines, *J. Reticuloendothelial Soc.* **27:**621.

Larrick, J. W., Fischer, D. G., Anderson, S. J., and Koren, H., 1980, Characterization of a human macrophage-like cell line stimulated *in vitro:* A model of macrophage functions, *J. Immunol.* **125:**6

Levy, J. A., Barrett, S. G., Leong, J. C., and Dirksen, E. R., 1981, Transformation of macrophages from NZB hybrid mice by simian virus 40, *J. Reticuloendothelial Soc.* **29:**35.

Männel, D. N., Moore, R. N., and Mergenhagen, S. E., 1980, Macrophages as a source of tumoricidal activity (TNF), *Infect. Immun.* **30:**523.

Moore, R. N., Oppenheim, J. J., Farrar, J. J., Carter, C. S., Waheed, A., and Shadduck, R. K., 1980, Production of lymphocyte-activating factor (interleukin 1) by macrophages activated with colony-stimulating factors, *J. Immunol.* **125:**1302.

Moore, R. N., Hoffeld, J. T., Farrar, J. J., Mergenhagen, S. E., Oppenheim, J. J., and Shadduck, R. K., 1981, Effects of colony-stimulating factor and other cytokines on macrophage function, *Lymphokines* **3:**168.

Murray, H. W., 1981, Interaction of *Leishmania* with a macrophage cell line: Correlation between intracellular killing and the generation of oxygen intermediates, *J. Exp. Med.* **153:**1690.

Muschel, R. J., Rosen, N., Rosen, O. M., and Bloom, B. R., 1977, Modulation of Fc-mediated phagocytosis by cyclic AMP and insulin in a macrophage-like cell line, *J. Immunol.* **119:**1813.

Nagao, K., Yokoro, K., and Aaronson, S. A., 1981, Continuous lines of basophil-mast cells derived from normal mouse bone marrow, *Science* **212:**333.

Nagata, K., Takahaski, E., Saito, M., Ono, J., Kuboyama, M., and Ogasa, K., 1976, Simultaneous induction of lysosomal enzymes and phagocytosis in a murine myeloid leukemia cell line, *Exp. Cell Res.* **100:**322.

Neumann, C., and Sorg, C., 1981, Independent induction of plasminogen activator and interferon in murine macrophages, *J. Reticuloendothelial Soc.* **30:**79.

Newman, W., Diamond, B., Flomenberg, P., Scharff, M. D., and Bloom, B. R., 1979, Response of a continuous macrophage-like cell line to MIF, *J. Immunol.* **123:**2292.

Norin, A. J., 1980, Macrophage cell line mutants deficient in phagocytosis have reduced pinocytic activity, in: *Genetic Control of Natural Resistance to Infection and Malignancy* (E. Skamene, P. A. L. Kungshavn, and M. Landy, eds.), pp. 531–536, Academic Press, New York.

Nozawa, R. T., Sekiguchi, R., and Yokota, T., 1980, Stimulation by conditioned medium of L-929 fibroblasts, *E. coli* lipopolysaccharide, and muramyl dipeptide of candidacidal activity of mouse macrophages, *Cell. Immunol.* **53:**116.

Okuma, M., Ichikawa, Y., Yamashito, S., Kitajima, K., and Numa, S., 1976, Studies on some lipogenic enzymes of cultured myeloid leukemic cells, *Blood* **47:**439.

Peiris, J. S. M., Gordon, S., Unkeless, J. C., and Porterfield, J. S., 1981, Monoclonal anti-Fc receptor IgG blocks antibody enhancement of viral replication in macrophages, *Nature (London)* **289:**189.

Pellus, L. M., Broxmeyer, H. E., Kurland, J. I., and Moore, M. A. S., 1979, Regulation of macrophage and granulocyte proliferation: Specificities of prostaglandin E and lactoferrin, *J. Exp. Med.* **150**:277.

Pfeifer, S., Kallio, A., Vaheri, A., Pettersson, R., and Oker-Blom, N., 1980, Stable bone marrow-derived cell line producing transforming avian acute leukemia virus OK 10, *Int. J. Cancer* **25**:235.

Pike, M. C., Fisher, D. G., Koren, H. S., and Snyderman, R., 1980, Development of specific receptors for N-formylated chemotactic peptides in a human monocyte cell line stimulated with lymphokines, *J. Exp. Med.* **152**:31.

Ralph, P., 1980, Functions of macrophage cell lines, in: *Mononuclear Phagocytes—Functional Aspects* (R. van Furth, ed.), pp. 439–456, Nijhoff, The Hague.

Ralph, P., 1981a, Continuous macrophage cell lines—Their use in the study of induced and constitutive macrophage properties and cytotoxicity, *Lymphokines* **4**:175.

Ralph, P., 1981b, Continuous cell lines with properties of mononuclear phagocytes, in: *Methods for Studying Mononuclear Phagocytes* (D. O. Adams, P. Edelson, and H. Koren, eds.), pp. 155–173, Academic Press, New York.

Ralph, P., 1983, Immunoglobulin class of antibody effective in macrophage ADCC, in: *Macrophage-Mediated Antibody-Dependent Cellular Cytotoxicity* (H. S. Koren, ed.), Dekker, New York, in press.

Ralph, P., and Nakoinz, I., 1977a, Direct toxic effects of immunopotentiators on monocytic, myelomonocytic, and histiocytic tumor cells in culture, *Cancer Res.* **37**:546.

Ralph, P., and Nakoinz, I., 1977b, Antibody-dependent killing of erythrocyte and tumor targets by monocyte related cell lines: Enhancement by PPD and LPS, *J. Immunol.* **119**:950.

Ralph, P., and Nakoinz, I., 1980, Environmental and chemical dissociation of antibody-dependent phagocytosis from lysis mediated by macrophages: Stimulation of lysis by sulfhydryl-blocking and esterase-inhibiting agents and depression by trypan blue and trypsin, *Cell. Immunol.* **50**:94.

Ralph, P., and Nakoinz, I., 1981, Diffierences in antibody-dependent cellular cytotoxicity and activated killing of tumor cells by macrophage cell lines, *Cancer Res.* **41**:3546.

Ralph, P., and Nakoinz, I., 1982, Augmentation of macrophage antibody-dependent killing of tumor targets by microtubule inhibitors, *Cell. Immunol.* **70**:321.

Ralph, P., and Nakoinz, I., 1983, Monoclonal antibodies of all murine IgG classes, but not IgM, mediate macrophage ADCC to tumor targets, *J. Immunol.* **131**:1028.

Ralph, P., Moore, M. A. S., and Nilsson, K., 1976, Lysozyme synthesis by established human and murine histiocytic lymphoma cell lines, *J. Exp. Med.* **143**:1528.

Ralph, P., Broxmeyer, H., and Nakoinz, I., 1977, Immunostimulators induce granulocyte/ macrophage colony-stimulating activity and block proliferation in a monocyte tumor cell line, *J. Exp. Med.* **146**:611.

Ralph, P., Broxmeyer, H., Nakoinz, I., and Moore, M. A. S., 1978a, Induction of myeloid colony-stimulating activity (CSA) in murine monocyte tumor cell lines by macrophage activators, and in a T cell line by Con A, *Cancer Res.* **38**:1414.

Ralph, P., Ito, M., Broxmeyer, H. E., and Nakoinz, I., 1978b, Corticosteroids block newly induced but not constitutive functions of macrophage cell lines: CSA production, latex phagocytosis, antibody-dependent lysis of RBC and tumor targets, *J. Immunol.* **121**:300.

Ralph, P., Nakoinz, I., Potter, J. E. R., and Moore, M. A. S., 1980a, Activity of macrophage cell lines in tumor cytotoxicity, in: *Genetic Control of Natural Resistance to Malignancy and Infection* (E. Skamene, P. A. S. Kongshavn, and M. Landy, eds.), pp. 519–530, Academic Press, New York.

Ralph, P., Nakoinz, I., Diamond, B., and Yelton, D., 1980b, All classes of murine IgG antibody mediate macrophage phagocytosis and lysis of erythrocytes, *J. Immunol.* **125**:1885.

Ralph, P., Williams, N., Sheridan, A., Nakoinz, I., Jackson, H., and Moore, M., 1980c, Effector cell functions in long-term culture of murine, prosimian and human bone marrow, in: *Mononuclear Phagocytes—Functional Aspects* (R. van Furth, ed.), pp. 363–372, Nijhoff, The Hague.

Ralph, P., Williams, N., Nakoinz, I., Jackson, H., and Watson, J. D., 1982a, Distinct signals for antibody-dependent and nonspecific killing of tumor targets mediated by macrophages, *J. Immunol.* **129**:427.

Ralph, P., Nakoinz, I., and Raschke, W. C., 1982b, Induction of differentiated functions coupled with growth inhibition in lymphocyte and macrophage tumor cell lines, in: *Maturation Factors in Cancer* (M. A. S. Moore, ed.), pp. 245–254, Raven Press, New York.

Ralph, P., Williams, N., Moore, M. A. S., and Litcofsky, P. B., 1982c, Induction of antibody-dependent and nonspecific tumor killing in human monocytic leukemia cells by nonlymphocyte factors and phorbol ester, *Cell. Immunol.* **71**:215.

Ralph, P., Ho, M.-K., Litcofsky, P. B., and Springer, T. A., 1983a, Expression and induction in vitro of macrophage-restricted antigens on murine cell lines, *J. Immunol.*, **130**:108.

Ralph, P., Nacy, C. A., Meltzer, M. S., Williams, N., and Nakoinz, I., 1983b, Different lymphokine factors activate macrophage cytotoxicity to *Leishmania*, sarcoma, and antibody-coated lymphoma targets, *Cell Immunol.* **76**:10.

Raschke, W. C., Baird, S., Nakoinz, I., and Ralph, P., 1978, Functional macrophage cell lines transformed by Abelson leukemia virus, *Cell* **15**:261.

Rosen, N., Piscitello, J., Schneck, J., Muschel, R., Bloom, B. R., and Rosen, O., 1979, Properties of protein kinase and adenylate cyclase-deficient variants of a macrophage-like cell line, *J. Cell. Physiol.* **98**:125.

Russell, S. W., Gillespie, G. Y., and Pace, J. L., 1980, Comparison of responses made to activating agents by mouse peritoneal macrophages and cells of the macrophage line RAW264, *J. Reticuloendothelial Soc.* **27**:607.

Sachs, L., 1978, Control of normal cell differentiation and the phenotypic reversion of malignancy in the myeloid leukaemia, *Nature (London)* **274**:535.

Sasada, M., and Johnston, R. B., 1980, Macrophage microbicidal activity: Correlation between phagocytosis-associated oxidative metabolism and the killing of *Candida* by macrophages, *J. Exp. Med.* **152**:85.

Schlesinger, J. J., and Brandriss, M. W., 1981, Growth of 17D yellow fever virus in a macrophage-like cell line, U937: Role of Fc and viral receptors in antibody-mediated infection, *J. Immunol.* **127**:659.

Snyderman, R. M., Pike, M. C., Fischer, D. G., and Koren, H. S., 1977, Biologic and biochemical activities of continuous macrophage cell lines P388D1 and J774.1, *J. Immunol.* **119**:2060.

Springer, T. A., 1980, Cell-surface differentation in the mouse: Characterization of "jumping" and "lineage" antigens using xenogeneic rat monoclonal antibodies, in: *Monoclonal Antibodies. Hybridomas: A New Dimension in Biological Analysis* (R. H. Kennett, T. J. McKearn, and K. B. Bechtol, eds.), pp. 185–218, Plenum Press, New York.

Stadecker, M. J., 1981, Comparison of pyrimidine and purine nucleoside secretion and nucleoside kinase expression in resident and elicited peritoneal macrophages, *J. Immunol.* **126**:1724.

Sündstrom, C., and Nilsson, K., 1976, Establishment and characterization of a human histiocytic lymphoma cell line (U-937), *Int. J. Cancer* **17**:565.

Sündstrom, C., and Nilsson, K., 1977, Cytochemical profile of human hematopoietic biopsy cells and derived cell lines, *Br. J. Haematol.* **25**:601.

Taniyama, T., and Holden, H. T., 1980, Cytolytic activity against tumor cells by macrophage cell lines and augmentation by macrophage stimulants, *Int. J. Cancer* **26**:61.

Testa, N. G., Dexter, T. M., Scott, D., and Teich, N. M., 1980, Malignant myelomonocytic cells after *in vitro* infection of marrow cells with Friend leukaemia virus, *Br. J. Cancer* **41**:37.

Thoman, M. L., Morgan, E. L., and Weigle, W. O., 1981, Fc fragment activation of T lymphocytes, *J. Immunol.* **126**:632.

Tsuchiya, S., Yamabe, M., Yamaguchi, Y., Kobayashi, Y., Konno, T., and Tada, K., 1980, Establishment and characterization of a human acute monocytic leukemia cell line (THP-1), *Int. J. Cancer* **26**:171.

Unkeless, J. C., 1979, Characterization of a monoclonal antibody directed against mouse macrophage and lymphocyte Fc receptors, *J. Exp. Med.* **150**:580.

van Loveren, H., van der Zeijst, B. A. M., De Weger, R. A., van Basten, C., Pijpers, H., and Den Otter, W., 1981, Identification of the neonatal liver cell line NCTC 1469 as a macrophage-like cell line, *J. Reticuloendothelial Soc.* **29**:433.

Walker, E. B., Lanier, L. L., and Warner, N. L., 1982, Concomitant induction of the cell surface expression of Ia determinants and accessory cell function by a murine macrophage cell line, *J. Exp. Med.* **155**:629.

Walker, W. S., and Gandour, D. M., 1980, Detection and functional assessment of complement receptors on two macrophage-like cell lines, *Exp. Cell Res.* **129**:15.

Wardley, R. C., Lawman, M. J., and Hamilton, F., 1980, The establishment of continuous macrophage cell lines from peripheral blood monocytes, *Immunology* **39:**67.

Werb, Z., Foley, R., and Munck, A., 1978, Glucocorticoid receptors and glucocorticoid-sensitive secretion of neutral proteinases in a macrophage cell line, *J. Immunol.* **121:**115.

Werb, Z., Banda, M. J., and Jones, P. A., 1980, Degradation of connective tissue matrices by macrophages, *J. Exp. Med.* **152:**1340.

Williams, N., 1979, Preferential inhibition of murine macrophage colony formation by prostaglandin E, *Blood* **53:**1089.

Williams, N., Eger, R. R., Moore, M. A. S., and Mendelsohn, N., 1978, Differentiation of mouse bone marrow precursor cells into neutrophil granulocytes by an activity separation from WEHI-3 cell-conditioned medium, *Differentiation* **11:**59.

Williams, N., Jackson, H., Ralph, P., and Nakoinz, I., 1981, Cell interactions influencing murine marrow megakaryocytes: Nature of the potentiator cell in bone marrow, *Blood* **57:**157.

Wing, E. J., Koren, H. S., Fischer, D. G., and Kelley, V., 1981, Stimulation of a human macrophage-like cell line (U937) to inhibit multiplication of an intracellular pathogen, *J. Reticuloendothelial Soc.* **29:**321.

Yung, Y.-P., Eger, R., Tertian, G., and Moore, M. A. S., 1981, Purification of a mast cell growth factor and its dissociation from TCGF, *J. Immunol.* **127:**794.

5

Immune Functions of Dendritic-Type Cells

JOHN G. TEW and RICHARD P. PHIPPS

1. INTRODUCTION

Over the last several years considerable evidence has accumulated indicating that cells with a dendritic morphology play important roles in a variety of immune functions. A list of the immunologically relevant dendritic-type cells (D cells) and the immune functions associated with each is presented in Table 1. As indicated in the footnotes in this table, a number of names have been used to describe and identify different D cells. The names and abbreviations used in the body of this table have been tentatively agreed upon by the RES committee on nomenclature.

A major question is how closely are the different D cells related to each other and to other lymphoid cells, especially macrophages. The final answer to this question probably will not be available until the ontogeny of the D cells has been clarified. Nevertheless, a few major points deserve comment. Occasionally some D cells have been referred to as "dendritic macrophages." However, none of the D cells have significant phagocytic activity. Furthermore, all cells in the D-cell series are irregularly shaped, their nuclei are irregularly shaped, and their cytoplasm is relatively devoid of major organelles. In contrast, macrophages tend to have a more regular shape, a more regular nucleus which is typically oval to reinform, and prominent cytoplasmic organelles like phagocytic vacuoles and lysosomes. In view of these differences in morphology and the lack of phagocytic activity in the D-cell series, it seems unreasonable at this time to refer to D cells as macrophages. However, like macrophages, some D cells can serve as accessory cells in a variety of immune responses. In this context the D cell–macrophage relationship may be compared with the macrophage–neutrophil relationship. Both macrophages and neutrophils are phagocytic but cytologically

JOHN G. TEW and RICHARD P. PHIPPS • Department of Microbiology and Immunology, Medical College of Virginia, Virginia Commonwealth University, Richmond, Virginia 23298.

TABLE 1. IMMUNE FUNCTIONS OF DENDRITIC-TYPE CELLS

Dendritic cell (abbreviation)	Immune functions
Follicular dendritic cells (FDCs)[a]	Trapping and retention of antigen–antibody complexes Formation of germinal centers Induction of B-memory cells Maintenance of antibody production
Lymphoid dendritic cells (LDCs)[b]	Stimulation of allogeneic and syngeneic mixed lymphocyte reactions Antigen presentation to T cells Accessory cells in T-cell-mediated cytotoxicity Accessory cells in oxidative mitogenesis Induction of contact allergy by intravenous injection of hapten-conjugated LDCs
Langerhans cells (LCs)[c]	Trapping of contact allergens Induction of contact allergy Antigen presentation to T cells Induction of mixed lymphocyte reactions

[a] Also known as antigen-retaining cells, follicular immune complex-retaining cells, follicular antigen-binding cells, follicular reticular cells, follicular dendritic reticulum cells, and Nossal's follicular dendritic reticulum cells.
[b] Also referred to as dendritic cells (DCs) and Steinman–Cohn's dendritic cells.
[c] The indeterminate dendritic cells in the skin and the interdigitating dendritic cells in the lymphatic organs are believed to be close relatives of Langerhans cells. The major difference is that Langerhans cells contain a Birbeck granule visible in sections used for electron microscopy. Certainly the presence or absence of the granule in cells with few granules is a function of which sections are examined.

they are quite different and the neutrophil lacks most accessory cell functions. On the other hand, macrophages and D cells share many accessory cell functions but cytologically they are quite different and D cells are nonphagocytic.

In the following sections of this chapter each of the D cells and associated immunological phenomena will be discussed. The sequence of the cells and a discussion of their immune functions will follow the sequence in which they are presented in Table 1.

2. IMMUNE FUNCTIONS OF FOLLICULAR DENDRITIC CELLS

2.1. ANTIGEN RETENTION AND THE FOLLICULAR DENDRITIC CELL

It is well known that the vast majority of an easily catabolizable antigen is degraded and eliminated from a normal animal in a few weeks. Innate clearance mechanisms are markedly enhanced with the initiation of specific antibody synthesis which mediates the immune elimination phenomena (Hawn and Janeway, 1947; Talmage *et al.*, 1951; Tew *et al.*, 1980b). Even though specific antibody facilitates removal of antigens in most locations, antibody facilitates the retention of a small portion of even simple protein antigens in lymphatic tissues (Franzl, 1962; Campbell and Garvey, 1963; Nossal and Ada, 1971; Tew *et al.*,

1979b). Antibody production thus results in an efficient elimination system for the majority of an antigenic challenge, yet mediates the retention of a small quantity of antigen in lymphatic tissue.

It has been known since the 1950s (Kaplan *et al.*, 1950) that the major anatomical site of antigen retention in lymphoid tissue is the lymphoid follicles. The investigations of White (1963; White *et al.*, 1967) described a characteristic "dendritic web" of antigen retention in chicken lymphoid follicles utilizing an immunofluorescent technique. The dendritic pattern of antigen localization differed markedly from the clearly intracytoplasmic distribution of labeled antigen within macrophages. Nossal and colleagues (1968, 1971) utilized radioiodinated *Salmonella adelaide* flagella to demonstrate antigen retention and localization in the popliteal lymph nodes of rats. Utilizing electron microscopic (EM) autoradiography, they demonstrated that antigen, believed to be localized as antigen–antibody (Ag–Ab) complexes, was retained at or near the surface processes of follicular dendritic cells (Nossal *et al.*, 1968). Follicular dendritic cells (FDCs) did not appear to be typical macrophages as evidenced by morphological criteria, nor was there any evidence of phagocytosis. Nossal *et al.* (1968) postulated that FDCs possessed surface receptors for the Fc portion of antibody which effected trapping of Ag–Ab complexes. Nonimmunogens, such as colloidal carbon, did not exhibit follicular localization, which argued against a nonspecific trapping mechanism. It was also noted that antigen retention occurred only in immunized animals or those possessing natural cross-reactive antibody, while tolerant animals failed to demonstrate follicular localization of antigen (Humphrey and Frank, 1967). Concurrent with Nossal and colleagues' work (1968), Hanna *et al.* (1967; Hanna and Szakal, 1968; Szakal and Hanna, 1968) described antigen retention in mouse spleen in EM studies. Antigen was retained in the dense lymphocytic sheaths surrounding secondary follicle germinal centers. Hanna and Szakal (1968; Szakal and Hanna, 1968) reported that radiolabeled antigen was associated with highly convoluted infoldings of the plasma membrane of FDCs. Sordat *et al.* (1970) and Chen *et al.* (1978) reported that horseradish peroxidase–anti-horseradish peroxidase complexes strictly localized to splenic lymphoid follicles. In EM studies immune complexes were located along thin sheets of cytoplasm which often folded and coiled into complex arrays (Chen *et al.*, 1978). The sheets of cytoplasm emanated from FDCs located in both the germinal center and the adjacent mantle region of murine spleen (Chen *et al.*, 1978).

The EM studies cited above revealed that antigen was associated with a type of "dendritic" cell apparently found only in primary or secondary lymphoid follicles. The nature of the association of antigen and FDCs could not be precisely determined because both EM autoradiography and histochemical techniques did not afford the resolution necessary to assess whether antigen is localized on FDC processes perhaps bound to an Fc or C3 receptor, or possibly sequestered just inside the cytoplasmic membrane. We recently (Mandel *et al.*, 1980, 1981) investigated antigen retention and localization utilizing ferritin as an immunogen in both actively and passively immunized mice. Since ferritin is electron dense, it can be directly visualized in the electron microscope. High-resolution examination of popliteal lymph node follicles clearly demonstrated that ferritin was localized in a patchy extracellular distribution. Even as long as 103 days after injection of ferritin, it remained localized in patchy aggregates, apparently attached to FDCs via antibody or complement.

The distinguishing characteristics of FDCs which we (Mandel *et al.*, 1980, 1981) and others (Nossal *et al.*, 1968; Hanna *et al.*, 1967; Hanna and Szakal, 1968; Chen *et al.*, 1978) have determined include the ability to retain antigen extracellularly and possession of an irregularly shaped large nucleus which appears lobulated and indented by its close association with follicular B cells. In addition FDCs contain relatively little perinuclear cytoplasm and the cell appears stellate with many dendritic processes extending away from the cell body. The FDC cytoplasm contains few organelles with the exception of an occasional centriole and a large well-developed Golgi region.

2.2. ROLE OF ANTIGEN RETAINED ON FOLLICULAR DENDRITIC CELLS AND GERMINAL CENTER ACTIVATION

There is little conclusive evidence concerning the role of antigen retained on FDCs and germinal center activation and development. Antigen may be retained in primary follicles which lack germinal centers (Mandel *et al.*, 1980, 1981; Phipps *et al.*, 1980), in T-cell-deficient mice (Tew *et al.*, 1979b; Klaus *et al.*, 1980), and in mice treated with certain immunosuppressants which lack recognizable follicles (Nettesheim and Hammons, 1970; Phipps *et al.*, 1981). A discrete primary, or secondary follicle with a germinal center is therefore not critical to the process of antigen localization and retention. However, the requirement for antigen localization to initiate germinal center development is more difficult to assess. Laissue *et al.* (1971) demonstrated that mice immunized in the hindfoot pads with Ag–Ab complexes developed popliteal lymph node germinal centers more rapidly than did mice which received antigen alone. In agreement with this finding, recent evidence presented by Klaus *et al.* (1980) showed a correlation between antigen localization effected by preformed Ag–Ab complexes and germinal center formation. Mice receiving an intravenous injection of Ag–Ab complex produced large numbers of splenic germinal centers 5 days later. Mice which received only antigen or antigen in adjuvant did not achieve a similar number of germinal centers until day 14. Furthermore, Klaus *et al.* (1980) noted that mice injected with Ag–Ab complexes produced larger germinal centers than did control groups.

The initiation of antigen localization in spleen and lymph node follicles of normal animals coincides with the appearance of specific antibody in the circulation. The overwhelming majority of antigen localizes well after antibody synthesis has begun (Van Rooijen, 1972). This is probably attributable to the fact that antibody is required to initiate follicular localization of antigen, possibly via C′-fixing properties. The fact that antigen does not localize until antibody production has begun and at this time germinal center development is well under way, argue against follicular antigen localization as responsible for germinal center development. It is not known, however, whether the localization of even picogram amounts of antigen, mediated by natural antibody, initiates the process of germinal center formation. Ag–Ab complexes could form in the circulation or in the lymph and rapidly localize to primary follicles whereby germinal center formation could be initiated and specific antibody production commenced. The initial antibody synthesis consisting primarily of IgM with some IgG would mediate the localization of a portion of the remaining antigen. Retained antigen could then accelerate germinal center development and antibody production.

2.3. FOLLICULAR DENDRITIC CELLS AND INDUCTION OF IMMUNOLOGICAL MEMORY

Recently, antigen retained in lymphoid follicles has been determined to be a critical component in the generation of B-cell memory. Klaus and Humphrey (1977) treated T-cell-deficient mice with antigen, and then cobra venom factor to destroy C3. They demonstrated that C3 was an absolute requirement to obtain primed B cells. Additional studies on the role of C3 clearly revealed that in decomplemented, normal, and T-cell-deficient mice, splenic follicular localization was severely impaired (Tew *et al.*, 1979b; Klaus and Humphrey, 1977). Complement fixation by Ag–Ab complexes appears to be a critical component in splenic follicular antigen localization and the subsequent development of B-cell memory.

Klaus (1979) predicted that if C′ were required for follicular localization of antigen and B-memory cell development, then those Ag–Ab complexes which best localized in splenic follicles and fixed C′ should elicit optimum B-cell memory. He found that Ag–Ab complexes formed with those isotypes which fixed C′ best also demonstrated maximum follicular localization and B-memory cell development. Complexes of Ag–IgG2 efficiently localized in splenic follicles and elicited substantial B-cell priming. Complexes formed with Ag–IgM did not activate murine C′, nor localize in follicles or elicit B-cell priming. This evidence supports the concept that follicular localization of antigen mediated by Ag–Ab–C′ complexes elicits B-memory cell production, even in the absence of T cells.

Antigen retained in follicles may not only be responsible for the generation of B-cell memory as pointed out above, but also for its maintenance many months after the initial antigen contact. Cerottini and Trnka (1970) suggested that persisting antigen manifested a central role in maintaining a population of memory cells in immunized mice. Elliott and Roszman (1975) investigated the regulatory role of persisting antigen on IgG precursor subpopulations in rabbit lymph node cultures undergoing a secondary response. They found that immunologic memory increased as time progressed after primary immunization. The increase in memory response was attributed to persisting antigen in the draining lymph nodes. They proposed that persisting antigen "selected" a variety of memory cells with respect to affinity, and maintained populations of both low- and high-affinity memory cells.

There are reports that the migration of lymphocytes to the lymph nodes draining the site of antigen injection is critical to the formation of antibody responses (Gowans, 1962; Ford and Gowans, 1967). Lymphocytes may become specifically trapped in those lymphoid organs containing the appropriate antigen. Sherr and Siskind (1977) demonstrated that high-avidity B cells localized in the draining lymph nodes, whereas the nondraining lymph nodes secured lower-avidity B cells. It was reasoned that antigen availability was a critical factor in trapping B cells with highly avid receptors. In agreement, Ponzio *et al.* (1977) presented evidence that B cells with highly avid receptors were trapped by persisting antigen. B-memory cells localized in highest numbers in lymph nodes containing the relevant persisting antigen. In splenectomized mice, additional B-cell trapping occurred in the draining lymph nodes presumably because there was no competition from the spleen for these cells. Persisting local memory was attributed to an accumulation of B-memory cells in the draining lymph nodes. In an extension of this work, Ponzio *et al.* (1980) recently demonstrated unilateral localization of B-memory cells in mice pretreated with cyclophosphamide, which inhibits humoral responses but does not cause a loss of retained antigen. It was proposed that antigen, localized on FDCs in the draining lymph nodes, acted as an immunosorbent to trap and sequester primed B cells. This would be a likely explanation, since Tew and Mandel (1978) calculated that even 7 weeks after injection of 1 μg of human serum albumin, there was still 30 pg of antigen remaining per 10^6 cells. This is enough antigen to coat 3000 FDCs with 10^5 antigen molecules. It does not therefore seem unreasonable to presume that retained antigen, present on a massive complex of FDC processes, could specifically trap and retain B-memory cells and furthermore maintain a population of high-avidity B-memory cells.

2.4. FOLLICULAR DENDRITIC CELLS IN THE MAINTENANCE AND REGULATION OF ANTIBODY LEVELS

Antigen can persist for months or even years in follicles of lymph nodes and spleen (Tew and Mandel, 1978, 1979; Mandel *et al.*, 1981; Tew *et al.*, 1979b; Phipps *et al.*, 1980). Once antigen has become localized in follicles on FDCs and a primary response initiated, little is known about the continuing role of persisting antigen. A number of investigations have suggested that retained antigen and specific antibody are major components in an antibody feedback system (Tew and Mandel, 1978; Britton *et al.*, 1968; Weigle, 1975; Bystryn *et al.*, 1970; Richter *et al.*, 1965; Tew *et al.*, 1980). A working hypothesis has been generated which focuses on retained antigen and the FDCs as the key components in the maintenance and regulation of humoral immune responses. The basic tenets of this hypothesis are presented in Fig. 1. When antigen contact first occurs, a primary response is generated and a portion of that antigen is retained on the FDCs (Tew *et al.*, 1979a, 1980a). At this time retained Ag–Ab–C′ complexes may be involved in the generation of B-memory cells. When high levels of specific antibody become present, the antigen bound to FDCs would be inactivated. A variety of

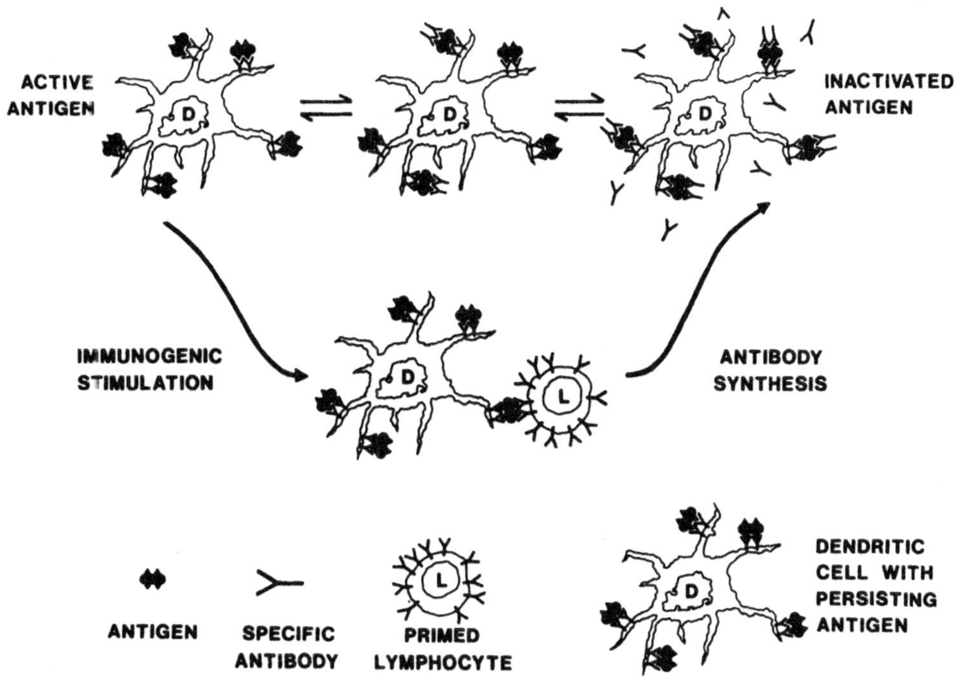

FIGURE 1. A model for feedback regulation of antibody synthesis during the maintenance phase of the immune response. The injection of antigen and the subsequent induction of the primary immune response results in the production of specific antibody, the generation of a population of primed lymphocytes, and a population of follicular dendritic cells with surface-associated persisting antigen. Later in the maintenance phase of the immune response, multiple dynamic equilibria are postulated to exist between persisting antigen, free specific antibody, and antigen–antibody complexes of various ratios in the lymphoid organs. The immunogenicity of the complexes is directly related to the antigen–antibody ratio, and alterations in serum antibody levels result in dissociation of these complexes When antibody levels in the circulation decline, antigenic determinants are exposed, memory B cells are stimulated, and a new cycle of antibody synthesis is induced. This newly produced antibody feeds back and terminates the immunogenic stimulus. Repetition of this cycle serves to maintain serum antibody levels within narrow limits for long periods of time. (From *Immunol. Rev.* **53**, 1980.)

dynamic equilibrium states can be postulated to occur between persisting antigen and antibody. The immunogenicity of the immune complexes is directly related to the Ag–Ab ratio, and alterations in serum antibody levels could result in the formation or dissociation of immune complexes. When relatively low levels of specific antibody are present in serum, antigenic determinants will be exposed and B-memory cells could be stimulated and a new cycle of antibody synthesis begun. The newly synthesized antibody could block the antigenic determinants and terminate the stimulus. Alternately, by cross-linking both antigen and Fc or C′ receptors on primed B cells, a negative signal may be generated and turn off the cells (Stockinger and Lemmel, 1978; Hoffman, 1980; Voisen, 1980). Klaus *et al.* (1980) recently proposed that immune complexes in follicles might stimulate the production of anti-idiotypic antibodies which may also play a role in the regulation of humoral immune responses. Since easily catabolized antigens like human serum albumin (HSA) are retained in lymphoid follicles and have a potential half-life of months (Tew and Mandel, 1979), the maintenance of humoral immune responses by persisting antigen might continue for months or even years. In fact, serum antibody directed against HSA is maintained at relatively high levels for months or years (Tew *et al.*, 1973; Kitces *et al.*, 1975).

If persisting follicular antigen is responsible for the maintenance of serum antibody, it follows that the removal of the draining lymph nodes containing persisting antigen should result in a dramatic decline in serum antibody levels. When this was tested, the removal of these organs resulted in a 50% decrease in serum antibody titers 2 weeks later. This decrease, in comparison to control mice, lasted at least 18 weeks.

Based upon the regulatory model presented in Fig. 1, one might predict that the removal of lymphoid organs from an *in vivo* environment rich in antibody, to an environment lacking specific antibody would result in the induction of an anamnestic response. This phenomenon does occur and is termed the "spontaneous antibody response." Evidence indicates that spontaneous responses, like secondary responses, require B, T, and accessory cells (Tew *et al.*, 1980). Some of the characteristics of the accessory cells responsible for the induction of the spontaneous response are listed in Table 2. The accessory cell is believed to be the FDC and its characteristics appear to be distinct from most macrophages.

Spontaneous antibody responses have occurred in a variety of systems (Tew *et al.*, 1980) including *in vitro* culture of organ fragments, adoptive transfer, and single-cell suspension cultures. Based on the assumption that persisting antigen is the stimulus for inducing spontaneous antibody responses, then those lymphoid organs containing the majority of persisting antigen should respond spontaneously by producing higher amounts of antibody. When this was tested

TABLE 2. CHARACTERIZATION OF THE ACCESSORY CELLS REQUIRED FOR SPONTANEOUS INDUCTION OF ANTIBODY PRODUCTION

Feature	Associated phenomena
Retains antigen for long periods *in vivo*	Follicular dendritic cells retain antigen for months or years
Circulation	Antigen-bearing FDCs do not circulate. Accessory cells capable of inducing the spontaneous response do not appear to circulate
Cellular site of antigen retention	*In vivo* antigen is on the surface of FDCs. *In vitro* antigen may be removed from accessory cells by gentle treatment with EDTA or trypsin indicating surface retention
Adherence	The accessory cell does not adhere to glass or plastic petri dishes or to glass bead columns
Density	The antigen-bearing cells are more dense than most macrophages but less dense than most lymphocytes
Velocity sedimentation	The antigen-bearing cells sediment faster than most lymphocytes but slower than most macrophages

both in single-cell suspension culture and in organ fragment culture, those lymph nodes with larger amounts of persisting antigen responded by producing the largest amount of antibody (Tew and Mandel, 1978). A high degree of correlation existed between the amount of retained antigen and the magnitude of the spontaneous response. The nondraining lymph nodes which contained little or no persisting antigen responded only if exogenous antigen was supplied. It was also found that the spontaneous antibody responses could be blocked if specific antibody was added to cultures during the induction phase (Tew *et al.*, 1973). If antibody was added to cultures after the induction phase, no inhibition occurred. Based on the model in Fig. 1, specific antibody inhibits during the induction phase of spontaneous responses by inactivating persisting antigen on FDCs.

3. IMMUNE FUNCTIONS OF LYMPHOID DENDRITIC CELLS

Lymphoid dendritic cells (LDCs) were first recognized as very irregularly shaped adherent cells found among the adherent macrophages after mouse spleen cells were incubated on glass or plastic surfaces (Steinman and Cohn, 1973, 1974, 1975; Steinman *et al.*, 1974). LDCs lack the classical markers of mouse lymphocytes like surface Ig, Thy 1, Fc receptor, C3b receptor, but they are rich in surface Ia alloantigen which appears to be linked to the *I-A* and *I-E* subregions (Steinman *et al.*, 1979; Steinman and Nussenzweig, 1980; Nussenzweig *et al.*, 1981). Using phase contrast microscopy, these adherent cells appear flattened, irregularly shaped, and exhibit numerous spherical phase-dense mitochondria (Steinman and Nussenzweig, 1980). When the cells are detached from the surface of the culture vessel, they remain irregular in shape with bulbous protrusions and may display large thin veils of cytoplasm which are especially striking when examined by scanning EM (Steinman and Nussenzweig, 1980). Transmission EM confirms the presence of numerous large mitochondria but reveals few lysosomal granules or polyribosomes (Steinman and Cohn, 1973). Physiologically, LDCs appear to be potent accessory cells and may play a variety of important roles in the afferent limb of the immune response. Many of these roles will be clarified in the following sections.

3.1. LYMPHOID DENDRITIC CELLS IN THE ALLOGENEIC AND SYNGENEIC MIXED LYMPHOCYTE REACTIONS

The most thoroughly studied immune function associated with LDCs is their ability to stimulate mixed lymphocyte reactions (MLR). The remarkable feature of MLRs stimulated by LDCs is that only 3×10^4 LDCs can maximally stimulate $4–5 \times 10^6$ responder cells in 4-day cultures (Steinman and Witmer, 1978; Steinman and Nussenzweig, 1980). Approximately 100 times this number of unfractionated spleen cells is required to achieve the same result (Steinman and Witmer, 1978). Using the same experimental conditions, Steinman and his colleagues found splenic macrophages to be totally inactive or very weakly stimulatory in primary MLRs (Steinman and Nussenzweig, 1980). Purified lymphocytes can stimulate, but 10^6 or more cells are needed and the responses are generally not as potent as those stimulated by LDCs (Steinman and Witmer, 1978).

Interestingly, mitomycin C-treated LDCs can stimulate syngeneic mouse T cells but not B cells to proliferate (Nussenzweig and Steinman, 1980). In contrast, mitomycin C-treated syngeneic macrophages, T cells, and B cells are inactive or are very weakly stimulatory in this T-cell proliferative response (Nussenzweig and Steinman, 1980). The syngeneic MLR appears to be Ia dependent since anti-Ia markedly inhibits the response even if the anti-Ia used is a monoclonal $F(ab')_2$ (Steinman and Nussenzweig, 1980). Furthermore, the syngeneic MLR normally obtained in unfractionated spleen cells can be markedly reduced by treatment with anti-Ia and complement. This reduced T-cell proliferative response can then be restored to normal by the addition of small numbers of LDCs (Steinman and Nussenzweig, 1980).

An interesting feature of the syngeneic MLR response is that the T cells form multicellular clusters around the LDCs in culture (Steinman and Nussenzweig, 1980). These clusters can be broken up by pipetting but reform again in a few hours. Furthermore, the multicellular clusters can be isolated and studied. It appears that the T cells forming clusters around LDCs during the first day of incubation eventually begin to proliferate and are responsible for the syngeneic MLR (Steinman and Nussenzweig, 1980). The intimate interaction between LDCs and T cells in the cluster is probably an important feature of the process leading to T-cell proliferation.

Syngeneic MLRs can also be demonstrated in human systems when irradiated non-T cells are added to T cells (Kuntz *et al.*, 1976). However, the biological significance of the syngeneic MLR remains to be clearly established. The potent primary allogeneic MLR stimulated by LDCs probably indicates that LDCs could contribute to transplantation reactions. Conceivably LDCs or their precursors could be among passenger leukocytes which may contribute to the rejection of a transplanted organ (Lafferty and Wollnough, 1977).

3.2. LYMPHOID DENDRITIC CELLS IN ANTIGEN PRESENTATION TO T CELLS

The ability of LDCs to present antigen was demonstrated when a potent lymphocyte proliferative response was measured after antigen plus LDCs was added to cultures of purified primed T lymphocytes. The appropriate controls indicated the LDCs served as the essential accessory cells (Sunshine *et al.*, 1980). The antigens used in this system included PPD, KLH, and the synthetic polypeptides GAT and (TG)AL. Genetic restriction was demonstrated using strains of mice that responded to the synthetic polypeptides and strains that were unable to respond. LDCs from nonresponder strains could not present antigen to the F_1 cross or a responder x nonresponder whereas LDCs from responder strain could. The data suggest that the LDCs may be the site of expression of the Ir gene product required in the stimulation process (Sunshine *et al.*, 1980).

3.3. LYMPHOID DENDRITIC CELLS AS ACCESSORY CELLS IN INDUCTION OF T-CELL-MEDIATED CYTOTOXICITY

The ability of LDCs to serve as accessory cells in the induction of a cytotoxic T-cell response was demonstrated when TNP-labeled stimulator cells were incubated with purified T cells. In the absence of LDCs, no T-cell-mediated cytotoxicity was demonstrable. However, the addition of 0.5–1 LDC/100 responding T cells induced a potent cytotoxic T-cell response against TNP-labeled targets (Nussenzweig *et al.*, 1980). Anti–Ia and complement inactivated accessory cells but had no effect on the responder cells. Interestingly, LDCs were sensitive to UV irradiation but were still functional in this system after 1000 rad of X irradiation. In contrast to the striking accessory cell activity of LDCs, macrophages were unable to induce T-cell-mediated cytotoxicity under the same experimental conditions. Even macrophages that contained a high level of surface Ia were inactive. In fact, the addition of macrophages to the LDC–T-cell preparations inhibited the accessory cell activity of the LDCs. However, the addition of indomethacin eliminated the macrophage-mediated inhibitory effect. Steinman and his colleagues concluded "that the development of anti-TNP CTL is an immune response in which (a) LDCs are the critical accessory cells; (b) Ia-bearing macrophages are weak or inactive; and (c) macrophages can inhibit LDC-mediated response by an indomethacin-sensitive mechanism" (Nussenzweig *et al.*, 1980).

3.4. LYMPHOID DENDRITIC CELLS AS ACCESSORY CELLS IN OXIDATIVE MITOGENESIS

Under appropriate conditions, exposure of lymphocytes from rats and mice to periodate and/or certain other oxidative agents, induces vigorous proliferative responses (O'Brien and Parker, 1976). This mitogenic response is accessory cell dependent since purified oxidized lymphocytes will not respond (Phillips *et al.*, 1980; Klinkert *et al.*, 1980). Interestingly, the addition of small numbers of LDCs to purified oxidized lymphocytes restores the proliferative response. The LDCs may be used in oxidized or unoxidized form and still provide the accessory cell activity. As expected, treatment of the accessory cells with anti-Ia abolished this mitogenic response (Phillips *et al.*, 1980).

3.5. LYMPHOID DENDRITIC CELLS AS ACCESSORY CELLS IN THE INDUCTION OF CONTACT ALLERGY BY HAPTENATED CELLS

When cells from a variety of sources including thymocytes and peritoneal exudate cells are conjugated with haptens and injected intravenously, the recipients become specifically tolerized. Subsequent painting of the specific hapten on the skin does not induce a delayed-type hypersensitivity response (DTH) (Ptak *et al.*, 1980). Normal controls exposed to the hapten under identical conditions respond normally. Furthermore, the tolerized animals respond normally to an immunologically unrelated hapten painted on the skin. Interestingly, intravenous injection of haptenated skin cells, which would include Langerhans cells, induces a DTH response in the recipient when assessed by ear swelling tests (Ptak *et al.*, 1980). Similarly, hapten-conjugated LDCs induce a DTH response rather than tolerance when injected intravenously (Steinman *et al.*, 1980).

4. IMMUNE FUNCTIONS OF LANGERHANS CELLS

Langerhans cells (LCs) were recognized over 100 years ago in the epidermal regions of human skin impregnated with gold salts (Langerhans, 1868). However, the immunological significance of these cells has only become apparent in the past few years. Immunological interest was kindled by observations that lymphocytes were in close apposition to LCs shortly after challenging a sensitive animal with a contact allergen (Silberberg, 1973). Further work indicated the LCs possessed important immunological markers including Fc and C3b receptors and surface Ia antigens (Stingl *et al.*, 1977, 1978a,b). In fact, they appear to be the only cells in the skin bearing these markers (Stingl *et al.*, 1978a). Subsequently, evidence has mounted indicating LCs play a variety of immunologically significant roles as will be explained in the following sections. In the skin, LCs may be identified by several special staining techniques (Wolff, 1972). The long dendritic processes of LCs appear to form an almost continuous network in the epidermal layer. Studies using transmission EM revealed a lobated nucleus and a relatively clear cytoplasm containing a unique organelle called the Birbeck granule or LC granule (Caputo *et al.*, 1976). LCs are distinguishable from keratinocytes or melanocytes in that they lack desmosomes, tonofilaments, melanosomes, and promelanosomes (Stingl *et al.*, 1980).

4.1. LANGERHANS CELLS AND THE TRAPPING OF CONTACT ALLERGENS

Shelley and Juhlin (1976, 1977) proposed that LCs with their long dendritic processes constitute a reticuloepithelial trap for contact allergens. This proposal was based on their observations that LCs selectively absorb compounds which have a known potential for causing contact allergy. These include formaldehyde, glutaraldehyde, paraphenylenediamine, ethylenediamine, toluenediamine, nickel, cobalt, chromium, mercury, and gold. Interestingly, when hapten-conjugated LCs were injected into previously unsensitized animals, the animals became specifically sensitized to the hapten as indicated by subsequent ear swelling tests for contact sensitization. In contrast, haptens conjugated to other cells including macrophages and lymphocytes failed to sensitize (Ptak *et al.*, 1980). These data indicate that LCs are peculiarly adept in presenting haptens to T cells responsible for contact allergy. Furthermore, these data support the concept that contact allergens picked up by LCs in the skin could be presented to the appropriate T cells and initiate contact allergy.

4.2. LANGERHANS CELLS AND THE INDUCTION OF CONTACT ALLERGY

The route of choice for experimentally administering contact allergens is by the skin. In fact, administering the contact allergen by other routes often results in specific unresponsiveness (Greene *et al.*, 1978). The possible relationship between LCs in the skin and induction of contact allergy was recently analyzed in a study by Toews *et al.* (1980). They found that the number of LCs in the skin site where the contact allergen was applied was directly related to the ability to induce contact sensitization in the animal. For example, mouse tail skin has about 100 LCs/mm^2 compared with about 800 LCs/mm^2 on the abdominal body wall or dorsal body wall. Application of a contact allergen (DNFB) to the abdominal body wall or dorsal body wall leads to contact sensitization as indicated by ear swelling responses. In contrast, application of the contact allergen to the tail skin failed to induce a response. In addition, UV irradiation of the dorsal body wall or abdominal body wall destroys LCs. Application of the contact allergen to UV-irradiated body wall skin also failed to induce contact allergy as indicated by the inability to subsequently demonstrate an ear swelling response. Furthermore, during the 15-day period required for the number of LCs in skin to return to normal, it was observed that the degree of sensitization was directly proportional to the number of LCs in the skin at the time the contact allergen was applied. More remarkably, animals whose first exposure to the contact allergen was through skin deficient in LCs (i.e., tail skin or UV-irradiated skin) were tolerant to a subsequent exposure to the allergen. Toews *et al.* (1980) concluded that "not only are Langerhans cells essential for induction of contact hypersensitivity to chemical allergens, but in their absence, exposure to these agents leads to specific unresponsiveness."

It would appear that if the contact allergen penetrates the skin and is presented by other lymphoid cells, the animal is tolerized. This view is supported by experiments of Ptak *et al.* (1980) who found that intravenous administration of contact allergens on macrophage-rich peritoneal exudate cells (PECs) induced suppressor cells and tolerized the animals. In contrast, intravenous administration of the allergens on skin cells induced contact allergy. When the allergens were presented on PECs and skin cells together, the animals had a positive contact allergic reaction. These results suggest that skin cells can sensitize if suppressors are not already present (Ptak *et al.*, 1980). Interestingly, PECs can elicit a short-lived or evanescent form of contact sensitivity if animals are pretreated with cyclophosphamide to diminish the suppressor cell response or if the PECs are administered by subcutaneous route which initially avoids splenic suppressors (Ptak *et al.*, 1980).

Interestingly, LCs are not restricted to skin although the epidermal layer of skin is certainly the primary site. Cells with LC granules have been found in lymphatic tissues including lymph nodes and thymus (Silberberg-Sinakin *et al.*, 1976a). Small number of LCs are generally present in lymph nodes; however, this number increases dramatically in the draining lymph node after exposure of skin to a contact allergen. Silberberg-Sinakin and Thorbecke (1980) believe that

LCs pick up the contact allergen in the skin and carry it by way of the dermal lymphatics to the draining lymph nodes. Some LCs are found in the paracortical region of the draining lymph nodes suggesting that sensitization of the T cells may occur at this site. Certainly subsequent to the sensitization, application of the contact allergen to the skin results in contact dermatitis and lymphocyte-like cells are found in apposition to LCs in the lesion (Silberberg, 1973). The LCs appear more active during episodes of contact dermatitis and may become damaged during the process (Silberberg-Sinakin *et al.*, 1977; Silberberg-Sinakin and Thorbecke, 1980).

4.3. LANGERHANS CELLS AND ANTIGEN PRESENTATION TO T CELLS

LCs may be separated from most other epithelial cells in an epithelial cell suspension by rosetting the LCs out using EA-IgG (Stingl *et al.*, 1978a). Since LCs have a receptor for IgG-Fc, the EA-IgG binds to LCs and the rosetted LCs can be separated on a Ficoll–Hypaque density gradient. Using rosette-enriched preparations of LCs from strain 2 guinea pigs, Stingl *et al.* (1978a) studied the ability of these cells to present antigen to primed T cells. The enriched LC preparations were as effective as macrophages in presenting antigen. Furthermore, the response was genetically restricted. That is, LCs and macrophages from strain 2 guinea pigs could present antigen to primed strain 2 T lymphocytes but not to primed strain 13 T lymphocytes. Conversely, LCs and macrophages from strain 13 guinea pigs could present antigen to primed strain 13 T lymphocytes but not to primed strain 2 T lymphocytes. Furthermore, this response could be abrogated by anti-Ia. Since LCs are the only Ia-positive cells in the skin, it appears antigen was presented by the LCs and not another epidermal contaminant (Stingl *et al.*, 1978a, 1980).

4.4. LANGERHANS CELLS AND THE INDUCTION OF MIXED LYMPHOCYTE REACTIONS

MLRs were studied using LCs separated from most other epidermal cells by the EA-IgG rosetting technique (Stingl *et al.*, 1978a). Appropriate cells from strain 2 and strain 13 guinea pigs were used for stimulators and responders. Epidermal cells enriched for LCs were as good as macrophages in stimulating MLRs in both guinea pig strains (Stingl *et al.*, 1978a, 1980). Again, anti-Ia plus complement eliminated the response. Furthermore, epidermal cells remaining after rosetting the LCs out were inactive (Stingl *et al.*, 1978a, 1980). These data indicate that LCs are the cells in skin capable of stimulating an MLR and suggest that LCs may play a major role in the process leading to rejection of transplanted skin. In fact, the high density of these cells in normal skin may explain why it is so difficult to avoid the rejection process and maintain grafted skin for long periods *in vivo*. Certainly the ability of small numbers of LCs and LDCs to stimulate potent MLRs suggests that these cells may be of major significance in transplantation biology.

5. CONCLUDING COMMENTS

The morphological features of D cells have been recognized for many years as a consequence of light and electron microscope studies of skin and lymphoid tissues. However, D cells remained morphological curiosities because data implicating these cells in functional roles were scant. In recent years, interest in D cells was kindled by evidence indicating that these cells have remarkable immunological features and functions. In fact, most of the immunological functions summarized in Table 1 have been reported in the past decade and many in the past two years. In some cases the data on the immune functions of D cells are so recent that they are based on a single report. We think it is reasonable to anticipate that the list of immunological features and functions of D cells will grow and some of the functions ascribed to D cells in this chapter may need to be modified as more information becomes available. However, we also believe it is clear that D cells are not simply morphological curiosities but that they represent important elements in the immune system. A decade ago, Nossal and Ada referred to the follicular dendritic cells in their book (*Antigens, Lymphoid Cells and the Immune Response*) as the Cinderella among lymphoid cells. This designation may yet prove to be apt for D cells in general. It may become feasible to modulate the immune response in important ways by manipulating D cells. In the future, immunotherapy may be based on an understanding of the basic biology of D cells. Certainly we anticipate that interest in D cells will be maintained and our knowledge base will grow rapidly over the next few years. We look forward to this prospect with interest and enthusiasm.

REFERENCES

Britton, S. T., Wepsic, T., and Moller, G., 1968, Persistence of immunogenicity of two complex antigens retained *in vivo*, *Immunology* **14**:491.

Bystryn, J. C., Graf, M. W., and Uhr, J. W., 1970, Regulation of antibody formation by serum antibody. II. Removal of specific antibody by means of exchange transfusion, *J. Exp. Med.* **132**:1279.

Campbell, D., and Garvey, J., 1963, Nature of retained antigen and its role in immune mechanisms, in: *Advances in Immunology* (F. J. Dixon and J. H. Humphrey, eds.), pp. 261–313, Academic Press, New York.

Caputo, R., Deluchetti, D., and Monti, M., 1976, Freeze-fracture of Langerhans granules: A comparative study, *J. Invest. Dermatol.* **66**:297.

Cerottini, J. C., and Trnka, Z., 1970, The role of persisting antigen in the development of immunological memory, *Int. Arch. Allergy Appl. Immunol.* **38**:37.

Chen, L. L., Adams, J. C., and Steinman, R. M., 1978, Anatomy of germinal centers in mouse spleen with special reference to "follicular dendritic cells," *J. Cell Biol.* **77**:148.

Elliott, L. H., and Roszman, T. L., 1975, Antigenic selection of IgG precursor populations, *J. Immunol.* **115**:495.

Ford, W. L., and Gowans, J., 1967, The role of lymphocytes in antibody formation. II. The influence of lymphocyte migration on the initiation of antibody formation in the isolated perfused spleen, *Proc. R. Soc. London Ser. B* **168**:244.

Franzl, R., 1962, The primary immune response in mice. III. Retention of sheep red blood cell immunogens by the spleen, *Infect. Immun.* **6**:469.

Gowans, J., 1962, The fate of parental strain small lymphocytes in F_1 hybrid rats, *Ann. N.Y. Acad. Sci.* **99**:432.

Greene, M. I., Sugimoto, M., and Benacerraf, B., 1978, Mechanisms of regulation of cell-mediated immune responses. I. Effect of the route of immunization with TNP-coupled syngeneic cells on the induction and suppression of contact sensitivity to picryl chloride, *J. Immunol.* **120**:1604.

Hanna, M. G., Jr., and Szakal, A. K., 1968, Localization of ^{125}I-labeled antigen in germinal centers of mouse spleen: Histologic and ultrastructural autoradiographic studies of the secondary immune reaction, *J. Immunol.* **101**:949.

Hanna, M. G., Jr., Makinodan, T., and Fisher, W. D., 1967, Lymphatic tissue germinal center localization of ^{125}I-labeled heterologous and isologous macroglobulins, in: *Germinal Centers in Immune Responses* (H. Cottier, N. Odartchenko, R. Schindler, and C. C. Congdon), p. 86, Springer-Verlag, Berlin.

Hawn, C., and Janeway, C., 1947, Histological and serological sequences in experimental hypersensitivity, *J. Exp. Med.* **85**:571.

Hoffman, M. K., 1980, Antibody regulates the cooperation of B-cells with helper cells, *Immunol. Rev.* **49**:79.

Humphrey, J. H., and Frank, M. M., 1967, The localization of nonmicrobial antigens in the draining lymph nodes of tolerant, normal and primed rabbits, *Immunology* **13**:87.

Kaplan, M. H., Coons, A. H., and Deane, H. W., 1950, Localization of antigen in tissue cells. III. Cellular distribution of pneumococcal polysaccharide type II and III in the mouse, *J. Exp. Med.* **91**:15.

Kitces, E. N., Tew, J. G., and Greene, E. J., 1975, Induction and maintenance of antibody responses by different forms of human serum albumin, *Immunol. Commun.* **4**:275.

Klaus, G. G. B., 1979, The generation of memory cells. III. Antibody class requirements for the generation of B-memory cells by antigen–antibody complexes, *Immunology* **37**:345.

Klaus, G. G. B., and Humphrey, J. H., 1977, The generation of memory cells. I. The role of C_3 in the generation of B memory cells, *Immunology* **33**:31.

Klaus, G. G. B., Humphrey, J. H., Kunkl, A., and Dongworth, D. W., 1980, The follicular dendritic cell: Its role in antigen presentation in the generation of immunological memory, *Immunol. Rev.* **53**:3.

Klinkert, W. E. F., Labadie, J. H., O'Brien, J. P., Beyer, D. F., and Powers, W. E., 1980, Rat dendritic cells function as accessory cells and control the production of a soluble factor required for mitogenic responses of T lymphocytes, *Proc. Natl. Acad. Sci. USA* **77**:5414.

Kuntz, M. M., Innes, J. B., and Weksler, M. E., 1976, Lymphocyte transformation induced by autologous cells. IV. Human T-lymphocyte proliferation induced by autologous or all geneic non-T lymphocytes, *J. Exp. Med.* **143**:1043.

Lafferty, K., and Woolnough, J., 1977, The origin and mechanism of allograft rejection, *Immunol. Rev.* **35**:231.

Laissue, J., Cotlier, H., Hess, M. W., and Stoner, R. D., 1971, Early and enhanced germinal center formation and antibody responses after primary stimulation with antigen–isologous antibody complexes as compared with antigen alone, *J. Immunol.* **107**:822.

Langerhans, P., 1868, Uber die nerven der menschlichen haut, *Virchows Arch. A* **44**:325.

Mandel, T. E., Phipps, R. P., Abbot, A. P., and Tew, J. G., 1980, The follicular dendritic cell: Long term antigen retention during immunity, *Immunol. Rev.* **53**:29.

Mandel, T. E., Phipps, R. P., Abbot, A. P., and Tew, J. G., 1981, Long term antigen retention by follicular dendritic cells in the popliteal lymph node of immunized mice, *Immunology* **43**:353.

Nettesheim, P., and Hammons, A. S., 1970, Effect of immunosuppressive agents on retention of antigen in the mouse spleen, *Proc. Soc. Exp. Biol. Med.* **133**:696.

Nossal, G. J. V., and Ada, G., 1971, *Antigens, Lymphoid Cells and the Immune Response*, Academic Press, New York.

Nossal, G. J. V., Abbot, A., Mitchell, J., and Lummus, Z., 1968, Antigens in immunity. XV. Ultrastructural features of antigen capture in primary and secondary lymphoid follicles, *J. Exp. Med.* **127:**277.

Nussenzweig, M. C., and Steinman, R. M., 1980, Contribution of dendritic cells to stimulation of the murine syngeneic mixed leukocyte reaction, *J. Exp. Med.* **151:**1196.

Nussenzweig, M. C., Steinman, R. M., Gutchinov, B., and Cohn, Z. A., 1980, Dendritic cells are accessory cells for the generation of anti-TNP cytotoxic T cells, *J. Exp. Med.* **152:**1070.

Nussenzweig, M. C., Steinman, R. M., Unkeless, J. C., Witmer, M. D., Gutchinov, B., and Cohn, Z., 1981, Studies of the cell surface of mouse dendritic cells and other leukocytes, *J. Exp. Med.* **154:**168.

O'Brien, R. L., and Parker, J. W., 1976, Oxidation-induced lymphocyte transformation, *Cell* **7:**13.

Phillips, M. L., Parker, J. A., Frelinger, J. A., and O'Brien, R. L., 1980, Characterization of responding cells in oxidative mitogen stimulation. II. Identification of an Ia-bearing adherent accessory cell, *J. Immunol.* **124:**2700.

Phipps, R. P., Mitchell, G. F., Mandel, T. E., and Tew, J. G., 1980, Antibody isotypes mediating antigen retention in passively immunized mice, *Immunology* **40:**459.

Phipps, R. P., Mandel, T. E., and Tew, J. G., 1981, Effect of immunosuppressive agents on antigen retained in lymphoid follicles and collagenous tissue of immune mice, *Cell. Immunol.* **57:**505.

Ponzio, N. M., Chapman-Alexander, J. M., and Thorbecke, G. J., 1977, Transfer of memory cells into antigen pretreated hosts. I. Functional detection of migration sites for antigen-specific B-cells, *Cell. Immunol.* **34:**79.

Ponzio, N. M., Baine, Y., and Thorbecke, G. J., 1980, Localization of functional memory B cells at sites of antigen localization and its relationship to local aspects of immunological memory, in: *Phylogeny of Immunological Memory* (M. J. Manning, ed.), p. 291, Elsevier, North-Holland.

Ptak, W., Rozycka, D., Askenase, P. W., and Gershon, R. K., 1980, Role of antigen-presenting cells in the development and persistence of contact hypersensitivity, *J. Exp. Med.* **151:**362.

Richter, M., Zimmerman, S., and Haurowitz, F., 1965, Relation of antibody titre to persistence of antigen, *J. Immunol.* **94:**938.

Shelley, W. B., and Juhlin, L., 1976, Langerhans cells form a reticuloepithelial trap for external contact allergens, *Nature (London)* **261:**46.

Shelley, W. B., and Juhlin, L., 1977, Selective uptake of contact allergens by the Langerhans cells, *Arch. Dermatol.* **113:**187.

Sherr, D. J., and Siskind, G. W., 1977, Studies on the control of antibody synthesis. XI. Effect of antigen on the localization of cells secreting different avidity antibody, *Proc. Soc. Exp. Biol. Med.* **155:**203.

Silberberg-Sinakin, I. Baer, R. L., and Thorbecke, J. G., 1980, Langerhana Cells: Role in contact hypersensitivity and relationship to lymphoid dendritic cells and to macrophages, *Immunol. Rev.*, **53:**203.

Silberberg, I., 1973, Apposition of mononuclear cells to Langerhans cells in contact allergic reactions: An ultrastructural study, *Acta Derm. Venereol.* **53:**1.

Silberberg-Sinakin, I., and Thorbecke, G. J., 1976, Contact hypersensitivity and Langerhans cells, *J. Invest. Dermatol.* **75:**61.

Silberberg-Sinakin, I., Thorbecke, G. J., Baer, R. L., Rosenthal, S. A., and Berezowsky, V., 1976, Antigen-bearing Langerhans cells in skin dermal lymphatics and in lymph nodes, *Cell. Immunol.* **25:**137.

Silberberg-Sinakin, I., Fecorko, M. E., Baer, R. L., Rosenthal, S. A., Berezowsky, V., and Thorbecke, G. J., 1977, Langerhans cells: Target cells in immune complex reactions, *Cell. Immunol.* **32:**400.

Sordat, B., Sordat, M., Hess, M. W., Stona, R. D., and Cottier, J., 1970, Specific antibody within lymphoid germinal center cells in mice after primary immunization with horseradish peroxidase: A light and electron microscopic study, *J. Exp. Med.* **131:**77.

Steinman, R. M., and Cohn, Z. A., 1973, Identification of a novel cell type in peripheral lymphoid organs of mice. I. Morphology, quantitation, tissue distribution, *J. Exp. Med.* **137:**1142.

Steinman, R. M., and Cohn, Z. A., 1974, Identification of a novel cell type in peripheral lymphoid organs of mice. II. Functional properties *in vitro*, *J. Exp. Med.* **139:**380.

Steinman, R. M., and Cohn, Z. A., 1975, Dendritic cells, reticular cells, and macrophages, in: *Mononuclear Phagocytes* (R. van Furth, ed.), p. 95, Blackwell, London.

Steinman, R. M., and Nussenzweig, M. C., 1980, Dendritic cells: Features and functions, *Immunol. Rev.* **53**:127.

Steinman, R. M., and Witmer, M., 1978, Lymphoid dendritic cells are potent stimulators of the primary mixed leukocyte reaction in mice, *Proc. Natl. Acad. Sci. USA* **75**:5132.

Steinman, R. M., Lustig, D. S., and Cohn, Z. A., 1974, Identification of a novel cell type in peripheral lymphoid organs of mice. III. Functional properties *in vivo*, *J. Exp. Med.* **139**:1431.

Steinman, R. M., Kaplan, G., Witmer, M., and Cohn, Z. A., 1979, Identification of a novel cell type in peripheral lymphoid organs of mice. V. Purification of spleen dendritic cells, maintenance *in vitro* and new surface markers of dendritic cells. *J. Exp. Med.* **149**:1.

Stingl, G., Wolff-Schreiner, E. C., Pichler, W. J., Eschnait, F., Knapp, W., and Wolff, K., 1977, Epidermal Langerhans cells bear Fc and C3 receptors, *Nature (London)* **268**:245.

Stingl, G., Katz, S., Clement, L., Green, I., and Shevach, E. M., 1978a, Immunologic functions of Ia-bearing epidermal Langerhans cells, *J. Immunol.* **131**:2005.

Stingl, G., Katz, S. I., Shevach, E. M., Wolff-Schreiner, E. C., and Green, I., 1978b, Detection of Ia antigens on Langerhans cells in guinea pig skin, *J. Immunol.* **120**:570.

Stingl, G., Tamaki, K., and Katz, S., 1980, Origin and function of Langerhans cells, *Immunol. Rev.* **53**:149.

Stockinger, B., and Lemmel, E., 1978, On the mechanism of antibody-mediated feedback regulation: Lack of inhibition in Fc receptor negative cells, *Cell. Immunol.* **40**:395.

Sunshine, G. H., Katz, D. R., and Feldman, M., 1980, Dendritic cells induce T-cell proliferation to synthetic antigens under Ir gene control, *J. Exp. Med.* **152**:1817.

Szakal, A. K., and Hanna, M. G., Jr., 1968, The ultrastructure of antigen localization and virus-like particles in mouse spleen germinal centers, *Exp. Mol. Pathol.* **8**:75.

Talmage, D., Dixon, F., Bukantz, S., and Dammin, C., 1951, Antigen elimination from the blood as an early manifestation of the immune response, *J. Immunol.* **67**:243.

Tew, J. G., and Mandel, T. E., 1978, The maintenance and regulation of serum antibody levels: Evidence indicating a role for antigen retained in lymphoid follicles, *J. Immunol.* **120**:1063.

Tew, J. G., and Mandel, T. E., 1979, Prolonged antigen half life in the lymphoid follicles of specifically immunized mice, *Immunology* **37**:67.

Tew, J. G., Self, C. H., Harold, W. W., and Stavitsky, A. B., 1973, The spontaneous induction of anamnestic antibody synthesis in lymph node cell cultures many months after primary immunization, *J. Immunol.* **111**:416.

Tew, J. G., Mandel, T. E., and Burgess, A. W., 1979a, Retention of intact HSA for prolonged periods in the popliteal lymph nodes of specifically immunized mice, *Cell. Immunol.* **45**:207.

Tew, J. G., Mandel, T. E., and Miller, G. A., 1979b, Immune retention: Immunological requirements for maintaining an easily degradable antigen *in vivo*, *Aust. J. Exp. Biol. Med. Sci.* **57**:401.

Tew, J. G., Phipps, R. P., and Mandel, T. E., 1980a, The maintenance and regulation of the humoral immune response: Persisting antigen and the role of follicular antigen binding dendritic cells as accessory cells, *Immunol. Rev.* **53**:175.

Tew, J. G., Mandel, T. E., and Rice, P. L., 1980b, Immune elimination and immune retention: The relationship between antigen retained in the foot and the elicitation of footpad swelling, *Immunology* **40**:425.

Toews, G. B., Bergstresser, P. R., and Streilein, J. W., 1980, Epidermal Langerhans cell density determines whether contact hypersensitivity or unresponsiveness follows skin painting with DNFB, *J. Immunol.* **124**:445.

Van Rooijen, N., 1972, Antigens in the spleen: The non-specificity of the follicles in the process of antigen trapping and the role of antibody, *Immunology* **22**:757.

Voisen, G. A., 1980, Role of antibody classes in the regulatory facilitation reaction, *Immunol. Rev.* **49**:3.

Weigle, W. O., 1975, Cyclical production of antibody as a regulatory mechanism in immune responses, *Adv. Immunol.* **21**:87.

White, R. G., 1963, *Functional Recognition of Immunologically Competent Cells by Means of the Fluorescent Antibody Technique*, Ciba Found. Study Group No. 16, p. 6.

White, R. G., French, V. I., and Stark, J. M., 1967, Germinal center formation and antigen localization in Malpighian bodies of the chicken spleen, in: *Germinal Centers in Immune Responses* (H. Cotlier, N. Odontchenki, R. Schindler, and C. C. Congdon, eds.), p. 131, Springer-Verlag, Berlin.

Wolff, K., 1972, The Langerhans cell, in: *Current Problems in Dermatology* (J. W. J. Mali, ed.), Vol. 4, p. 79, Karger, Basel.

6

Utilization of Monoclonal Antibodies in the Characterization of Monocyte-Macrophage Differentiation Antigens

ROBERT F. TODD, III, and STUART F. SCHLOSSMAN

1. INTRODUCTION

Cells of the monocyte-macrophage lineage perform diverse functions ranging from phagocytosis of microorganisms and other foreign substances, killing of antibody-coated erythrocytes or tumor cells (antibody-dependent cellular cytotoxicity, ADCC) (Poplack *et al.*, 1976; Levy *et al.*, 1979), spontaneous killing of unsensitized tumor cells (natural killing, NK) (Mantovani *et al.*, 1979; de Vries *et al.*, 1980; and Fischer *et al.*, 1981), uptake and presentation of antigenic material in a form that is stimulatory to helper T lymphocytes (Unanue, 1978), suppression of immune responses (Allison, 1978), and secretion of certain complement components and other stimulatory products (Nathan *et al.*, 1980; Beatty *et al.*, 1981).

Given the contribution of these cells to the integrity of both afferent and efferent limbs of the immune response, a considerable research effort has been undertaken to better understand their origin, differentiation, and function. Until recently, these efforts have been hindered by the lack of well-defined surface markers which could be used to identify members of the monocyte-macrophage lineage. Monocytic-macrophage markers could be useful in (1) determining the number of macrophages in cell suspensions (e.g., calculating the purity of mononuclear cell populations); (2) depleting macrophages from other mono-

ROBERT F. TODD, III, and STUART F. SCHLOSSMAN • Division of Tumor Immunology, Dana-Farber Cancer Institute, and Department of Medicine, Harvard Medical School, Boston, Massachusetts 02115.

nuclear cells (e.g., by complement-mediated lysis, cell sorting, or by rosette techniques; (3) selecting out pure populations of macrophages to be used in functional and biochemical studies; (4) identifying macrophage progenitor cells sharing common antigens; and (5) serologic diagnosis and specific immunotherapy of reticuloendothelial disorders originating from the macrophage lineage (e.g., monocytic leukemia, histiocytic medullary reticuloendotheliosis, Gaucher's disease, etc.).

Monoclonal antibody technology (Kohler and Milstein, 1975) has facilitated the development of antibodies directed against cell surface antigens. These reagents have several advantages over conventional heteroantisera in that their monospecificity does not require extensive absorption, they are generally high-titered, and they can be produced in almost limitless quantities. We and other investigators have taken advantage of these techniques and have directed our efforts toward identifying antigenic markers on the surface of cells within the macrophage lineage. To date, several unique nonpolymorphic determinants have been described both in the human and murine systems, and it is the purpose of this review to summarize the accomplishments achieved thus far. We have placed particular emphasis on work carried out in man and will touch only briefly on the polymorphic Ia antigen system which is shared between macrophages and B cells. Tables 1–4 serve as a summary of the results of pertinent investigations.

2. MONOCLONAL ANTIBODIES WITH RELATIVE SPECIFICITY FOR HUMAN MONOCYTES AND MACROPHAGES

2.1. Mo2

Mo2 is a monocyte-specific antigen characterized by our laboratory (Todd *et al.*, 1981a; Todd and Schlossman, 1982). It is defined by a lytic IgM monoclonal antibody which binds selectively to peripheral blood monocytes, macrophages derived from cultured monocytes, and peritoneal macrophages. Mo2 is not expressed by other circulating human cells (including T, B, and null cells, granulocytes, platelets, or red cells), nor is it found on any human cultured cell line tested. Among myeloid leukemias cells, Mo2 is found on 45% of patients whose malignant cells express monocyte characteristics (e.g., acute monocytic or myelomonocytic variants) while it is rarely expressed on immature blast forms (Todd *et al.*, 1981a, Todd and Schlossman, 1983). The antigen, which is sensitive to proteolytic treatment of monocytes with trypsin or papain, has a glycoprotein structure with a molecular weight of 55K (Todd and Schlossman, 1982; Todd *et al.*, 1982). Sorted Mo2-positive cells bear the morphological, histochemical, and functional characteristics of monocytes; Mo2-negative cells are devoid of these features (Todd *et al.*, 1981a, 1983). In other functional studies, treatment of human mononuclear cells with anti-Mo2 and complement diminishes the subsequent primary *in vitro* antibody response to DNP-KLH and the secondary proliferative response to tetanus toxoid which can be restored by appropriate numbers of monocytes (Morimoto *et al.*, 1981; Todd *et al.*, 1983). This indicates that Mo2-positive cells serve as antigen-presenting monocytes in the primary and secondary responses to soluble antigen. Treatment of monocytes with anti-Mo2 in the absence of complement has no effect on other monocyte functions (e.g., Fc receptor-mediated binding to IgG-sensitized erythrocytes) (Todd *et al.*, 1981a).

2.2. Mac-120

Raff and co-workers have reported the development of a lytic monoclonal antibody which binds selectively to a subset of human peripheral blood monocytes (37% by complement lysis; 60–95% by immunofluorescence) to the exclusion of other circulating cells as well as certain cultured human cell lines (U937 and HL60) (Hausman *et al.*, 1980; Raff *et al.*, 1980; T. Gonwa *et al.*, unpublished). Preliminary biochemical analysis has shown that this antigen consists of a polypeptide chain of 120K. Most significantly, complement-mediated lysis of the subset of monocytes bearing this antigen abrogates proliferation by the remaining cells in response to Con A and soluble antigen. Thus, Mac-120-positive cells, which are included within the larger Ia (HLA-DRw)-positive subset, appear to define a subpopulation of monocytes which have antigen-presenting accessory function. Furthermore, the Mac-120-positive subset has greater stimulatory potential in autologous MLR (but not allogeneic MLR). To date, this represents the first report of a serologically defined, functionally distinct macrophage subset either in the murine or human system (excluding the well-documented requirement of Ia expression by antigen-presenting cells).

2.3. UC-45

Using indirect immunofluorescence, Hogg and co-workers have recently characterized the reactivity of an IgM monoclonal antibody, UC-45, which is reactive with an antigen found on the fibrous processes of spreading human monocytes, and the neurofilaments of neurons (Hogg *et al.*, 1981). Among circulating cells, UC-45 is monocyte specific and is negative on all human hematopoietic cell lines tested. Its specificity is unique to spreading monocytes, since monocytes in suspension are generally negative. On biochemical analysis, UC-45 reacts with a single polypeptide chain of 45K. Its expression on spreading monocytes and neurons does not relate to other chemical structures known to be shared between these cells.

2.4. Mo3

We have recently identified an antigenic determinant defined by an IgM monoclonal antibody which is weakly expressed by freshly harvested peripheral blood monocytes but which becomes strongly expressed by the majority of cells which have been cultured overnight at 37°C (Todd and Schlossman, 1982). This dramatic increase in antigen expression appears unrelated to monocyte spreading (occurring when monocytes are cultured on polypropylene surfaces to which they do not adhere), is temperature dependent, and is blocked by puromycin. Among circulating cells, Mo3 is restricted to monocytes; except for the histiocytic lymphoma cell line U937, human hematopoietic cell lines are negative. Like Mo2, Mo3 is protease sensitive but is resynthesized by cultured monocytes. The expression of Mo3 can be induced on HL60 promyelocytes stimulated toward macrophage differentiation by phorbol diester or lymphokines.

2.5. D5D6 AND C10H5

Linker-Israeli and co-workers have described two lytic monoclonal antibodies, D5D6 and C10H5, which are reactive with human peripheral blood monocytes but not granulocytes or other normal circulating cells (Linker-Israeli *et al.*, 1981). Raised by immunization with acute myelogenous leukemia (AML) cells, D5D6 and C10H5 are lytic for blast cells of patients (88% and 33%, respectively) with this disease (malignant cells from patients with chronic myelogenous leukemia or lymphocytic leukemias being negative). Among human cultured cell lines, only the HL60 promyelocytic leukemic line is positive. Significantly, D5D6 and C10H5 are cytotoxic for bone marrow stem cells in the CFU-C assay (Pike and Robinson, 1970), which may limit their usefulness for possible immunotherapy.

2.6. MϕP-15, MϕP-7, AND MϕR-17

Dimitriu-Bona and colleagues have recently reported their experience with a series of six monoclonal reagents reactive with monocytes and macrophages from various sources (Dimitriu-Bona *et al.*, 1981, 1983). Three of these antibodies, MϕP-15, MϕP-7, and MϕR-17 are relatively specific for this lineage; MϕP-15 demonstrates moderate immunofluorescent staining for the majority of PB monocytes (~ 70%) but intense staining for fluid phase macrophages (pleural, peritoneal, and synovial). MϕP-7 and MϕR-17 bind to distinct antigens expressed in low density on peripheral blood monocytes (approx. 35% of cells stained), pleural and peritoneal macrophages, but demonstrating high antigen density on synovial fluid phagocytes. Although other circulating cells are unreactive, both of these antibodies bind to activated T-cell blasts (low density).

2.7. MY3

Griffin and co-workers have characterized a series of four monoclonal antibodies reacting with human myeloid cells (Griffin *et al.*, 1981). One of these,

MY3, is found on the majority of peripheral blood monocytes but is negative on other circulating cells (except for a small subpopulation of granulocytes of questionable significance). It is also negative on all human hematopoietic cell lines except for weak expression on HL60. Among acute leukemia cells, it is found on monoblasts from most patients with monocytic or myelomonocytic leukemia (95%) and on a lesser fraction (12%) of patients with myeloblastic leukemia; malignant lymphoid cells are negative. Its expression can be augmented on HL60 promyelocytes if these cells are induced to differentiate by DMSO or lymphokines.

2.8. B44.1

B44.1 is an IgM monoclonal antibody reactive with peripheral blood monocytes as well as bone marrow promonocytes (and possibly a small fraction of promyelocytes, myelocytes, and metamyelocytes) (Perussia *et al.*, 1982). The expression of the antigen reactive with B44.1 is not induced by treatment of HL60 promyelocytes with lymphokines or DMSO (Dayton *et al.*, 1983).

2.9. 4F2

Eisenbarth and co-workers have produced an IgG2a monoclonal antibody by immunization with human T-cell line HSB-2, which is reactive not only with the immunizing cell but with all peripheral blood monocytes to the exclusion of other normal circulating cells (excluding a 5% fraction of SRBC rosette-positive cells of questionable significance) (Eisenbarth *et al.*, 1980). However, after MLR or mitogen activation, a large subset (70%) of T lymphoid cells becomes positive for the 4F2 antigen. 4F2 binds to several hematopoietic cell lines of T- and B-cell lineage as well as U937 and erythrocytic line K562. On biochemical analysis, 4F2 precipitates a 120K structure, which, under reducing conditions, consists of two subunits of 40 and 80K. The antigen is resistant to treatment with trypsin, pronase, and neuraminidase (Haynes *et al.*, 1981). Functionally, 4F2 (in the absence of complement) does not inhibit NK, ADCC, or cytolytic T-cell killing. It does, however, produce a partial inhibition of mitogen-induced proliferation by human mononuclear cells (Haynes *et al.*, 1981).

2.10. 61D3

Nunez and colleagues have characterized an IgG1 monoclonal reagent, 61D3, that is specific for peripheral blood monocytes (unlike 63D3 which has weak reactivity for granulocytes) (Nunez *et al.*, 1982). This antibody binds to a 75K structure that is gradually lost from the monocyte surface with prolonged culture, and is also absent from pulmonary alveolar macrophages.

2.11. 1D5

In a report dealing with human monocyte differentiation *in vitro*, Kaplan and Gaudernack refer to their development of a monoclonal antibody, 1D5, that is specific for peripheral blood monocytes and monocytes cultured on collagen matrices, but is unreactive with other circulating elements (Kaplan and Gaudernack, 1982).

2.12. OKM5

Shen and co-workers, in a recent paper evaluating the possibility of functional monocyte heterogeneity (Shen *et al.*, 1983), allude to the characterization of an IgG1 monoclonal antibody, OKM5, defining an 88K antigen that is expressed by 60–80% of peripheral blood monocytes (along with the majority of bone marrow monocytes). In their functional analysis, they have used both OKM1 and OKM5 to define a small subset of monocytes (E−, OKM1−, OKM5+) that is responsible for presenting self-antigens in the autologous mixed leukocyte reaction.

2.13. PHM3

PHM3 is an IgG2a monoclonal reagent raised against thymocytes that binds to a 50K antigenic structure expressed on most peripheral blood monocytes as well as peritoneal macrophages and Kupffer cells (Becker *et al.*, 1981). While it is also found on thymocytes, it is not borne by circulating T lymphocytes or any other blood element.

3. MONOCLONAL ANTIBODIES WHOSE SPECIFICITY IS SHARED BY HUMAN MONOCYTES AND OTHER PERIPHERAL BLOOD ELEMENTS

3.1. OKM1

OKM1 is an IgG2b monoclonal antibody reactive for all peripheral blood monocytes, granulocytes, and a population of non-T, non-B lymphoid cells operationally defined as null cells. T and B lymphoid cells are negative as are various hematopoietic human cell lines (Breard *et al.*, 1980). Malignant cells from patients with myelomonocytic leukemia tend to express the OKM1 antigen. Functionally, Breard and co-workers have reported that treatment of mononuclear cells with OKM1 and complement abrogates subsequent proliferation to soluble antigen, suggesting the depletion of antigen-presenting monocytes. Also, several investigators have shown that complement-mediated OKM1 lysis diminishes both ADCC and NK activity of human mononuclear cells (Kay and

Horowitz, 1980; Zarling and Kung, 1980; Breard *et al.*, 1981) possibly by killing off a null-cell population thought to be responsible for these activities (Brier *et al.*, 1975; Ozer *et al.*, 1979). Preliminary biochemical analysis indicates that the cell surface antigen precipitated by OKM1 antibody consists of two polypeptide subunits of 94 and 155K (Todd *et al.*, 1982).

3.2. Mo1

Mo1 is an antigen defined by a lytic IgM antibody whose reactivity appears identical to that of OKM1 (positive on monocytes, granulocytes, and null cells) (Todd *et al.*, 1981a). A recent biochemical study indicates that both antibodies detect antigenic sites on the same molecule of 94 and 155K (Todd *et al.*, 1982). The possibility of separate antigenic sites is suggested by the fact that binding of OKM1 does not block the subsequent binding of Mo1 (Todd *et al.*, 1982) although differences in antibody affinity for the same site could also explain this observation. Mo1, unlike Mo2, is resistant to proteolysis by trypsin and papain. The antigen is expressed by a majority of myeloid bone marrow cells (from myelocyte to mature granulocyte), but has not been detected on the stem cell CFU-C (Todd and Schlossman, 1983; Griffin *et al.*, 1982). Mo1 is found on malignant cells from a majority of patients with acute monocytic or myelomonocytic leukemia (80%) but is absent from lymphoid leukemia cells (Todd *et al.*, 1981a; Todd and Schlossman, 1983). Expression of Mo1 can be induced by stimulation of HL60 promyelocytes with phorbol diester or lymphokines (Todd *et al.*, 1981b). In recent functional studies, anti-Mo1 treatment of normal monocytes and granulocytes blocks C3bi binding and inhibits the phagocytosis of opsonized particles (Arnaout *et al.*, 1983). The inhibitory effect of anti-Mo1 on phagocytosis by normal cells parallels the cellular defects seen in a patient whose monocytes and granulocytes lack Mo1 (Dana *et al.*, 1983).

3.3. Mac-1

Mac-1 is an antigen defined by a rat IgG2b antibody (M1/70) raised against nonadherent mitogen-activated mouse splenocytes (Springer *et al.*, 1979). In the murine system, the antigen is expressed by resident and exudate peritoneal macrophages, monocytes, and granulocytes, 44% of bone marrow cells, and murine macrophage cell lines $P388D_1$ and J744. In man, it has a distribution of cellular expression identical with that of OKM1 and Mo1 (Ault and Springer, 1981). Likewise, further analysis has indicated the expression of Mac-1 on the human mononuclear cells responsible for natural killing. Biochemical studies have demonstrated that on murine cells, Mac-1 exists as a two-polypeptide structure of 105 and 190K but attempts to immunoprecipitate the cross-reacting human molecule have been unsuccessful (probably due to relatively weak antibody affinity for the corresponding human structure). Anti-Mac-1 antibody, like anti-Mo1, blocks C3bi rosetting (Beller *et al.*, 1982).

3.4. MY4, MY7, AND MY8

In addition to MY3, Griffin and co-workers have produced three additional antibodies whose binding is shared among cells within the myeloid lineage (monocytes, granulocytes, and their progenitors), but not lymphoid cells (Griffin *et al.*, 1981). MY4 is expressed by most peripheral blood monocytes and a subset of peripheral blood granulocytes (28%). In normal bone marrow, it is expressed by a significant fraction of adherent cells; among leukemic cells, its expression is nearly identical to MY3 with a predilection for cells demonstrating monocytic features. Of all cultured hematopoietic cell lines tested, it is weakly expressed by U937 and HL60. MY7 is found on a subset of peripheral blood monocytes (21%) but a majority of granulocytes (72%). It is strongly positive on myeloid cell lines HL60, KG1, and U937, as well as myeloblasts from most patients with all forms of myeloid leukemia. It is expressed by the CFU-C stem cell (Griffin *et al.*, 1983). MY8 is found on the majority of peripheral blood monocytes and granulocytes and all peroxidase-positive bone marrow cells. U937 and HL60 are strongly and weakly reactive, respectively. The CFU-C is MY8 negative (Griffin, *et al.*, 1982).

3.5. B9.8, B13.4, B34.3, AND B43.4

Perussia and co-workers have reported the characterization of a series of monoclonal antibodies all reactive with peripheral blood monocytes and granulocytes as well as bone marrow myeloid cells of varying degrees of maturation (B43.4, B9.8, B13.4, and B43.4 antigens arising in sequence on promyelocytes, myelocytes, metamyelocytes, and granulocytes) (Perussia *et al.*, 1981, 1982). B43.4 is also expressed by null cells (Perussia *et al.*, 1982) giving it a distribution of expression identical to that of Mo1 and OKM1. All four antibodies are unreactive for unstimulated HL60 promyelocyte cells but, with the exception of B34.3, the expression of these antigenic determinants can be elicited by differentiation induced by exposure to various activating agents (TPA, DMSO, retinoic acid, or lymphokines) (Perussia *et al.*, 1981; Dayton *et al.*, 1983).

3.6. TA-1

TA-1 is a monoclonal IgG2a antibody raised against the human T-cell line HSB-2 (cf. 4F2), which in addition to peripheral blood T cells is reactive for all peripheral blood monocytes (LeBien and Kersey, 1980). It is unreactive with peripheral blood B cells (except for a 10% fraction of questionable significance) and granulocytes but is positive for MLR-activated T-cell blasts, and approximately 13% of nucleated bone marrow cells. Among leukemic cells, TA-1 is positive for approximately 50% of T-cell ALLs but negative on null cell ALLs. It is reactive for the myelomonocytic variant of acute myelogenous leukemia but negative for myeloblastic leukemia. The antigen defined by TA-1 (a two-subunit protein of 95 and 170K) thus appears to be shared between both T- and monocyte-macrophage lineages (LeBien *et al.*, 1983).

3.7. Mo4

In addition to Mo1, 2, and 3, we have recently described our experience with a fourth monoclonal antibody raised by immunization with human monocytes (Todd and Schlossman, 1982). It reacts with an antigen, Mo4, which is expressed by a variable fraction of peripheral blood monocytes (40–80%) and platelets. T, B, and null lymphoid cells, as well as granulocytes and erythrocytes are negative. Mo4 (MW = 100K) is protease sensitive (both trypsin and papain) and its expression can be induced on HL60 promyelocytes by lymphokine exposure. Like Mo1-3, Mo4 is infrequently expressed on leukemic cells from patients with myeloblastic leukemia but is present on the malignant cells of approximately 35% of patients with monocytic or myelomonocytic leukemia (Todd and Schlossman, 1983).

3.8. Mo5

Mo5 is a 95K protein antigen defined by an IgG2a monoclonal antibody developed by our laboratory (Todd and Schlossman, 1983). It is similar in its distribution of expression to MY8, being found on all peroxidase positive myeloid precursors (promyelocyte stage on) and mature monocytes and granulocytes (null cells are negative as is the CFU-C cell). Mo5 is resistant to both trypsin and papain treatment; the antigen modulates from the cell surface after exposure to anti-Mo5 antibody. It is expressed by 30% of patients with AML and 54% of individuals with AMML or AMoL.

3.9. AML-2-23 AND PM-81

Ball and co-workers have reported the characterization of two monoclonal reagents, AML-2-23 and PM-81, that define distinct determinants found on most peripheral blood monocytes and granulocytes, as well as bone marrow myeloid cells beyond the CFU-C (Ball and Fanger, 1983; Ball *et al.*, 1982, 1983). The PM-81 antigen is expressed on a wide variety of myeloid cell lines (e.g., HL60, KG-1, K562, U937) while AML-2-23 demonstrates weak reactivity for HL60 (antigen expression augmented after exposure of HL60 cells to activating substances) (Graziano *et al.*, 1983). Among leukemias, AML-2-23 shows relative specificity for M4 and M5 cells with monocytoid features, while PM-81 binds to the majority of patients with all stages of acute nonlymphocytic leukemia plus a limited number of patients with ALL, and CML.

3.10. 5F1

5F1 is a lytic IgM reagent raised against AMML cells that reacts with the majority of peripheral blood monocytes and platelets as well as most bone marrow monocytes and erythroid precursors (Bernstein *et al.*, 1982). The antigen is expressed by the malignant cells of a significant proportion of patients with AMML and AML but is not found on ALL cells or a variety of lymphoid and myeloid cell lines.

3.11. 1G10

In addition to 5F1, Bernstein and co-workers have reported the development of 1G10, an IgM antibody binding to an antigen expressed in high density on granulocytes, but in low concentration on a subset of monocytes (approx. 20%) (Bernstein *et al.*, 1982). In normal bone marrow, the IG10 antigen is found on most myeloid precursors; among leukemic forms, IG10 is expressed by cells of all stages of myeloid maturation (ALL cells are negative).

3.12. 63D3

Ugolini et al. have produced an antibody, 63D3, which is specific for a 200K antigen expressed by human peripheral blood monocytes and, to a much lesser extent, peripheral blood granulocytes (Ugolini *et al.*, 1980). T and B lymphocytes are negative as are endothelial cells and various human cultured cell lines including U937 and HL60 (but positive on HL60 cells exposed to agents inducing monocytic differentiation, Graziano *et al.*, 1983). 63D3 is in the IgG1 subclass and requires a second anti-immunoglobulin antibody for complement mediated lysis (greater than 80% of peripheral blood monocytes lysed). On cell sorter analysis, 63D3 positive cells have the morphology and size distribution of monocyte-enriched adherent cells and, in contrast to the 63D3 negative fraction, are able to phagocytize antibody-coated erythrocytes (Rosenberg *et al.*, 1981).

Isolated 63D3 positive or negative mononuclear cells are unable to proliferate in response to pokeweed mitogen; however, mitomycin C-treated 63D3 positive cells can serve as accessory cells in restoring mitogen-induced proliferation (Rosenberg *et al.*, 1981).

3.13. MPA

Burckhardt and colleagues have reported a monoclonal IgG2a antibody reactive with peripheral blood monocytes, platelets, and bone marrow megakaryocytes (Burckhardt *et al.*, 1982). Hematopoietic human cell lines including U937 and HL60 are also positive as are malignant cells from a limited number of patients with monocytic leukemia. The antigen, on preliminary biochemical analysis, consists of two subunits of 93 and 35K; it is trypsin resistant but pronase sensitive.

3.14. M206

M206 is an IgG2a antibody raised against U937 that defines an 180 K antigen found on peripheral blood monocytes, and, in low surface density, on granulocytes, (Maruyana *et al.*, 1983). In an analysis of a limited number of patients with leukemia, the antigen tends to be expressed on AMoL cells but not cells from patients with ALL or CLL. Functional studies indicate that the M206 antigen is borne by the accessory cell required in the proliferative response to PWM.

3.15. MφP-9, MφS-1, and MφS-39

Besides the three previously mentioned anti-monocyte/macrophage reagents, Dimitriu-Bona and co-workers have reported the development of a series of three additional antibodies binding to distinct antigens expressed by peripheral blood monocytes and certain fluid-phase macrophages (Dimitriu-Bona *et al.*, 1983). These reagents demonstrate intense immunofluorescent staining on most monocytes as well as peritoneal, pleural, and synovial macrophages, with much weaker staining for granulocytes (setting them apart from the antibodies in Table 1). Other circulating elements, the cell lines U937 and K562, and myelomonocytic leukemia cells are negative.

3.16. PHM2

PHM2 is an IgG2a monoclonal antibody (raised against peritoneal macrophages) characterized by Becker et al. that is specific for a 52K antigen whose distribution of expression is similar to PHM3 except that it is also found on the surface of a small subset of circulating T lymphocytes (6–9%) (Becker *et al.*, 1981).

3.17. MMA

Hanjan and colleagues (Hanjan *et al.*, 1982) have reported the development of MMA, a lytic antibody that binds to most monocytes, granulocytes, and activated T lymphoblasts (and to several T-cell lines). In complement depletion experiments, MMA is cytotoxic for peripheral blood accessory cells involved in antigen and mitogen proliferation and for the bone marrow CFU-C. The antigen is found on the malignant cells of a small series of patients with AML and CML, but is absent from individuals with ALL and CLL.

4. RAT MONOCLONAL ANTIBODIES DIRECTED AGAINST MURINE MACROPHAGE ANTIGENS

Springer (1981a) has recently reviewed the current progress in defining differentiation antigens on murine macrophages. The following is a brief resume.

4.1. Mac-1

Springer and co-workers' characterization of differentiation antigen, Mac-1, represents the first report of a monoclonal antibody with unique specificity for phagocytic cells (Springer *et al.*, 1979). As outlined above, Mac-1 is an antigen expressed by murine phagocytes (peritoneal macrophages and peripheral blood monocytes and granulocytes) as well as 44% of bone marrow cells. The rat IgG2b antibody (M1/70) that defines this antigen cross-reacts with a human antigenic structure found on monocytes, granulocytes, and null cells (Ault and Springer, 1981). As noted above, Mac-1 is closely associated with the C3bi receptor (CR3) in that Mac-1 blocks the binding of this complement component to murine phagocytes (Beller *et al.*, 1982). Another monoclonal antibody, 1.2IJ, reported by Mellman *et al.* (1980), is similar if not identical to M1/70.

4.2. Mac-2, 3, AND 4

Subsequent to their description of Mac-1, Springer and co-workers characterized three additional antigens expressed by thioglycollate-induced peritoneal macrophages (all are negative on lymphoid cells in lymph node and thymus) (Springer, 1981b). The antibodies defining these structures are novel in that they were raised by immunization of rats with purified macrophage glycoproteins (instead of whole cells) in an attempt to exclude hybridoma clones reactive for more immunodominant but less restrictive cell surface antigens (Springer, 1981c). On biochemical analysis, Mac-2, 3, and 4 are single polypeptide structures of 32, 110, and 180K respectively. Unlike Mac-1, none of these antigens is expressed on bone marrow cells, which, due to a lack of reactivity for granulocyte progenitors, indicates their restriction to the monocyte-macrophage lineage.

LeBlanc and co-workers have independently developed an IgG2a monoclonal antibody that appears to be detecting the same antigenic structure as Springer's anti-Mac-4 (M3/37) (LeBlanc *et al.*, 1980).

4.3. F4/80

Austyn and Gordon have characterized a monoclonal antibody (F4/80) precipitating a single polypeptide structure of 160K expressed by murine peripheral blood monocytes, resident and induced peritoneal macrophages, and macrophage cell lines (lymphoid cells are negative) (Austyn and Gordon, 1981).

4.4. 2.4G2

2.4G2 is an IgG monoclonal antibody developed by Unkeless which is specific for the protease-resistant Fc receptor II (FcRII) expressed by murine macrophages, B lymphocytes, granulocytes, and macrophage cell lines (Unkeless, 1979). Functionally, this antibody blocks mouse macrophage FcRII binding to mouse IgG1- and IgG2b-coated erythrocytes. On biochemical analysis, 2.4G2 precipitates a two-subunit polypeptide structure of 47 and 60K (Mellman and Unkeless, 1980). The characterization of this antibody is significant because it represented the first monoclonal reagent defining a macrophage surface structure of known function.

5. IMMUNE RESPONSE-ASSOCIATED ANTIGENS ON MACROPHAGES

In mouse, guinea pig, and human systems, it has become clear that the polymorphic system of immune response-associated (Ia) antigens (HLA-D or DRw antigens in man) play a significant role in macrophage accessory function (for review see Niederhuber, 1978; Rosenthal, 1978; Schwartz *et al.*, 1978). Namely, only the Ia-positive subset of macrophages is capable of presenting antigen in a form that is stimulatory to helper T lymphocytes. This macrophage–lymphocyte collaboration is genetically restricted in that the antigen-presenting cell in a secondary (recall) immune response must bear the same Ia genotype as the antigen-presenting macrophage in the primary response to a given antigen (Pierce *et al.*, 1976; Thomas and Shevack, 1976). To account for the participation of Ia antigens in antigen presentation, two hypotheses have been advanced: (1) macrophage-processed antigen becomes physically bound to Ia antigens to form a structure that is stimulatory to the appropriate helper T cell; or (2) the Ia antigen, as a physically separate entity, provides a necessary second signal to consummate the interaction.

Structurally, human Ia antigens have been found to consist of two polypeptide subunits of 29 and 34K (Springer *et al.*, 1977). Conventional isoantisera have identified 10 genetic variants of this molecule (Albert *et al.*, 1981) which is shared among monocytes, B lymphocytes, and activated (but not resting) T lymphocytes. As in mouse and guinea pig experimental systems, these anti-Ia antibodies can block antigen presentation (Breard *et al.*, 1979; Bergholtz and Thorsby, 1978; Rodey *et al.*, 1979; Geha *et al.*, 1980) and T–macrophage binding which precedes T-lymphocyte proliferation (Todd and Schlossman, 1980; Geha *et al.*, 1981). Monoclonal mouse anti-human Ia antibodies are frequently produced by immunization with human mononuclear cells, but these tend to react with a common (invariant) portion of the molecule (Charron and McDevitt, 1979; Reinherz *et al.*, 1979; Nadler *et al.*, 1981a). Recently, however, antibodies with recognition for polymorphic or variants have been reported (Truco *et al.*, 1979; Zola *et al.*, 1980; Nadler *et al.*, 1981a,b; Quaranta *et al.*, 1981) as have reagents for non-DR Ia loci (reviewed in Trowsdale *et al.*, 1983).

While in the murine system there exist distinct subsets of macrophages which are Ia positive or Ia negative, in man the majority of peripheral blood monocytes bear these antigens (Smith and Ault, 1981; Nunez and Stastny, 1983). One report suggests that the density of Ia increases with time in culture (Smith and Ault, 1981).

6. DISCUSSION

Mouse monoclonal antibodies have been produced by immunization with human-derived tissues which are reactive with nonpolymorphic antigens borne by cells of the monocyte-macrophage lineage. To date, at least 16 reagents detect antigens which, among circulating normal cells, appear to be relatively specific for monocytes (antigens in Table 1). Among these, Mo2, D5D5, C10H5, MϕP-15, MY3, B44.1, 4F2, 61D3, 1D5, OKM5, and PHM3 are found on the majority of freshly harvested peripheral blood monocytes. Mac-120, MϕP-7, and MϕR-17 identify subsets within the circulating monocyte pool, which, in the case of Mac-120, is reported to be functionally significant. UC-45 is negative on monocytes kept in suspension but is positive on spreading adherent cells. Mo3 is weakly expressed on freshly harvested monocytes but increases substantially in antigen density after culture. Several of these antigens can be further distinguished one from another by virute of molecular weight estimations: Mo2 = 55K; Mac-120 = 120K; UC-45 = 45K; 4F2 = 40 + 80K; 61D3 = 75K; OKM5 = 88K; and PHM3 = 50K. Other antigens demonstrate distinctive coexpression on various hematopoietic cell lines; Mo3 is expressed on U937; D5D6 and C10H5 are expressed by HL60; 4F2 is found on HSB-2 and SB cells. Whereas none of these reagents define a molecule of known function (e.g., Fc or complement receptors), Mo2, Mac-120, 4F2, and OKM5 identify accessory cells that are active in the proliferative response to antigen and/or mitogen.

Twenty-four mouse anti-human monoclonal antibodies define antigens that are shared between monocytes and other circulating blood elements (antigens in Table 2). In addition to their monocyte-reactivity, OKM1, Mo1, Mo5, MY7, MY8, B13.4, B9.8, B43.4, B34.3, PM-81, MMA, AML-2-23, IG10, (MY3?), MY4, 63D3, MϕS-39, MϕP-9, MϕS–1, and M206 are expressed by granulocytes (variable degrees of antigen density). TA-1 and PHM2 are borne by resting T lymphocytes (~ 100% and ~ 8%, respectively) while activated T-cell blasts bear TA-1, MMA, 4F2, MϕR-17, and MϕP-7. Mo4, MPA, and 5F1 are found on platelets. MY4 is distinctive in its expression on 28% of granulocytes, while MY7 and 1G10 are likewise unique in their delineation of a similar proportion of monocytes (both expressed on the majority of granulocytes). Among this group of 24 reagents, certain other clear similarities exist: OKM1, Mol, and B43.4 (found on monocytes, granulocytes, and null cells); and MY8 and Mo5 (monocytes, granulocytes, and all peroxidase positive bone marrow cells) suggesting reactivity for antigens expressed on identical or related structures. A recent international workshop (Bernard and Boumsell, in press) has taken a first step in organizing the monocyte-myeloid reagents to define overlapping or distinctive reactivities.

The OKM1, Mol, Mac-1 antibodies, (the latter, a rat monoclonal reactive with both murine and human phagocytes) all having similar molecular weight characteristics and a cellular distribution that includes null cells, have been particularly useful in studies identifying the cells responsible for natural killing and antibody-dependent cellular cytotoxicity. Moreover, recent studies have suggested a functional role for the molecular species identified by this group. Both Mo1 and Mac-1 reagents selectively inhibit the binding of C3bi-coated particles to phagocytic cells, suggesting the possibility that Mo1 and Mac-1 represent the receptor for this complement component (CR3). However, anti-Mo1 also blocks the phagocytosis of IgG and C3-opsonized particles (zymosan and sheep erythrocytes) which closely parallels the functional defect seen in the monocytes and granulocytes of a patient who lacks Mo1 (but whose phagocytes appear to rosette with C3bi-coated erythrocytes normally). Further work is ongoing to resolve the precise functional role of this class of surface molecules.

In the murine system, six rat anti-mouse monoclonal antibodies define four structurally distinct antigens expressed on macrophages alone (Mac 2, 3, and 4 and F4/80) and three antibodies are reactive for antigens shared among myeloid cells (Mac-1 and 2.4G2) (see Table 3). 2.4G2 has a clear functional importance binding specifically to the protease-resistant Fc receptor II found on murine macrophages, B cells, and granulocytes.

Of clinical significance is the fact that many of the mouse anti-human reagents are reactive for myeloid leukemia cells (reactivity varying with the degree of macrophage differentiation) as distinguished from malignant cells within the lymphoid lineage. This finding may facilitate diagnosis of myeloid leukemia when conventional methods (morphology or histochemistry) are equivocal. Moreover, it is conceivable that these reagents will become useful in specific immunotherapy of "benign" and malignant disorders of the reticuloendothelial system (Groopman and Golde, 1981).

The potential usefulness of these monoclonal antibodies in studying the ontogeny of the myeloid lineage is highlighted in Table 4. It will be noted that certain antigens are shared by peripheral blood monocytes and granulocytes which represent the end products of two developmental pathways sharing the same progenitor, the CFU-C (Moore *et al.*, 1972). That many of these antigens are also borne by immature myeloid forms resident in the bone marrow (monocytic and granulocytic precursors) may indicate that the expression of these markers occurs early at a common sequence during the differentiation of both granulocytic and monocytic series. Other shared antigens are more prevalent on either granulocytes or monocytes (e.g., MY7 and 1G10; MY4, respectively) while still other markers are restricted to monocytes alone (antigens underlined). Among these "monocyte-specific" antigens are those that represent late differentiation markers since they are not found on morphologically identifiable granulocytic precursors; other antigens may arise earlier because of their expression on immature myeloid forms but are selectively retained only by mature mono-

TABLE 1. MOUSE MONOCLONAL ANTIBODIES WITH RELATIVE SPECIFICITY FOR HUMAN MONOCYTES

Antibody/antigen designation	Antibody subclass	Antigen[a] MW (Kd)	Immunizing cells	Cellular distribution: Reactive	Cellular distribution: Nonreactive	Distinguishing features functional studies	References
Mo2	IgM	55	PB monocytes	PB monocytes; cultured[b] monocytes; perit. Mϕ; 45% AMML/AMoL Pt's; 16% AML Pt's	T, B, and null cells; RBC; PMN; platelets; U937; HL60; CLL, ALL Pt's	C' lysis blocks antigen proliferation; protease sensitive; lymphokine-induced HL60 Mo2+	Todd and Schlossman (1982, 1983), Morimoto *et al.* (1981), Todd *et al.* (1981a, 1982, 1983)
Mac-120	IgM	120	PB monocytes	60–90% PB monocytes	T and B cells; PMN; U937; HL60	C' lysis blocks antigen proliferation; Mac-120+ cells stimulate AMLR	Hausman *et al.* (1980), Raff *et al.* (1980)
UC-45	IgM	45	AMoL cells	Spreading PB monocytes; neurofilaments	Monocytes in suspension; T and B cells; PMN; platelets; RBC; cell lines	UC-45 antigen expressed on neural tissue	Hogg *et al.* (1981)
Mo3	IgM	NR	PB monocytes	Cultured monocytes; 14% AMML/AMoL Pt's; U937	T, B, and null cells; RBC; PMN; platelets; fresh monocytes (weak); HL60; AML, ALL Pt's	Protease sensitive; lymphokine or TPA-induced HL60 Mo3+	Todd and Schlossman (1982)
D5D6	IgM	NR	AML cells	PB monocytes; 88% AML Pt's; HL60	T and B cells; PMN; CML, CLL and ALL Pt's	CFU-C, D5D6+; BFU-E, D5D6−	Linker-Israeli *et al.* (1981)
C10H5	IgM	NR	AML cells	PB monocytes; 33% AML Pt's	Same as D5D6	Same as D5D6	Linker-Israeli *et al.* (1981)
MϕP-15	IgG1	NR	PB monocytes	70% PB monocytes; peritoneal, pleural, synovial Mϕ	T and B cells; PMN; RBC; platelets; U937; K562	NR	Dimitriu-Bona *et al.* (1983)
MϕP-7 MϕP-17	IgG1 NR	NR NR	PB monocytes PB monocytes	35% PB monocytes (weak); peritoneal and pleural Mϕ (weak); synovial Mϕ (strong); T-cell blasts (weak)	T and B cells; PMN; RBC; platelets; U937; K562	NR	Dimitriu-Bona *et al.* (1983)

MY3	IgM	NR	AMML cells	PB monocytes; 8% PMN; HL60 (weak); 95% AMoL and AML Pt's	T, B, and null cells; most PMN; RBC; platelets; U937	NR	Griffin *et al.* (1981)
B44.1	IgM	NR	PB monocytes	PB monocytes	T and B cells; PMN; platelets, RBC; KG1; HL60; K562	Lymphokine or DMSO-induced HL60 B44.1+	Perussia *et al.* (1982), Dayton *et al.* (1983)
4F2	IgG2a	40 80	HSB-2 cells	PB monocytes; HSB-2; SB; K562, U937; 70% activated T cells	T, B and null cells; RBC; PMN; splenocytes	Protease and neuraminidase resistant; C' lysis blocks mitogen proliferation	Eisenbarth *et al.* (1980), Haynes *et al.* (1981)
61D3	IgG1	75	PB monocytes	PB monocytes	T and B cells; PMN; cult. monocytes; PAM; U937	NR	Nunez *et al.* (1982)
1D5	NR	NR	PB monocytes	PB monocytes; cultured monocytes	T and B cells; PMN; U937; T and B cell lines	NR	Kaplan and Gaudernack (1982)
OKM5	IgG1	88	NR	PB monocytes; BM monocytes	T, B and null cells; PMN	$E^-OKM1^-OKM5^+$ cells present self-antigens in AMLR	Shen *et al.* (1983)
PHM3	IgG2a	50	Thymocytes	PB monocytes; thymocytes; Kupffer cells; peritoneal Mϕ	T, B and null cells; PMN; RBC	NR	Becker *et al.* (1981)

[a]Reducing conditions.

[b]Abbreviations: ADCC, antibody-dependent cellular cytotoxicity; ALL, acute lymphoblastic leukemia; AML, acute myeloblastic leukemia; AMML, acute myelomonocytic leukemia; AMoL, acute monocytic leukemia; AMLR, autologous mixed leukocyte response; BFU-E, burst-forming unit, erythroid; BM, bone marrow (pro's, promyelocytes; myelo's, myelocytes; metamyelo's, metamyelocytes); C', complement; CFU-C, colony-forming unit; CLL, chronic lymphocytic leukemia; CML, chronic myelogenous leukemia; DMF, dimethyl foramide; E^+, sheep RBC rosette +; Mϕ, macrophage; NK, natural killing; NR, not reported; PB, peripheral blood; PAM, pulmonary alveolar macrophage; PMN, granulocytes; Pt's, patients; RA, retinoic acid; RBC, erythrocytes; TPA, phorbol diester.

TABLE 2. MOUSE MONOCLONAL ANTIBODIES WITH SPECIFICITY FOR HUMAN MONOCYTES AND OTHER CIRCULATING CELLS[a]

Antibody/antigen designation	Antibody subclass	Antigen MW (Kd)	Immunizing cells	Cellular distribution: Reactive	Cellular distribution: Nonreactive	Distinguishing features functional studies	References
OKM1	IgG2b	94 155	E^+ cells	PB monocytes; PMN; null cells; most AMoL/AMML Pt's; U937 (weak)	T and B cells; K562; HL60	C′ lysis blocks antigen proliferation and NK/ADCC effector function	Kay and Horowitz (1980), Zarling and Kung (1980), Breard *et al.* (1980, 1981), Todd *et al.* (1982)
Mol	IgM	94 155	PB monocytes	PB monocytes; PMN; null cells; BM myelo's, metamyelo's, bands; 80% AMML/AMoL, 38% AML Pt's; U937 (weak); peritoneal MΦ	T and B cells; CLL and ALL Pt's; platelets; RBC; K562; HL60	Inhibition of C3bi binding and phagocytic function; protease-resistant; TPA and lymphokine-induced HL60 cells Mol^+; CFU-C Mol−	Todd and Schlossman (1982, 1983), Todd *et al.* (1981a,b, 1982), Arnaout *et al.* (1983), Dana *et al.* (1983)
(Mac-1)	See Table 3						
MY4	IgG2a	NR	AMML cells	PB monocytes; 28% PMN; 95% AMML/AMoL, 14% AML Pt's; HL60 and U937 (weak)	T, B and null cells; RBC; platelets; CML, ALL, and CLL Pt's	NR	Griffin *et al.* (1981)
MY7	IgG1	NR	AMML cells	21% PB monocytes; PMN; 84% AML, 74% AMoL/AMML, 50% CML Pt's.; HL60; KG-1; U937	T, B and null cells; RBC; platelets; ALL and CLL Pt's	CFU-C $MY7^+$	Griffin *et al.* (1981, 1983)
MY8	IgG2b	NR	AMML cells	PB monocytes; PMN; peroxidase + BM cells; 79% AMML/AMoL, 41% AML, 44% CML Pt's; U937; HL60	T, B and null cells; RBC; platelets; ALL and CLL Pt's	CFU-C MY8−	Griffin *et al.* (1981, 1982)
B13.4	IgM	NR	PB cells	PB monocytes; PMN; BM metamyelo's, bands	T and B cells; RBC; platelets; eos.; HL60; KG-1; K562; ALL Pt's	RA-induced HL60 cells B13.4+	Perussia *et al.* (1981, 1982), Dayton *et al.* (1983)
B9.8	IgM	NR	PB cells	Similar to B13.4 plus BM myelocytes	Similar to B13.4	Lymphokine, RA, and DMSO induced HL60 cells, B9.8+	Perussia *et al.* (1981, 1982), Dayton *et al.* (1983)
B34.3	IgG1	NR	PMN	PB monocytes; PMN	T and B cells; RBC; platelets; HL60; KG-1 K562; ALL, AML Pt's	No induced expression on HL60 cells	Perussia *et al.* (1981, 1982), Dayton *et al.* (1983)
B43.4	IgG2a	NR	PB monocytes	PB monocytes; PMN; null cells; BM pro's, myelo's, and metamyelo's; KG-1, HL60	T and B cells; RBC; platelets; K562; T- and B-cell lines	Lymphokine and DMSO-induced HL60 B43.4+	Perussia *et al.* (1981, 1982), Dayton *et al.* (1983)

TA-1	IgG2a	95 170	HSB-2	PB monocytes, T cells; 67% thymocytes; activated T cells; 13% BM cells; 55% T ALL and AMML Pt's	PMN; RBC; platelets; AML and CLL Pt's	NR	LeBien and Kersey (1980), LeBien *et al.* (1983)
Mo4	IgM	100	PB monocytes	40–80% PB monocytes; platelets; megakaryocytes; 35% AMML/AMoL Pt's	T, B and null cells; PMN; RBC; ALL Pt's; K562; HL60	Protease sensitive; lymphokine-induced HL60 Mo4+	Todd and Schlossman (1982, 1983)
Mo5	IgG2a	94	AMoL cells	PB monocytes; PMN; BM myeloid precursors; U937; 30% AML, 54% AMML/AMoL Pt's	T, B and null cells; RBC; platelets	Protease resistant; modulates; CFU-C is Mo5−	Todd and Schlossman (1983)
AML-2-23	IgG1	NR	AMML cells	PB monocytes; PMN; AMML/AMoL Pt's; HL60 (weak)	Lymphoid cells; RBC; platelets; CEM; Daudi; U937; K562; KG-1	Lymphokine, DMSO, DMF, and RA-induced HL60 AML-2-23+; CFU-C, BFU-E, AML-2-23−	Ball and Fanger (1983), Ball *et al.* (1982), Graziano *et al.* (1983)
PM-81	IgM	NR	HL60	PB monocytes; PMN; BM myeloid precursors; eosinophils; ALL, AML, CML Pt's; HL60; K562; KG-1; U937; HSB-2	Lymphoid cells, null cells; RBC; platelets; CEM: Daudi	CFU-C, BFU-E PM-81−	Ball *et al.* (1983)
5F1	IgM	NR	AMML cells	PB monocytes; platelets; BM erythroid precursors; AML/AMML Pt's	Lymphoid cells; PMN; myeloid precursors; ALL Pt's; K562; HL60	NR	Bernstein *et al.* (1982)
1G10	IgM	NR	AMML cells	20% PB monocytes (weak) PMN; BM pro's, myelo's, metamyelo's; AML, AMML, AMoL Pt's; HL60	T and B cells; platelets; RBC; erythroid precursors; thymocytes; K562; ALL Pt's	NR	Bernstein *et al.* (1982)
63D3	IgG1	200	PB monocytes	PB monocytes; PMN (weak)	T and B cells; endothelial cells; cultured monocytes; PAM; U937; HL60	C′ lysis blocks PWM proliferation	Ugolini *et al.* (1980), Rosenberg *et al.* (1981)
MPA	IgG2a	93 135	E+ cells	PB monocytes; platelets; megakaryocytes; U937; HL60	T and B cells; PMN	Trypsin-resistant; Pronase-sensitive	Burckhardt *et al.* (1982)
M206	IgG2a	180	U937	PB monocytes, PMN (weak); U937; AMoL Pt's	T and B cells; K562; ALL and CLL Pt's	C′ lysis blocks PWM proliferation	Maruyana *et al.* (1983)
MϕP-9 MϕS-1 MϕS-39	IgG2b IgG2a IgG2a	NR NR NR	PB monocytes Pleural Mϕ Pleural Mϕ	PB monocytes; peritoneal, pleural, and synovial Mϕ; PMN (weak)	T, B and null cells; RBC; platelets; U937; K562	NR	Dimitriu-Bona *et al.* (1983)
PHM2	IgG1	52	Peritoneal Mϕ	PB monocytes; T cells (8%); Kupffer cells; peritoneal Mϕ	Most T cells; B cells; PMN; RBC	NR	Becker *et al.* (1981)
MMA	IgM	NR	U937	PB monocytes; PMN; AML CML Pt's; HSB-2; Molt-3,4; U937; K562; activated T cells	T and B cells; platelets; RBC; ALL and CLL Pt's	C′ lysis blocks antigen, mitogen proliferation; CFU-C is MMA+	Hanjan *et al.* (1982)

[a]See Table 1 for abbreviations.

TABLE 3. RAT MONOCLONAL ANTIBODIES SPECIFIC FOR MURINE MACROPHAGE ANTIGENS[a]

Antibody/antigen designation	Antibody subclass	Antigen MW (Kd)[b]	Immunizing cells	Cellular distribution: Reactive	Cellular distribution: Nonreactive	Distinguishing features functional studies	References
Mac-1	IgG2b	105 190	NA[c] spleen cells	Resident and exudative peritoneal macrophages; splenic histiocytes; 44% BM cells; PB monocytes PMN; J774; P388d_1	T and B cells; RBC; thymocytes; LN cells; most spleen cells	Binds to human PB monocytes; PMN; NK; anti-Mac-1 blocks C3bi rosetting	Ault and Springer (1981), Ho and Springer (1982a), Springer *et al.* (1979), Beller *et al.* (1982)
Mac-2	IgG2a IgM	32	Macrophage membrane	Peritoneal exudate macrophages	Lymphoid cells; BM cells	NR	Springer (1981b,c), Ho and Springer (1982b)
Mac-3	IgG1	110	Macrophage membrane	Peritoneal resident and exudate macrophages; PAM; Kupffer cells	Lymphoid cells; BM cells	NR	Springer (1981b,c), Ho and Springer (1981c)
Mac-4	NR	180	Macrophage membrane	Peritoneal exudate macrophages	Lymphoid cells; BM cells	NR	Springer (1981b,c), LeBlanc *et al.* (1980)
F4/80	NR	160	Peritoneal macrophages	PB monocytes; resident and induced macrophages; J774; P815	Lymphoid cells	NR	Austyn and Gordon (1981)
2.4G2	IgG	47 60	J774	Macrophages; PMN; B cells; J774	T lymphocytes	Blocks binding of IgG1 and IgG2b Fc to FcRII; protease-resistant	Unkeless (1979), Mellman and Unkeless (1980)

[a]Adapted from Springer, 1981a.
[b]Reducing conditions.
[c]Abbreviations: NA, nonadherent; BM, bone marrow cells; PMN, granulocytes; RBC, erythrocytes; LN, lymph node; PB, peripheral blood; NK, natural killers; NR, not reported.

TABLE 4. HUMAN MYELOMONOCYTIC ANTIGENS EXPRESSED ON CELLS WITHIN THE MYELOID LINEAGE DEFINED BY MOUSE MONOCLONAL ANTIBODIES

Bone Marrow		Peripheral Blood				Extravascular space	
Monocytic precursors[a]		Monocyte				Macrophage	
Mo1	TA-1	Mo2[c]	4F2	Mo1	B9.8	Mo1	MφS-1
Mo2	1G10	Mac-120	PHM3	Mo5	B43.4	Mo2	MφS-39
Mo5	MPA	1D5	*Mo3*	MY3	B34.3	Mo4	MφP-15
MY3	AML-2-23	61D3	*MφP-7*[d]	MY4	5F1	PHM3	MφP-7
MY4	M206	UC-45	*MφR-17*	MY8	AML-2-23	PHM2	MφP-17
MY7	PM-81	B44.1	*1G10*	TA-1	MPA	MφP-9	
MY8	5F1	D5D6	*MY7*	MMA	MφP-9		
		C10H5	Mo4	M206	MφS-1		
		MφP-15	63D3	PHM2	MφS-39		
		OKM5	OKM1	B13.4	PM-81		
CFU-GM							
MY7							
D5D6							
C10H5							
MMA							
Granulocytic precursors[b]		Granulocyte					
Early	Late	OKM1	MMA				
Mo5	Mo5	Mo1	AML-2-23				
MY8	MY8	Mo5	1G10				
1G10	1G10	MY7	*MY4*				
AML-2-23	AML-2-23	MY8	*63D3*				
B43.4	B43.4	B13.4	*MY3*				
PM-81	PM-81	B9.8	*MφS-39*				
MY7	B13.4	B43.4	*MφP-9*				
	B9.8	B34.3	*MφS-1*				
	Mo1	PM-81	*M206*				
Megakaryocyte		Platelet					
Mo4		Mo4					
MPA		MPA					
		5F1					
Erythroid precursors							
5F1							

[a]Expressed by myelomonocytic leukemia cells.
[b]Expressed by normal bone marrow cells; early (blasts, promyelocytes); late (myelocytes, metamyelocytes, bands).
[c]UNDERLINE indicates relative specificity for monocytes and macrophages (unstimulated hematopoietic cells only).
[d]*ITALICS* indicates weak reactivity (low antigen density).

cytes and not granulocytes (D5D6, C10H5). Further along the path of monocyte differentiation, Mo3 and UC-45 (expressed on cultured and spreading monocytes, respectively) may represent antigens that signal the morphological and biochemical changes that occur during the transformation from monocyte to macrophage. Other markers are clearly expressed by fully differentiated macrophages isolated from peritoneal, pleural, and synovial fluids as well as tissue histiocytes (e.g., Kupffer cells). Among these antigens, MϕP-7 and MϕR-17 are preferentially expressed by synovial macrophages relative to monocytes and phagocytic cells from other sources. Apart from the distribution of the myelomonocytic antigens on normal (or malignant) human tissue, their acquired expression on myeloid cell lines (e.g., HL60) induced to transform into macrophage-like cells as a result of activating factors, provides an *in vitro* model of myeloid differentiation.

In summary, monoclonal methodology has allowed the identification of differentiation antigens which distinguish members of the monocyte-macrophage lineage. These markers have facilitated the study of macrophage function and ontogeny and could become employed as tools for the diagnosis or therapy of diseases of the reticuloendothelial system. In the future, it may be possible to identify additional functionally distinct subsets of monocytes-macrophages and to characterize membrane structures which perform other macrophage-specific functions.

ACKNOWLEDGMENTS The authors wish to thank Ms. Bonnie Frisard for her help in the preparation of the manuscript and Dr. James Griffin for his critical review. Supported in part by National Institutes of Health Grant CA 33555-02.

REFERENCES

Albert, E., Amos, D. B., Bodmer, W. F., Ceppellini, R., Dausset, J., Kissmeyer-Nielsen, F., Mayr, W., Payne, R., vanRood, J. J., and Terasaki, P. I., 1981, WHO Report, Nomenclature for factors of the HLA system, 1980, *Eur. J. Immunol.* **11**:350.

Allison, A. C., 1978, Mechanisms by which activated macrophages inhibit lymphocyte responses, *Immunol. Rev.* **40**:3.

Arnaout, M. A., Todd, R. F., III, Dana, N., Melamed, J., Schlossman, S. F., and Colten, H. R., 1983, Inhibition of phagocytosis of complement C3 or IgG coated particles and of C3bi binding by monoclonal antibodies to a monocyte-granulocyte membrane glycoprotein (Mo1), *J. Clin. Invest.*, **72**:171.

Ault, K. A., and Springer, T. A., 1981, Cross-reaction of a rat anti-mouse phagocyte-specific monoclonal antibody (anti-Mac-1) with human monocytes and natural killer cells, *J. Immunol.* **126**:359.

Austyn, J. M., and Gordon, S., 1981, F4/80—A monoclonal antibody directed specifically against the mouse macrophage, *Eur. J. Immunol.* **11**:805.

Ball, E. D., and Fanger, M. W., 1983, The expression of myeloid-specific antigens on myeloid leukemia cells: Correlations with leukemia subclasses and implications for normal myeloid differentiation, *Blood* **61**:456.

Ball, E. D., Graziano, R. F., Shen, L., and Fanger, M. W., 1982, Monoclonal antibodies to novel myeloid antigens reveal human neutrophil heterogeneity, *Proc. Natl. Acad. Sci. U.S.A.* **79**:5374.

Ball, E. D., Graziano, R. F., and Fanger, M. W. 1983, A unique antigen expressed on myeloid cells and acute leukemia blast cells defined by a monoclonal antibody, *J. Immunol.* **130**:2937.

Beatty, D. W., Davis, A. E., Cole, F. S., Einstein, L. P., and Colten, H. R., 1981, Biosynthesis of complement by human monocytes, *Clin. Immunol. Immunopathol.* **18**:334.

Becker, G. J., Hancock, W. W., Kraft, N., Lanyon, H. C., and Atkins, R. C., 1981, Monoclonal antibodies to human macrophage and leukocyte common antigens, *Pathol.* **13**:669.

Beller, D. I., Springer, T. A., and Schreiber, R. D. 1982, Anti-Mac-1 selectively inhibits the mouse and human type three complement receptor, *J. Exp. Med.* **156**:1000.

Bergholtz, B. O., and Thorsby, E., 1978, HLA-D restriction of the macrophage-dependent response of immune human T lymphocytes to PPD in vitro: Inhibition by anti-HLA-DR antisera, *Scand. J. Immunol.* **8**:63.

Bernard, A., and Boumsell L., (eds.) Human Leukocyte Markers Detected by Monoclonal Antibodies. Springer-Verlag, Berlin, in press.

Bernstein, I. D., Andrews, R. G., Cohen, S. F., and McMaster, B. E., 1982, Normal and malignant human myelocytic and monocytic cells identified by monoclonal antibodies, *J. Immunol.* **128**:876.

Breard, J., Fuks, A., Friedman, S. M., Schlossman, S. F., and Chess, L., 1979, The role of p23,30-bearing human macrophages in antigen-induced T lymphocyte responses, *Cell. Immunol.* **45**:108.

Breard, J., Reinherz, E. L., Kung, P. C., Goldstein, G., and Schlossman, S. F., 1980, A monoclonal antibody reactive with human peripheral blood monocytes, *J. Immunol.* **124**:1943.

Breard, J., Reinherz, E. L., O'Brien, C., and Schlossman, S. F., 1981, Delineation of an effector population responsible for natural killing and antibody-dependent cellular cytotoxicity in man, *Clin. Immunol. Immunopathol.* **18**:145.

Brier, A. M., Chess, L., and Schlossman, S. F., 1975, Human antibody dependent cellular cytotoxicity: Isolation and identification of a subpopulation of peripheral blood lymphocytes which kill antibody-coated autologous target cells, *J. Clin. Invest.* **56**:1580.

Burckhardt, J. J., Anderson, W. H. K., Kearney, J. F., and Cooper, M. D., 1982, Human blood monocytes and platelets share a cell surface component, *Blood* **60**:767.

Charron, D. J., and McDevitt, H. O., 1979, Analysis of HLA-D region associated molecules with monoclonal antibody, *Proc. Natl. Acad. Sci. USA* **76**:6567.

Dana, N., Todd, R. F., III, Pitt, J., Springer, T. A., and Arnaout, M. A., 1983, Deficiency of a surface membrane glycoprotein (Mo1) in man, *J. Clin. Invest.*, in press.

Dayton, E. T., Perussia, B., and Trinchieri, G., 1983, Correlation between differentiation, expression of monocyte-specific antigens and cytotoxic function in human promyelocytic cell lines treated with leukocyte-conditioned medium, *J. Immunol.* **130**:1120.

deVries, J. E., Mendelsohn, J., and Bont, W. S., 1980, Requirement for monocytes in the spontaneous cytotoxic effects of human lymphocytes against non-lymphoid target cells, *Nature (London)* **283**:574.

Dimitriu-Bona, A., Burmester, G. R., Waters, S. J., and Winchester, R. J., 1981, Lineage and differentiation antigens on human mononuclear phagocytes, *Fed. Proc.* **40**:988.

Dimitriu-Bona, A., Burmester, G. R., Waters, S. J., and Winchester, R. J., 1983, Human mononuclear phagocyte differentiation antigens. I. Patterns of antigenic expression on the surface of human monocytes and macrophages defined by monoclonal antibodies, *J. Immunol.* **130**:145.

Eisenbarth, G. S., Haynes, B. F., Schroer, J. A., and Fauci, A. S., 1980, Production of monoclonal antibodies reacting with peripheral blood mononuclear cell surface differentiation antigens, *J. Immunol.* **124**:1237.

Fischer, D. G., Hubbard, W. J., and Koren, H. S., 1981, Tumor cell killing by freshly isolated peripheral blood monocytes, *Cell. Immunol.* **58**:426.

Geha, R., Milgrom, H., Broff, M., Alpert, S., Martin, S., and Yunis, E. J., 1980, Effect of anti-HLA antisera on macrophage–T cell interaction, *Proc. Natl. Acad. Sci. USA* **76**:4038.

Geha, R. S., Jonsen, M. E., Ault, B. H., Yunis, E. J., and Broff, M. D., 1981, Macrophage–T cell interaction in man: Binding of antigen-specific human proliferating and helper T cells to antigen-pulsed macrophages, *J. Immunol.* **126**:781.

Graziano, R. F., Ball, E. D., and Fanger, M. W., 1983, The expression and modulation of human myeloid-specific antigens during differentiation of the HL60 cell line, *Blood* **61**:1215.

Griffin, J. D., Ritz, J., Nadler, L. M., and Schlossman, S. F., 1981, Expression of myeloid differentiation antigens on normal and malignant myeloid cells, *J. Clin. Invest.* **68**:932.

Griffin, J. D., Beveridge, R. P., and Schlossman, S. F., 1982, Isolation of myeloid progenitor cells from peripheral blood of chronic myelogenous leukemia patients, *Blood* **60**:30.

Griffin, J. D., Ritz, J., Beveridge, R. P., Lipton, J. M., Daley, J. F., and Schlossman, S. F., 1983, Expression of MY7 antigen on myeloid precursor cells, *Int. J. Cell Cloning* **1**:33.

Groopman, J. E., and Golde, D. W., 1981, The histiocytic disorders: A pathophysiologic analysis, *Ann. Intern. Med.* **94**:95.

Hanjan, S. N. S., Kearney, J. F., and Cooper, M. D., 1982, A monoclonal antibody (MMA) that identifies a differentiation antigen on human myelomonocytic cells, *Clin. Immunol. Immunopathol.* **23**:172.

Hausman, P. B., Raff, H. V., Gilbert, R. C., Picker, L. J., and Stobo, J. D., 1980, T cells and macrophages involved in the autologous mixed lymphocyte reaction are required for the response to conventional antigen, *J. Immunol.* **125:**1374.

Haynes, B. F., Hemler, M. E., Mann, D. L., Eisenbarth, G. S., Shelhamer, J., Mostowski, H. S., Thomas, C. A., Strominger, J. L., and Fauci, A. S., 1981, Characterization of a monoclonal antibody (4F2) that binds to human monocytes and to a subset of activated lymphocytes, *J. Immunol.* **126:**1409.

Ho, M.-K., and Springer, T. A., 1982a, Mac-1 antigen: Quantitative expression in macrophage populations and tissues, and immunofluorescent localization in spleen, *J. Immunol.* **128:**2281.

Ho, M.-K., and Springer, T. A., 1982b, Mac-2, a novel 32,000 M_r mouse macrophage subpopulation-specific antigen defined by monoclonal antibodies, *J. Immunol.* **128:**1221.

Ho, M.-K., and Springer, T. A., 1982c, Tissue distribution, structural characterization, and biosynthesis of Mac-3, a macrophage surface glycoprotein exhibiting molecular weight heterogeneity, *J. Biol. Chem.* **258:**636.

Hogg, N., Slusarenko, M., Cohen, J., and Reiser, J., 1981, Monoclonal antibody with specificity for monocytes and neurons, *Cell* **24:**875.

Kaplan, G., and Gaudernack, G., 1982, *In vitro* differentiation of human monocytes: Differences in monocyte phenotypes induced by cultivation on glass or on collagen. *J. Exp. Med.* **156:**1101.

Kay, H. D., and Horowitz, D. A., 1980, Evidence by reactivity with hybridoma antibodies for a myeloid origin of peripheral blood cells active in natural cytoxocity and antibody-dependent cell-mediated cytotoxicity, *J. Clin. Invest.* **66:**847.

Kohler, G., and Milstein, C., 1975, Continuous cultures of fused cells secreting antibody of predefined specificity, *Nature (London)* **256:**495.

LeBien, T. W., and Kersey, J. H., 1980, A monoclonal antibody (TA-1) reactive with human T lymphocytes and monocytes, *J. Immunol.* **125:**2208.

LeBien, T. W., Bradley, J. G., and Koller, G., 1983, Preliminary structural characterization of the leukocyte cell surface molecule recognized by monoclonal antibody TA-1, *J. Immunol.* **130:**1833.

LeBlanc, P. A., Katz, H. R., and Russell, S. W., 1980, A discrete population of nonnuclear phagocytes detected by monoclonal antibody, *Infect. Immun.* **8:**520.

Levy, P. C., Shaw, G. M., and Lobuglio, A. F., 1979, Human monocyte, lymphocyte and granulocyte antibody-dependent cell-mediated cytotoxicity toward tumor cells. I. General characteristics of cytolysis, *J. Immunol.* **123:**594.

Linker-Israeli, M., Billing, R. J., Foon, K. A., and Terasaki, P. I., 1981, Monoclonal antibodies reactive with acute myelogenous leukemia cells, *J. Immunol.* **127:**2473.

Mantovani, A., Jerrells, T. R., Dean, J. H., and Herberman, R. B., 1979, Cytolytic and cytostatic activity on tumor cells of circulating human monocytes, *Int. J. Cancer* **23:**18.

Maruyana, S., Naito, T., Kakita, H., Kishimoto, S., Yamamura, Y., and Kishimoto, T., 1983, Preparation of a monoclonal antibody against human monocyte lineage, *J. Clin. Immunol.* **3:**57.

Mellman, I. S., and Unkeless, J. C., 1980, Purification of a functional mouse Fc receptor through the use of a monoclonal antibody, *J. Exp. Med.* **152:**1048.

Mellman, I. S., Steinman, R. M., Unkeless, J. C., and Cohn, Z. A., 1980, Selective iodination and polypeptide composition of pinocytic vesicles, *J. Cell. Biol.* **86:**712.

Moore, M. A. S., Williams, N., and Metcalf, D., 1972, Purification and characterization of the *in vitro* colony forming cells in monkey hemopoietic tissue, *J. Cell. Physiol.* **79:**283.

Morimoto, C., Todd, R. F., III, Distaso, J. A., and Schlossman, S. F., 1981, The role of macrophage in *in vitro* primary anti-DNP antibody production in man, *J. Immunol.* **127:**1137.

Nadler, L. M., Stashenko, P., Hardy, R., Pesando, J. M., Yunis, E. J., and Schlossman, S. F., 1981a, Monoclonal antibodies defining serologically distinct HLA-D/DR related Ia-like antigens in man, *Hum. Immunol.* **1:**77.

Nadler, L. M., Stashenko, P., Hardy, R., Tomaselli, K. J., Yunis, E. J., Schlossman, S. F., and Pesando, J. M., 1981b, Monoclonal antibody identifies a new Ia-like (p 29, 34) polymorphic system linked to the HLA-D/DR region, *Nature (London)* **290:**591.

Nathan, D. F., Murray, H. W., and Cohn, Z. A., 1980, The macrophage as an effector cell, *N. Engl. J. Med.* **303:**622.

Niederhuber, J. E., 1978, The role of I region gene products in macrophage–T lymphocyte interaction, *Immunol. Rev.* **40**:28.

Nunez, G., Ugolini, V., Capra, J. D., and Stastny, P., 1982, Monoclonal antibodies against human monocytes. II. Recognition of two distinct cell surface molecules, *Scand. J. Immunol.* **16**:515.

Nunez, G., and Stastny, P., 1983, Cytofluorometric analysis of major histocompatibility antigens on human monocytes using monoclonal antibodies, *Human Immunol.* **6**:1.

Ozer, H., Strelkaskas, A. J., Callery, R. T., and Schlossman, S. F., 1979, The functional dissection of human peripheral null cells with respect to antibody-dependent cellular cytotoxicity and natural killing, *Eur. J. Immunol.* **9**:112.

Perussia, B., Lebman, D., Ip, S. H., Rovera, G., and Trinchieri, G., 1981, Terminal differentiation surface antigens of myelomonocytic cells are expressed in human promyelocytic leukemia cells (HL60) treated with chemical inducers, *Blood* **58**:836.

Perussia, B., Trinchieri, G., Lebman, D., Jankiewicz, L., Lang, B., and Rovera, G., 1982, Monoclonal antibodies that detect differentiation surface antigens on human myelomonocytic cells, *Blood* **59**:382.

Pierce, C W., Knapp, J. A., and Benacerraf, B., 1976, Regulation by the H-2 gene complex of macrophage–lymphoid cell interactions in secondary antibody responses *in vitro*, *J. Exp. Med.* **144**:371.

Pike, B. L., and Robinson, W. A., 1970, Human bone marrow colony growth in agar-gel, *J. Cell. Physiol.* **76**:77.

Poplack, D. G., Bonnard, G. D., Holiman, B. J., and Blaese, R. M., 1976, Monocyte-mediated antibody-dependent cellular cytotoxicity: A clinical test of monocyte function, *Blood* **48**:809.

Quaranta, V., Pellegrino, M. A., and Ferrone, S., 1981, Serologic and immunochemical characterization of the specificity of four monoclonal antibodies to distinct antigenic determinants expressed on subpopulations of human Ia-like antigens, *J. Immunol.* **126**:548.

Raff, H. V., Picker, L. J., and Stobo, J. D., 1980, Macrophage heterogeneity in man: A subpopulation of HLA-DR-bearing macrophages required for antigen-induced T-cell activation also contains stimulators for autologous-reactive T-cells, *J. Exp. Med.* **152**:581.

Reinherz, E. L., Kung, P. C., Goldstein, G., and Schlossman, S. F., 1979, Ia determinants on human T cell subsets defined by monoclonal antibody: Activation stimuli required for expression, *J. Exp. Med.* **150**:1472.

Rodey, G. E., Luehrman, L. K., and Thomas, D. W., 1979, *In vitro* primary immunization of human peripheral blood lymphocytes to KLH: Evidence for HLA-D region restriction, *J. Immunol.* **123**:2250.

Rosenberg, S. A., Ligler, F. S., Ugolini, V., and Lipsky, P. E., 1981, A monoclonal antibody that identifies human peripheral blood monocytes recognizes the accessory cells required for mitogen-induced T lymphocyte proliferation, *J. Immunol.* **126**:1473.

Rosenthal, A. S., 1978, Determinant selection and macrophage function in genetic control of the immune response, *Immunol. Rev.* **40**:134.

Schwartz, R. H., Yano, A., and Paul, W. E., 1978, Interaction between antigen-presenting cells and primed T lymphocytes: An assessment of Ia gene expression in the antigen-presenting cell, *Immunol. Rev.* **40**:152.

Shen, H. H., Talle, M. A., Goldstein, G., and Chess, L., 1983, Functional subsets of human monocytes defined by monoclonal antibodies: A distinct subset of monocytes contains the cells capable of inducing mixed lymphocyte culture, *J. Immunol.* **130**:698.

Smith, B. R., and Ault, K. A., 1981, Increase in surface Ia-like antigen expression on human monocytes independent of antigenic stimuli, *J. Immunol.* **127**:2020.

Springer, T. A., 1981a, Monoclonal antibodies as tools for the study of mononuclear phagocytes, in: *Methods for Studying Mononuclear Phagocytes* (D. Adams, P. Edelson, and H. Koren, eds.), p. 305, Academic Press, New York.

Springer, T. A., 1981b, Mac-1, 2, 3 and 4: Murine macrophage differentiation antigens identified by monoclonal antibodies, in: *Heterogeneity of Mononuclear Phagocytes* (O. Forster, ed.), p. 37, Academic Press, New York.

Springer, T. A., 1981c, Monoclonal antibody analysis of complex biological systems, *J. Biol. Chem.* **256**:3833.

Springer, T. A., Kaufman, J. F., Terhorst, C., and Strominger, J. L., 1977, Purification and structural characterization of human HLA-linked B cell antigens, *Nature (London)* **268**:213.

Springer, T., Galfre, G., Secher, D. S., and Milstein, C., 1979, Mac-1: A macrophage differentiation antigen identified by monoclonal antibody, *Eur. J. Immunol.* **9**:301.

Thomas, D. W., and Shevack, E. M., 1976, Nature of the antigenic complex recognized by T lymphocytes. I. Analysis with an *in vitro* primary response to soluble protein antigen, *J. Exp. Med.* **144**:1263.

Todd, R. F., III, and Schlossman, S. F., 1980, Human macrophage–lymphocyte interaction in proliferation to soluble antigen. II. Characterization of lymphocyte binding to antigen-pulsed macrophage monolayers, *Cell. Immunol.* **56**:205.

Todd, R. F., III, and Schlossman, S. F., 1982, Analysis of antigenic determinants on human monocytes and macrophages, *Blood* **59**:775.

Todd, R. F., III, and Schlossman, S. F., 1983, Differentiation antigens on human monocytes and macrophages defined by monoclonal antibodies, in: *Mononuclear Phagocyte Biology* (A. Volkman, ed.), Marcel Dekker, New York, in press.

Todd, R. F., III, Nadler, L. M., and Schlossman, S. F., 1981a, Antigens on human monocytes identified by monoclonal antibodies, *J. Immunol.* **126**:1435.

Todd, R. F., III, Griffin, J. D., Ritz, J., Nadler, L. M., Abrams, T., and Schlossman, S. F., 1981b, Expression of normal monocyte-macrophage differentiation antigens on HL-60 promyelocytes undergoing differentiation induced by leukocyte conditioned medium or phorbol diester, *Leuk. Res.* **5**:491.

Todd, R. F., Van Agthoven, A., Schlossman, S. F., and Terhorst, C., 1982, Structural analysis of differentiation antigens Mo1 and Mo2 on human monocytes, *Hybridoma* **1**:329.

Todd, R. F., III, Leeman, E. L., Daley, J. F., and Schlossman, S. F., 1983, Mo2: Functional properties of antigen-bearing cells, *Clin. Immunol. Immunopath.* **26**:118.

Trowsdale, J., Lee, J., and McMichael, A., 1983, HLA-DR bouillabaisse, *Immunology Today* **4**:33.

Truco, M. M., Garotta, G., Stocker, J. W., and Ceppellini, R., 1979, Murine monoclonal antibodies against HLA structures, *Immunol. Rev.* **47**:219.

Ugolini, V., Nunez, G., Smith, R. G., Stastny, P., and Capra, J. D., 1980, Initial characterization of monoclonal antibodies against human monocytes, *Proc. Natl. Acad. Sci. USA* **77**:6764.

Unanue, E. R., 1978, The regulation of lymphocyte functions by the macrophage, *Immunol. Rev.* **40**:227.

Unkeless, J. C., 1979, Characterization of a monoclonal antibody directed against mouse macrophage and lymphocyte Fc receptors, *J. Exp. Med.* **150**:1048.

Zarling, J. M., and Kung, P. C., 1980, Monoclonal antibodies which distinguish between human NK cells and cytotoxic T lymphocytes, *Nature (London)* **288**:394.

Zola, H., Bradley, J., MacArdle, P., McEvoy, R., and Thomas, M., 1980, A hybridoma antibody which reacts with human cells carrying the DRw4 tissue type: Evidence for heterogeneity of DRw4, *Transplantation* **29**:72.

7

The Role of Mononuclear Phagocytes as Accessory Cells in Lymphocyte Responses

HENRY C. STEVENSON

1. INTRODUCTION

For some time it has been known that certain immunologic functions of lymphocytes require the addition of mononuclear phagocytes in order to be operative. Historically, Mosier and Coppleson (1968) initially described a need for adherent cells in animal *in vitro* primary immune responses. As the supportive role of adherent cells in immune responses became apparent, efforts were made to identify the lineage of this accessory cell. The evidence to date indicates that although a number of cells can function as accessory cells, mononuclear phagocytes are the predominant accessory cell type operational in many current immunologic assay systems. Mononuclear phagocytes have been employed as accessory cells in both their blood monocyte and tissue macrophage forms; both animal and human research systems abound.

Recent immunologic research has emphasized the complicated cell-to-cell interactions required for the initiation and modulation of specific immune responses. Following the description of the basic subsets of mononuclear immunologic effector cells (mononuclear phagocytes, B lymphocytes, T lymphocytes, and null cells), it has become quite clear that subsets of each of these groups exist as identified on the basis of function, cell markers, or both criteria. Perhaps no major group of cells has a greater number of distinct functions than does the mononuclear phagocyte series (see Table 1); there is an ever-emerging literature about the existence of mononuclear phagocyte subsets as defined by functional studies and cell marker analysis (reviewed elsewhere in this volume). Exactly which of various documented mononuclear phagocyte functions can be considered *accessory* in nature is not entirely clear. In a general sense it can be stated

HENRY C STEVENSON • Clinical Investigations Section, Biologic Response Modifiers Program, National Cancer Institute, National Institutes of Health, Frederick, Maryland 21701.

TABLE 1. PARTIAL LIST OF THE VARIOUS FUNCTIONS OF MONONUCLEAR PHAGOCYTES

Antigen presentation
Cytotoxic function (ADCC and spontaneous killing)
Production of complement components
"Scavenger" function of clearing cellular debris and senescent red blood cells
Antimicrobial activity
Antiviral activity—secretion of interferons
Scores of other secreted soluble products (monokines)
Suppressor function of various lymphocyte functions

that mononuclear phagocytes function as accessory cells *when they support* (promote) *the function of other immunologic effector cells* (T lymphocytes, B lymphocytes, and null cells). If an analogy can be made between mononuclear phagocyte accessory cell function and T-cell-subset functions, one could best visualize mononuclear phagocytes (when they function in an accessory cell fashion) as being analogous to those T lymphocytes known as the helper T-cell subset. To carry the T-cell-subset analogy even further, it should be noted that mononuclear phagocytes can also exert profound suppression on various lymphocyte functions (reviewed elsewhere in this volume); this function of mononuclear phagocytes is analogous to the function of the suppressor T-cell subset. Table 2 illustrates the general groups of functions of the mononuclear phagocyte which can be considered as accessory in nature; antigen presentation, support functions ascribed to specific monokines, and other support functions not yet ascribed to specific monokines (possibly dependent on cell-to-cell interactions). This chapter will only focus on the last two mechanisms of the accessory cell function of mononuclear phagocytes, since the antigen-presenting role of the mononuclear phagocyte has been reviewed elsewhere in this series. It is important to bear in mind that mononuclear phagocytes are not the only cells which have been described to have accessory cell function; endothelial cells (Ashida *et al.*, 1981), dendritic cells (Steinman and Nussenzweig, 1980), and many other cell types have been found to be supportive of several lymphocyte effector functions. Since this review will only focus on the accessory cell function of mononuclear phagocytes, the reader is referred to excellent reviews of the accessory cell function of other cell types (Tew *et al.*, 1980; Stavitsky, 1980).

TABLE 2. MONONUCLEAR PHAGOCYTE ACCESSORY CELL FUNCTION: POSSIBLE MECHANISMS FOR HELPER MODULATORY FUNCTION OF MONONUCLEAR PHAGOCYTES ON EFFECTOR LYMPHOCYTES

Antigen processing
Helper support not related to monokine release
Release of helper monokines for lymphocyte function
Release of monokines which inhibit suppressor cells of lymphocyte function

The cell types that comprise the mononuclear phagocyte system are the promonocyte, the monocyte, and the various forms of tissue macrophages. The promonocyte ordinarily only exists in the bone marrow and has been little utilized in studies of the accessory cell function of mononuclear phagocytes. The exclusive source of monocytes in animals and humans is the peripheral blood. The studies summarized in this review regarding blood monocytes use the following general cell identification criteria in both animal and humans: phagocytic capability, possession of esterase and/or peroxidase enzymes, and adherency. There is still lack of uniform agreement about the presence of certain membrane receptors, possession of DR antigens, specific size criteria, and possession of unique membrane antigens (as defined by monoclonal antibodies) by monocytes, and thus it is not yet possible to define monocytes on the basis of these other criteria alone. Human and animal macrophage experiments utilize a variety of sources: splenic, lymph node, liver, lung, and peritoneal macrophages predominantly. There is also an increasing use of macrophages that have been cultivated *in vitro* from blood monocytes (Stevenson *et al.*, 1981). Two types of macrophages obtained from the skin are also employed in experimental systems: Langerhans cells and skin blister-fluid macrophages. Although Langerhans cells have distinctive morphological and functional characteristics, it is felt that they are part of the mononuclear phagocyte lineage (Stingl *et al.*, 1980). Blister-fluid macrophages from skin have also been studied, including macrophages elicited by the skin irritant cantharidin (Chang and Yao, 1979). Tissue macrophages are usually identified by the same criteria as are blood monocytes, although it is generally agreed that monocytes and macrophages possess distinct biochemical and functional differences (Johnson *et al.*, 1977; Stevenson *et al.*, 1981). The reader should bear in mind the functional differences between monocytes and macrophages obtained by this wide array of different techniques and also remember that we possess a very incomplete understanding about the correlation between animal and human experimentation in this area. The subsequent pages will review the accessory cell function of mononuclear phagocytes as they affect the three main groupings of effector lymphocytes: T lymphocytes, B lymphocytes, and null cells.

2. MONONUCLEAR PHAGOCYTES AS ACCESSORY CELLS IN T-LYMPHOCYTE RESPONSES

Following activation, T lymphocytes proliferate into five major functional groups: cytotoxic cells, helper cells, suppressor cells, lymphokine-secreting cells, and memory cells. As previously discussed, all aspects of antigen-specific T-cell responses have a mononuclear phagocyte requirement for antigen presentation, including T-cell memory (Burckhardt, 1979). The five functional groups of T cells are defined somewhat artificially, since there exists considerable overlap between groups: Cytotoxic T cells may have suppressor cell capability and all T-cell subsets may have lymphokine-secreting capabilities. Mononuclear phagocytes appear to function as accessory cells beyond their role as antigen-presenting cells in at least four of the five T-cell subsets.

When antigens are used as stimuli for T-cell activation, it becomes very difficult to dissect the antigen-processing function of the mononuclear phagocyte from the other accessory functions of the cell. For this reason, polyclonal activators of T lymphocytes by means of mitogenic stimulation have been utilized in various *in vitro* assay systems in an attempt to delineate the other roles of mononuclear phagocytes in the T-lymphocyte activation process. The most frequent assays of mitogen-triggered T-cell activation have been cell proliferation assays. Mononuclear phagocytes are required for T-cell proliferative responses to Con A. This phenomenon has been noted in the mouse (Habu and Raff, 1977; Kammer and Unanue, 1980; Satoh *et al.*, 1980), rat (Munthe-Kass, 1980), rabbit (Schuyler and Todd, 1980), and man (Raff *et al.*, 1978). Similarly, the T-cell lymphoproliferative responses to PHA exhibit a mononuclear–phagocyte dependence in mice (Kammer and Unanue, 1980; Habu and Raff, 1977; Satoh *et al.*, 1980) and guinea pigs (Gorenberg and Daniele, 1978; Rogoff and Lipsky, 1979). A consistent finding with these mitogens is that T-cell proliferation in the peripheral blood and lymph nodes is more dependent on mononuclear phagocytes than are splenic T cells. This observation has been found to be secondary to the accessory cell function of splenic dendritic cells which complement the accessory function of splenic macrophages in mitogen proliferation systems (Satoh *et al.*, 1980).

The role of mononuclear phagocytes in pokeweed mitogen (PWM)-driven systems has probably been best studied in man. PWM stimulates the proliferation of both T lymphocytes and B lymphocytes in a polyclonal fashion. The proliferative response of human T cells to PWM is absolutely dependent on the presence of mononuclear phagocytes as accessory cells (Rosenberg *et al.*, 1981; Stevenson *et al.*, 1983; Rosenberg and Lipsky, 1981). The exact role of monocytes in these *in vitro* T-lymphocyte proliferation systems is not entirely clear, but some intriguing details of this accessory function have been recently demonstrated. Monocytes must be alive in order to stimulate T-lymphocyte proliferation following PWM exposure and cell-to-cell contact appears critical (Rosenberg and Lipsky, 1981); these observations suggest that monocytes do not function in a passive fashion (nor can they be completely replaced by soluble factors) during the process of T-cell activation by PWM. Further evidence for a direct role of monocytes in PWM-driven systems comes from the observation that PWM appears to preferentially bind to monocytes at those concentrations which best promote lymphocyte activation (Stevenson *et al.*, 1983). As seen in Fig. 1, this interaction of PWM with human monocytes is sugar-specific since monocyte-bound PWM can be competitively displaced with *N*-acetylglucosamine.

The mixed lymphocyte response (MLR) is another potent polyclonal stimulus of T-lymphocyte proliferation. Mononuclear phagocytes are required for the initiation of and maintenance of MLRs in both animal (Lutz and Fitch, 1979) and human (Geier and Cresswell, 1980) systems.

Mononuclear phagocytes appear to be required both for the initiation and maintenance of cytotoxic T cells. In animals, alloreactive cytolytic T lympho-

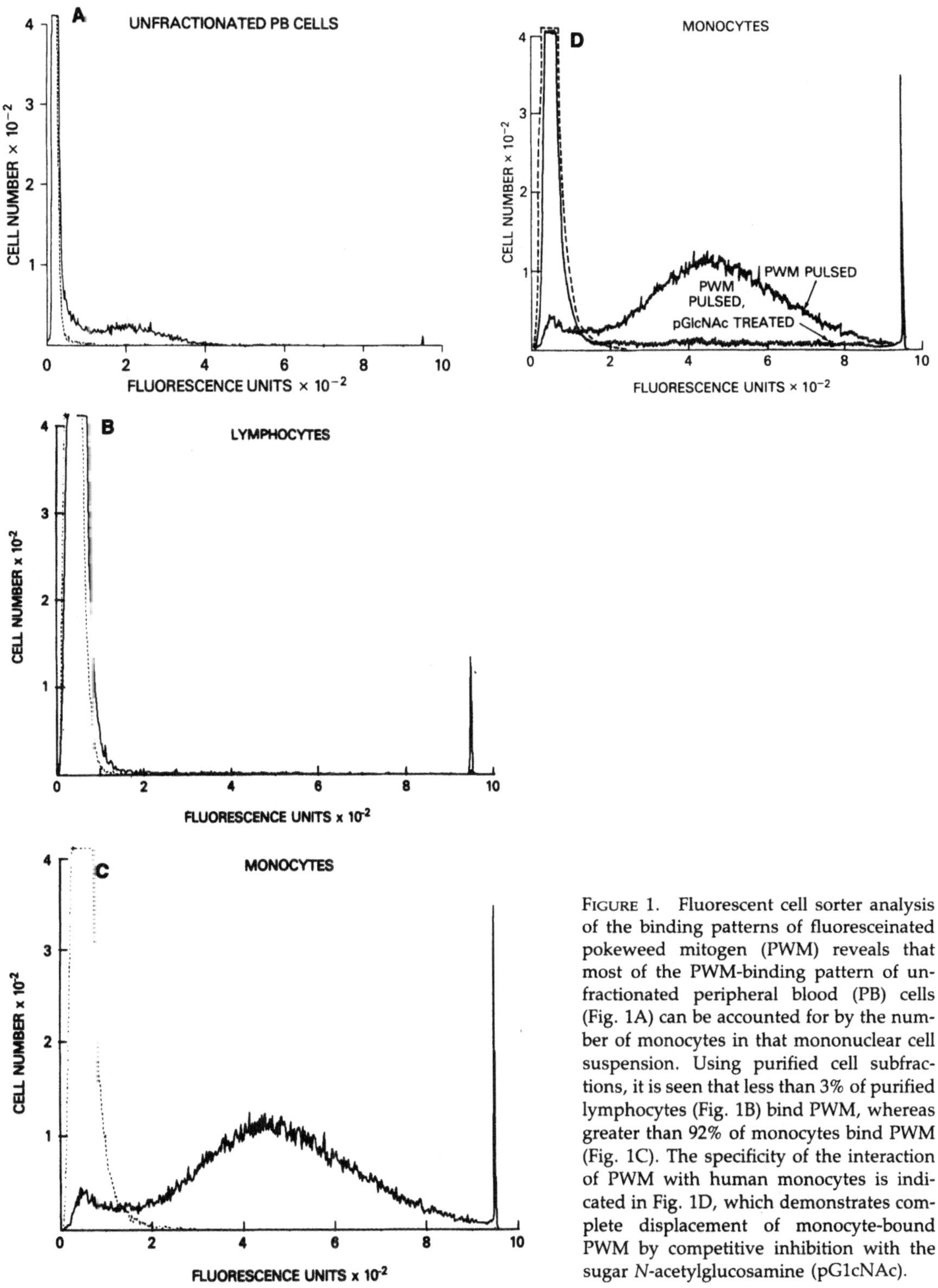

FIGURE 1. Fluorescent cell sorter analysis of the binding patterns of fluoresceinated pokeweed mitogen (PWM) reveals that most of the PWM-binding pattern of unfractionated peripheral blood (PB) cells (Fig. 1A) can be accounted for by the number of monocytes in that mononuclear cell suspension. Using purified cell subfractions, it is seen that less than 3% of purified lymphocytes (Fig. 1B) bind PWM, whereas greater than 92% of monocytes bind PWM (Fig. 1C). The specificity of the interaction of PWM with human monocytes is indicated in Fig. 1D, which demonstrates complete displacement of monocyte-bound PWM by competitive inhibition with the sugar *N*-acetylglucosamine (pG1cNAc).

cytes do not respond to allogeneic tumor cells unless macrophages are added to the culture (Lutz and Fitch, 1979). The growth requirement of cloned cytolytic T-cell lines for macrophages can be replaced with soluble factors (Lutz *et al.*, 1981). Macrophages are necessary for the *in vitro* generation of cytolytic T cells for C-type viruses: This process is dependent on Ia matching between the presenting macrophage and responding T cell, but part of the accessory cell function can be replaced with interleukin-1 (IL-1) (Gomard *et al.*, 1981).

Mononuclear phagocytes appear capable of functioning as accessory cells in the generation of helper and suppressor T-cell subsets. Macrophages produce a soluble factor which allows for the development of helper T cells of a variety of functions (Mishell *et al.*, 1980; Lee, 1977); this soluble factor can be replaced by 2-mercaptoethanol and its release appears to be inhibited by corticosteroids (Lee, 1977). The generation of low-dose Con A-induced human suppressor T cells is also a mononuclear phagocyte-dependent process (Raff *et al.*, 1978).

The ability of most antigens and mitogens to induce lymphokine secretion by T cells appears to require mononuclear phagocytes as accessory cells. The release of T-cell growth factor by lymphocytes requires that these cells first be primed by IL-1 which is derived from mononuclear phagocytes (Oppenheim *et al.*, 1979). Immune interferon production by T cells is similarly a macrophage-dependent process in certain mitogen-driven systems (Farrar *et al.*, 1981). The *in vitro* treatment of human T cells with monoclonal antibodies (OKT3) has been shown to induce cellular proliferation and lymphokine release; this process has been shown to be monocyte dependent (VanWauwe and Goosens, 1982).

3. MONONUCLEAR PHAGOCYTES AS ACCESSORY CELLS IN B-LYMPHOCYTE RESPONSES

As with T-lymphocyte activation, mononuclear phagocytes clearly are required for the antigen-processing component of the B-cell activation process. In addition, however, the mononuclear phagocyte has other accessory cell functions which increase B-lymphocyte proliferation, differentiation, and/or immunoglobulin release. Murine B-cell proliferation in response to polyclonal activators exhibits a dependence on a macrophage soluble factor which can be replaced with 2-mercaptoethanol (Wood and Staruch, 1981). Macrophages also secrete a soluble B-lymphocyte colony-stimulating factor which cannot be replaced by 2-mercaptoethanol (Kurland, 1978). Macrophages secrete soluble factors in response to LPS stimulation that enhance B-cell differentiation to immunoglobulin-secreting cells (Unanue, 1978); these factors are only active in the presence of antigen and are not mitogenic (Hoffmann *et al.*, 1979). In the human B-cell activation response to PWM, monocytes are an absolute requirement (Stevenson *et al.*, 1983; Rosenberg and Lipsky, 1981): Both cell-to-cell interactions and the release of IL-1 appear necessary for the generation of immunoglobulin-secreting cells in response to PWM (Rosenberg and Lipsky, 1981). When B cells are directly activated by anti-immunoglobulin treatment, a need for mononuclear phagocytes still exists (Mongini *et al.*, 1978). Macrophages also appear capable of up-regulating the rate of immunoglobulin secretion following exposure of the cells to immunoglobulin Fc fragments (Morgan and Weigle, 1981).

4. MONONUCLEAR PHAGOCYTES AS ACCESSORY CELLS IN NULL-CELL RESPONSES

Null cells (cells bearing no markers for B or T lymphocytes) appear to be a very heterogeneous population of cells probably consisting of pre-T cells, pre-B cells, premonocytes, and other cell types. The role of mononuclear phagocytes as accessory cells for null-cell functions has probably best been studied in the case of the natural killer (NK) cell. The NK cell is a lymphocyte without surface immunoglobulin, but possessing low-affinity sheep erythrocyte receptors, Fc receptors, distinct cytoplasmic granules and a variety of cell surface antigens (some shared with other cell types, such as the OKM1 antigen). The NK cell appears capable of killing a wide variety of tumor targets both spontaneously and in antibody-dependent cellular cytotoxicity (ADCC). Animal *in vivo* models demonstrate a need for macrophages in order to generate functional NK cells (Keissling *et al.*, 1977; Djeu *et al.*, 1979). Similarly, *in vitro* models of mouse and rat NK cell function demonstrate a need for macrophages; the ability of macrophages to induce NK cell function is related to their ability to release interferon (Reynolds and Herberman, 1981). In contrast, although human NK cell function can be enhanced with interferon, *in vitro* tumor target lysis by NK cells takes place very efficiently in the absence of mononuclear phagocytes (Reynolds *et al.*, 1981).

5. CONCLUSION

Mononuclear phagocytes are needed for the initiation and maintenance of a variety of lymphocyte effector cell functions. Other than in the case of antigen presentation, there is no unified theory to date which explains the myriad of other accessory functions of the mononuclear phagocyte. Certain mitogens appear to be preferentially "focused" on the mononuclear phagocyte (Stevenson *et al.*, 1983). A portion of the interaction between certain mitogens and mononuclear phagocytes may center around the Ia antigens on the membranes of these cells (Habu and Raff, 1977). Other investigators report that Ia-negative cell lines can replace mononuclear phagocytes in mitogen-driven systems (Fagnani *et al.*, 1983). Certain of the accessory cell functions that are found in soluble factors produced by mononuclear phagocytes are closely linked to their similarities to the reducing agent 2-mercaptoethanol (Ellner *et al.*, 1976). More attention has been paid recently to specific monokines (soluble mononuclear phagocyte products) which when released have the capability of directly activating the various subpopulations of effector lymphocytes (Diamantstein *et al.*, 1979).

This last area of research is still in its infancy and holds promise for a much greater understanding of mononuclear phagocyte accessory cell function in the near future.

REFERENCES

Ashida, E. R., Johnson, A. R., and Lipsky, P. E., 1981, Human endothelial cell–lymphocyte interaction: Endothelial cells function as accessory cells necessary for mitogen-induced human T lymphocyte activation *in vitro*, *J. Clin. Invest.* **67**:1490.

Burckhardt, J. J., 1979, Rat memory thymus-derived lymphocytes. II. Differences in macrophage dependent activation shown by *Actinomyces viscosus* antigens and by mitogens using silica *in vitro*, *Scand. J. Immunol.* **10**:229.

Chang, Y., and Yao, C., 1979, Investigation of the human macrophage. I. Collection and *in vitro* cultivation, *Eur. J. Immunol.* **9**:577.

Diamantstein, T., Oppenheim, J. J., Unanue, E. R., Wood, D. D., Handschumacher, R. E., Rosenstreich, D. L., and Waksman, B. H., 1979, Nonspecific "lymphocyte activating" factors produced by macrophages, *Cell. Immunol.* **46**:422.

Djeu, J. Y., Heinbaugh, J. A., Vieira, W. D., Holden, H. T., and Herberman, R. B., 1979, The effect of immunopharmacological agents on mouse natural cell-mediated cytotoxicity and on its augmentation by poly I, poly C, *Immunopharmacology* **1**:231.

Ellner, J. J., Lipsky, P. E., and Rosenthal, A. S., 1976, Phytohemagglutinin-induced proliferation of guinea pig thymus-derived lymphocytes. II. Accessory cell function, *J. Immunol.* **116**:876.

Fagnani, R., Zicht, R. R., Bonnard, G. D., and Herberman, R. B., 1983, Accessory cell functions of the human leukemic cell line K562, submitted for publication (personal communication).

Farrar, W. L., Johnson, H. M., and Farrar, J. J., 1981, Regulation of the production of immune interferon and cytotoxic T lymphocytes by interleukin 2, *J. Immunol.* **126**:1120.

Geier, S. S., and Cresswell, P., 1980, Monocytes as accessory cells in the human mixed lymphocyte response: Lack of requirement high cell densities, *Cell. Immunol.* **49**:190.

Gomard, E., Wybier-Franqui, T., and Levy, T. P., 1981, Accessory cells in the *in vitro* generation of type C virus specific T killer lymphocytes. I. Role of macrophages in primary anti-FMR reaction, *J. Immunol.* **126**:891.

Gorenberg, D. T., and Daniele, R. P., 1978, The alveolar macrophage: Its capacity to act as an accessory cell in mitogen-stimulated proliferation of guinea pig lymphocytes, *Cell. Immunol.* **36**:115.

Habu, S., and Raff, M. C., 1977, Accessory cell dependence of lectin-induced proliferation of mouse T lymphocytes, *Eur. J. Immunol.* **7**:451.

Hoffmann, M. K., Koenig, S., Mittler, R. S., Oettgen, H. F., Ralph, P., Galanos, C., and Hämmerling, V., 1979, Macrophage factor controlling differentiation of B cells, *J. Immunol.* **122**:497.

Johnson, W. D., Mei, B., and Cohn, Z. A., 1977, The separation, long-term cultivation and maturation of the human monocyte, *J. Exp. Med.* **146**:1613.

Kammer, G. M., and Unanue, E. R., 1980, Accessory cell requirement in the proliferation response to T lymphocytes to hemocyanin, *Clin. Immunol. Immunopathol.* **15**:434.

Keissling, R., Hochman, P. S., Haller, O., Shearer, G. M., Wigzell, H., and Cudkowicz, G., 1977, Evidence for a similar or common mechanism for natural killer cell activity and resistance to haemopoietic grafts, *Eur. J. Immunol.* **7**:655.

Kurland, J. I., 1978, Regulatory interactions of the macrophage in B lymphocyte proliferation, *J. Reticuloendothelial Soc.* **24**:19.

Lee, K. C., 1977, Cortisone as a probe for cell interactions in the generation of cytotoxic T cells. I. Effect on helper cells, cytotoxic T cell precursors and accessory cells, *J. Immunol.* **119**:1836.

Lutz, C. T., and Fitch, F. W., 1979, Accessory cell requirements for the generation of cytolytic T lymphocytes, *J. Immunol.* **122**:2598.

Lutz, C. T., Glasebrook, A. L., and Fitch, F. W., 1981, Alloreactive cloned T cell lines. III. Accessory cell requirements for the growth of cloned cytolytic T lymphocytes, *J. Immunol.* **126**:1404.

Mishell, R. I., Shiigi, J. M., Mishell, B. B., Grabstein, K. H., and Shiigi, S. M., 1980, Prevention of the immunosuppressive effects of glucocorticosteroids by cell-free factors from adjuvant activated accessory cells, *Immunopharmacology* **2**:233.

Mongini, P., Fredman, S., and Wortiz, H., 1978, Accessory cell requirement for anti-IgM-induced proliferation of B lymphocytes, *Nature (London)* **276**:709.

Morgan, E. L., and Weigle, W. O., 1981, Regulation of the immune response. III. The role of macrophages in the potentiation of the immune response by Fc fragments, *J. Immunol.* **126**:1302.

Mosier, D. C., and Coppleson, L. W., 1968, A three cell interaction required for the induction of the primary immune response *in vitro, Proc. Natl. Acad. Sci. USA* **61**:542.

Munthe-Kass, A. C., 1980, The accessory cell effects of liver macrophages in concanvalin A stimulation of rat spleen lymphocytes, *Scand. J. Immunol.* **11**:523.

Oppenheim, J. J., Mizel, S. B., and Meltzer, M. S., 1979, Comparison of lymphocyte and mononuclear phagocyte derived mitogenic "amplification" factors, in: *Biology of the Lymphokines* (S. Cohen, E. Pick, and J. J. Oppenheim, eds.), Academic Press, New York.

Raff, H. V., Cochrum, K. C., and Stobo, J. D., 1978, Macrophage–T cell interactions in the Con A induction of human suppressive T cells, *J. Immunol.* **121**:2311.

Reynolds, C. W., and Herberman, R. B., 1981, *In vitro* augmentation of rat natural killer (NK) cell activity, *J. Immunol.* **126**:1581.

Reynolds, C. W., Brunda, M., J., Holden, H. T., and Herberman, R. B., 1981, Role of macrophages in *in vitro* augmentation of rat, mouse and human natural killer activities, *J. Natl. Cancer Inst.* **66**:837.

Rogoff, T. M., and Lipsky, P. E., 1979, Characterization of isolated guinea pig Kupffer cells: Accessory cell function in mitogen-induced T lymphocyte activation, *J. Immunol.* **123**:1920.

Rosenberg, S. A., and Lipsky, P. E., 1981, The role of monocytes in pokeweed mitogen-stimulated human B cell activation: Separate requirements for intact monocytes and a soluble monocyte factor, *J. Immunol.* **126**:1341.

Rosenberg, S. A., Ligler, F. S., Ugolini, V., and Lipsky, P. E., 1981, A monoclonal antibody that identified human peripheral blood monocytes recognizes the accessory cells required for mitogen-induced T lymphocyte proliferation, *J. Immunol.* **126**:1473.

Satoh, J., Rikiishi, H., Nagahashi, M., Ohuchi, E., and Kumagai, E., 1980, Mitogen responsiveness of various immune tissues: Heterogeneity of accessory cells and susceptibility to suppression by macrophages, *Cell. Immunol.* **56**:1.

Schuyler, M. R., and Todd, L. S., 1981, Accessory cell function of rabbit alveolar macrophages, *Am. Rev. Respir. Dis.* **123**:53.

Stavitsky, A. B., 1980, Induction, maintenance, and regulation of antibody responses due to persistent antigen and accessory cell, *Immunol. Rev.* **53**:87.

Steinman, R. M., and Nussenzweig, M. C., 1980, Dendritic cells: Features and functions, *Immunol. Rev.* **53**:127.

Stevenson, H. C., Katz, P., Wright, D. G., Contreras, T. J., Jemionek, J. F., Hartwig, V. M., Flor, W. J., and Fauci, A. S., 1981, Human blood monocytes: Characterization of negatively selected human monocytes and their suspension cell culture derivatives, *Scand. J. Immunol.* **14**:243.

Stevenson, H. C., Miller, P. J., Waxdal, M. J., Haynes, B. F., Thomas, C. A., and Fauci, A. S., 1983 Interaction of pokeweed mitogen with monocytes in the initiation of the human lymphocyte activation process, *Immunology* **49**:633.

Stingl, G., Tamaki, K., and Katz, S. I., 1980, Origin and function of epidermal Langerhans cells, *Immunol. Rev.* **53**:149.

Tew, J. G., Phipps, A. P., and Mandel, T. E., 1980, The maintenance and regulation of the humoral immune response: Persisting antigen and the role of follicular antigen-binding dendritic cells as accessory cells, *Immunol. Rev.* **53**:175.

Unanue, E. R., 1978, The regulation of lymphocyt function by the macrophage, *Immunol. Rev.* **40**:227.

VanWauwe, J., and Goosens, J., 1981, Mitogenic actions of OKT3 on human peripheral blood lymphocytes: Effects of monocytes and serum components, *J. Immunopharmacol.* **44**:865.

Wood, D. D., and Staruch, M. J., 1981, Control of the mitogeneicity of muramyl dipeptide, *J. Immunopharmacol.* **3**:31.

8

Role of the Reticuloendothelial System in T-Helper Cell Induction

DAVID R. KATZ, GEOFFREY H. SUNSHINE, MARC FELDMANN, and PETER ERB

1. INTRODUCTION

The development of *in vitro* culture systems and cell separation methods has provoked increasing interest in understanding the role of RES accessory cells (AC) in immune induction. As the relevant technology was improved, AC were found to be important in every immune function assayed, such as antibody production *in vitro* (Mosier, 1969), killer cell induction (Wagner *et al.*, 1972), mixed leukocyte reaction (MLR) (Greineder and Rosenthal, 1975), T-cell proliferation (Rosenwasser and Rosenthal, 1978), etc. Apparent exceptions early on (Diener *et al.*, 1970) were almost certainly reflections of the different types and numbers of AC required for various responses, and also of the inefficiency of AC depletion by conventional adherence procedures which are usually only maintained for the depletion of classical macrophages. Accordingly we were not surprised that T-cell help *in vitro* required macrophages (Erb and Feldmann, 1975a).

The major RES AC type is the macrophage (Mϕ), present typically in peritoneal washout, but also found in lymph node medulla and red pulp of spleen, which is phagocytic and has Fc and C3 receptors. In recent years, heterogeneity of the Mϕ-like AC pool has been uncovered, and its full extent is still not known. Nossal and Ada (1971) and Humphrey and his colleagues (Klaus *et al.*, 1980) found dendritic cells (with long processes) in the follicles and germinal centers. These cells retained antigen for prolonged periods of time, depending on Fc and

DAVID R. KATZ, GEOFFREY H. SUNSHINE, and MARC FELDMANN • Imperial Cancer Research Fund, Tumour Immunology Unit, Department of Zoology, University College London, London, England. PETER ERB • Institute for Microbiology and Hygiene, The University of Basel, Basel, Switzerland.

C3 receptors for their function. These cells are not phagocytic and so are not defined as "macrophages." Steinman and Cohn (1973) isolated a novel cell from the spleen of mice, which had long processes, and was not phagocytic, but did not have Fc or C3 receptors. This cell, termed "dendritic cell," was recognized as being distinct from the "dendritic follicular cell," and was subsequently shown to be very strikingly Ia positive, the most potent cell at inducing the MLR (Sunshine *et al.*, 1981) and T-cell proliferation to antigen, and involved in Ir gene control (Sunshine *et al.*, 1980). By morphological and enzymatic criteria, these appear to be related to the Langerhans cells of the skin (Stingl *et al.*, 1980), the interdigitating cells of the lymph node paracortical region (Verrman, 1974), and the veiled cells of the lymph (Drexhage *et al.*, 1979), suggesting a traffic pattern of some AC.

That these different cells are as direct influence on RES–T-helper cell responses specifically has been highlighted by Humphrey and Grennan (1981) who have shown that certain thymus-independent (TI) antigens of neutral charge such as Ficoll and hydroxyethyl starch are taken up selectively by macrophages with long processes in the marginal zone of the spleen and not by those of the red pulp. These were termed "marginal zone macrophages." Negatively charged antigens such as pneumococcal capsular polysaccharide are taken up by both marginal zone and red pulp cells. Cell separation procedures have also shown that there are different AC for different TI antigens (Gorczynski, 1977).

Currently we do not know the full extent of RES influence and of AC heterogeneity on T-helper responses. Even within each of the cell types described above there may be further heterogeneity: for example, there are Ia^+ and Ia^- macrophages, which may reflect either stages of differentiation or of activation (Scher *et al.*, 1980).

Recently several technical advances have allowed us to study RES–T_H relationships in more detail. The genetic restriction in this interaction is clearly a crucial step in directing responses to antigen (Vogt *et al.*, 1981). The isolation of long-term T_H clones (Schreier *et al.*, 1981) provides a unique opportunity to examine the influence of RES cells on T_H cells. Furthermore, the role of soluble factors as mediators of RES–T_H interaction is now amenable to analysis using improved reagents. These are among the most interesting aspects of current RES–T_H research; in this review we concentrate on these three elements and indicate how they can be interpreted into an overall concept of immune mechanisms in which the T_H immune induction step is a pivotal point of immunoregulation.

2. MACROPHAGE-LIKE CELLS IN T_H CELL INDUCTION

The prototype of *in vitro* induction of T_H cells with any antigen requires the participation of Mϕ-like AC which can be found in various anatomical sites, e.g., peritoneum, spleen, bone marrow. Similarly, the restimulation of antigen-specific memory T_H is equally AC dependent (Klaus *et al.*, 1980).

For convenience, peritoneal exudate cells (PEC) of normal or nonspecifically stimulated mice (e.g., 2% solution of starch injected intraperitoneally 3–4 days prior to use) or *in vitro* cultured Mϕ derived from bone marrow (BMMϕ) are usually taken as the source of AC. Both these AC populations represent a mixture of various different cell types. Therefore we have examined the precise phenotype of the cell in the PEC or BMMO pool is responsible for the activation of a given T-cell function. To do this we have separated PEC or BMMϕ into Fc receptor-positive and -negative cells, into phagocytic and nonphagocytic cells, and into Ia-positive and Ia-negative cells. Each fraction can then be compared to see their relative capacity to induce T_H to soluble antigens. The results obtained demonstrated that only Fc receptor-bearing, phagocytic, and Ia-positive cells can induce T_H. Furthermore, the relevant cells were adherent to glass or plastic, radioresistant, and positive for staining with nonspecific esterases (Erb *et al.*, 1980). Thus, the characteristics of the PEC are typical of Mϕ.

For successful T–Mϕ interaction leading to the *in vitro* generation of T_H, the Mϕ and T cells had to be identical at the *I-A* subregion of the *H-2* complex (Erb and Feldmann, 1976). This observation confirmed previous findings made in the guinea pig by Rosenthal and Shevach (1973) who demonstrated the requirement for *I* region identity between Mϕ and T cells in antigen-induced T-cell proliferation assays. The results also raise the question as to whether genetic restriction of T–Mo interaction is induced by the priming event (Pierce *et al.*, 1976) or is already manifest prior to priming. Restimulation of F_1 hybrid T cells was only effective with parental Mϕ of that type used for priming, implying that restriction can indeed be induced by priming. However, T cells of chimeric mice have been used to establish that restriction is also present prior to priming (Erb *et al.*, 1980). For example, T cells of F_1(A × B) A chimeras, constructed by reconstituting lethally irradiated A mice with anti-Thy = 1 + C′-treated bone marrow of F_1 mice, only became T_H if stimulated with antigen presented by F_1 or A-type Mϕ but not B-type Mϕ. If genetic restriction would have been induced by priming, B-type Mϕ should have been just as effective as F_1 or A-type Mϕ. Using the reciprocal chimeric combination, A F_1(A × B), it was found that for restimulation of primed T_H there was restriction of cooperation with A-type Mϕ, unless the chimeric mice were repopulated with Mϕ of the B haplotype at the time of priming. These later experiments indicated a critical role of the presenting Mϕ in selecting which T cells differentiate and/or are maintained in the peripheral T-cell pool (Table 1).

Thus, the hypothesis was proposed that there are two stages in the genesis of immunocompetence of T_H; one is a "permissive" stage which occurs in the environment where T stem cells differentiate and determines the potential T-cell repertoire, the other is a "selective" or proliferative stage and determines which of the potential repertoires is expressed at detectable frequency in the peripheral T-cell pool. This later stage is dependent on Mϕ-like AC (Erb *et al.*, 1979a). Subsequent data with nude mice have confirmed this (Zinkernagel *et al.*, 1980).

Genes located within the *I* region govern the interaction between Mϕ–AC and T_H cells. Since genes in the same region also control the immune response to a number of antigens, the *in vitro* T_H system enables one to study whether

TABLE 1. HELPER CELL INDUCTION WITH PRIMED ($P \rightarrow F_1$) CHIMERAS[a,b,c]

Helper cell induction: $b \rightarrow (k \times b)F_1T$ *In vivo* priming[d]	*In vitro* priming[e]	Cooperation[f]: HC added	F$_1$B cells	Antigen (μg/culture)	Anti-DNP response[g] AFC/10^5: IgM	IgG
KLH	KLH	+	+	TNP-KLH 0.05	75 ± 10	125 ± 55
"	" + F$_1$ Mϕ	+	+	"	485 ± 28	585 ± 105+
"	" + B10 Mϕ (a)	+	+	"	640 ± 25	890 ± 150
"	" + CBA Mϕ (b)	+	+	"	188 ± **	185 ± 5*
"	" + B10·D2 Mϕ (c)	+	+ (+ B10·D2 Mϕ)	"	58 ± 18***	65 ± 15**
		a + b[h]	+	"	495 ± 30	760 ± 10
		a + c	+	"	450 ± 80	920 ± 20
KLH + CBA Mϕ	KLH	+	+	"	75 ± 0	175 ± 5
" "	" + F$_1$ Mϕ	+	+	"	298 ± 97+	465 ± 25+
" "	" + B10 Mϕ (d)	+	+	"	360 ± 25	785 ± 75
" "	" + CBA Mϕ	+	+	"	295 ± 15	505 ± 15
" "	" + B10·D2 Mϕ (e)	+	+ (+ B10·D2 Mϕ)	"	88 ± 42**	40 ± 10***
		d + e	+	"	273 ± 8	575 ± 25

KLH + B10·D2 MΦ		KLH		+	+	″	3 ± 3	3 ± 3
″	″	″ + F_1 MΦ	(f)	+	+	″	95 ± 10	113 ± 27
″	″	″ + B10 MΦ	(g)	+	+	″	215 ± 50+	283 ± 13+
″	″	″ + CBA MΦ	(h)	+	–	″	48 ± 8	68 ± 3***
″	″	″ + B10·D2 MΦ	(i)	+	+	″	18 ± 8**	3 ± 3***
					(B10·D2 MΦ)			
				g + h	+	″	158 ± 23	195 ± 10
				f + i	+	″	105 ± 10	133 ± 18
NIL	NIL	NIL	NIL	–	+	″	65 ± 5	15 ± 5
″	″	″	″	–	+	DNP-CGG 0.05	965 ± 115	2555 ± 45
″	″	″	″	–	+	NIL	53 ± 32	20 ± 0

[a]Reprinted with permission from Erb *et al.* (1979b).
[b]Mice used were B10 → F_1 (B10 × CBA).
[c]H-2 typing:

	Percent killing
Anti-H-2^b (D-2)	96
Anti-H-2^k (D-32)	3
Control	<4

[d]Mice were primed *in vivo* with KLH (100 μg), KLH and 5 × 10^6 cultured CBA bone marrow cells as a source of macrophages, or KLH and anti-Thy-l and C′-treated B10·D2 PE cells induced with starch 4 days previously.
[e]Nylon wool-purified T cells of the primed chimeras were restimulated *in vitro* with KLH (0.1 μg) and 5 × 10^4 macrophages of the strains as indicated for 4 days.
[f]10^4 living cells of the first cultures (HC cells) were added to 1 × 10^6 DNP-CGG-primed F_1 B cells and incubated with TNP-KLH (0.05 μg/culture) for 5 days.
[g]IgM as well as IgG-AFC were measured and given as numbers of AFC/10^6 input B cells. For detecting IgG-AFC an enhancing serum (rabbit anti-mouse IgG) to develop IgG plaques and an anti-μ serum to depress IgM plaques were added to the assay system.
[h]To test for suppressor cells 10^5 cells of cultures (a), (d), (f), or (g) were mixed with 5 × 10^4 cells of cultures (b), (c), (e), (h), or (i) and tested for helper activity in the cooperation culture.
*$P < 0.05$; **$P < 0.01$; ***$P < 0.005$.
+Positive control.

both phenomena—genetic control of cell interactions and of the immune response (Ir)—are based on the same principle. One way to pursue that problem is to locate the cellular sites of Ir gene function. Rosenthal and co-workers provided the first evidence in the guinea pig that Ir genes function at the level of Mϕ. This has been confirmed by many groups including ourselves (Erb *et al.*, 1981). For example, we showed that the activation of T cells of $F_1(b \times k)$ mice, a hybrid between a responder (b) and a nonresponder (k) to bovine insulin (Erb, 1980), was only possible with bovine insulin presented by responder F_1 or b-type Mϕ, but not nonresponder k-type Mϕ. It was concluded that Mϕ of nonresponder mice do not function due to an Ir gene defect. However, these results did not exclude other possible sites; Ir genes might also function at the T-cell level or at the level of generation of the T-cell repertoire. Chimeric mice again yielded one approach to study such predictions. Using different antigens, under Ir gene control such as (T,G)-A-L, or the natural hormone, insulin of beef or pork origin, we found that stem cells of nonresponder (NR) genotype differentiated into T cells that were of responder (R) phenotype in an R environment, judged by their capacity to become functional T_H in the presence of Mϕ of responder T genotype (Erb *e al.*, 1981). However, stem cells of NR genotype did not differentiate into R antigen-presenting Mϕ in an R environment. In the reverse situation where T cells of R animals differentiated in an NR host, T_H could not be generated from chimeric T cells even with Mϕ from R animals. Analogous observations have been made by many groups using other systems, e.g., cell-mediated cytolysis (Von Boehmer *et al.*, 1978). Thus, the results suggest that Ir genes are also expressed in the host where T stem cells differentiate and, moreover, that there is no need for a responder Ir gene to be present in T cells.

Taken together, the chimeric data propose that Ir genes are expressed in Mϕ and in the host, and thus that both host and Mϕ but not T cells (intrinsically) and Mϕ must have identical Ir gene sets in order to allow the induction of T_H. The role of the host's Ir gene set would be to instruct or select maturing T cells to respond to certain Ir gene products (which are presumably Ia antigens), while the peripheral Mϕ might select out the appropriate antigenic determinants for presentation to T cells. Ir gene defects at either site would result in nonresponsiveness of the animal. According to that hypothesis, it is apparent that the genetic control of cell cooperation and Ir gene regulation of the immune response are two phenomena with the same underlying mechanism.

3. OTHER RES CELLS INVOLVED IN T_H INDUCTION

The involvement of accessory cells with Mϕ-like characteristics in T_H induction has been discussed in the previous section. Cells with the characteristics of an Mϕ subpopulation (FcR^+, phagocytic, radioresistant, and I-A^+) are required for the differentiation of unprimed T cells to T_H cells (Erb *et al.*, 1981). What is not as clear is whether the other RES AC are involved in the selective induction of other types of T_H cell response, such as second T_H responses, or whether more than one AC type can elicit the same kind of T-cell help.

One candidate which must be considered for involvement in T_H induction is the dendritic cell (Steinman and Cohn, 1973). Its role in syngeneic and allogeneic T-cell proliferation systems (which are considered to be partial analogs of T_H induction) has been discussed previously (Feldmann *et al.*, 1983). Recently, we have been particularly interested in the possible role of dendritic cells in the induction of function of primed and unprimed T_H cells *in vitro.*

We are studying whether the dendritic cell population can present antigen to unprimed T_H cell precursors, a necessarily more complex phenomenon as at least two distinct T subpopulations are involved (Feldmann *et al.*, 1975). If we preincubate soluble antigens such as insulin or chicken gamma globulin with either Mϕ or dendritic cells in the presence of purified unprimed spleen T lymphocytes there is relatively little induction of T help. However, a combined dendritic cells and Mϕ population coincubated with T cell and antigen will induce T_H cells. These preliminary experiments suggest the possibility that two distinct AC are required for the induction of T-cell help. On present evidence we do not know whether the two RES cells are activating different T-cell subsets in this system, since a T–T cell interaction has been demonstrated (Erb *et al.*, 1979b). It is tempting to speculate that the twin requirement for Mϕ and dendritic cell in this system may reflect different aspects of antigen processing and presentation: the phagocytic Mϕ perhaps processing the antigen and breaking it down into fragments which a specialized Ia^+ presenting cell, the dendritic cell, then presents to the T cell. Tentative support for such a model has come from recent observations (Inaba *et al.*, 1981) which suggest that both Ia^- and Ia^+ AC are required for the induction of antibody responses to sheep red cells.

4. RES CELLS IN ACTIVATION OF T-CELL CLONES

The previous discussion has illustrated that there is a definite AC role in the induction of T_H cells, but that this role is incompletely defined at present. One of the limiting features of many experiments mentioned is that the T-cell compartment is very heterogeneous, making it difficult to differentiate between the RES–T cell interaction and T–T cell interaction in the complex pools of spleen or lymph node T cells. Even the best fractionated T cells may suffer the problem of carryover of small numbers of AC among them.

Homogeneous T-cell populations of the T_H phenotype have now been isolated in numerous laboratories (Watson, 1979; Schreier and Tees, 1980). These T cells and clones enable one to analyze the RES component in more detail. The range of clones now available includes both T helpers to red cell antigens and to soluble antigens (Schreier *et al.*, 1982).

These experiments employ an *in vivo* priming step to induce the T_H cell population; for these T cells the RES influence is not different from that already discussed. This cell population is cultured in the presence of antigen for a variable period of time. The cell density at this stage may be critical: spleen cells are grown at lower density than lymph node cells, which may in fact reflect higher syngeneic RES-presenting cell fraction in the spleen cell suspension

(Schreier *et al.*, 1981). This phase may also be critical in selecting the type of RES AC to which the cells will give on optimal response subsequently.

At the next phase of culture when the cells are used to form a continuous line (rather than a clone) there is an obligatory requirement for irradiated spleen cells in addition to antigen. The precise inducer cells in the spleen population which produce this effect are not known. Broadly speaking they are considered to be Mϕ by virtue of their radioresistance.

At the crucial cloning step there is also a requirement for a splenic radioresistant cell or for a peritoneal washout cell. At this stage TCGF (interleukin-2) is required as a supplement in the culture medium. After the cloning step the cells can be maintained without either "filler" cells or antigen, but if the growth rate falls, then radioresistant spleen cells and antigen are again required to restore the responsiveness to TCGF (Schreier *et al.*, 1980).

From the point of view of the AC, these findings are based upon empirical observations on what makes the system work. There are, however, general principles about RES–T interactions which can be extrapolated. These relate to the questions of antigen presentation, to genetic restriction, and to the role of TCGF.

Antigen is required at two different stages of these T-cell cloning and testing systems. Firstly, antigen forms a part of this proliferative drive and secondly, it is an intrinsic part of the test system of helper cell function. An AC-antigen combination is especially crucial at those stages of isolation at which maximal proliferative drive is required, such as during cloning itself. However, the fact that the AC are radioresistant cells does not mean merely that irradiation of the feeder layer is useful to stop unwanted irrelevant proliferating cells overgrowing the desired clone. The radioresistant cells commonly used will have distinctive features which include many classic macrophage characteristics such as phagocytosis and lysosomal enzyme secretion. The peritoneal cell and antigen combination which is optimum for most clones raises the possibility that an antigen-presenting step is required of these cells at some point and that their function must not be regarded as purely filler, nutritional, or disposal.

Recently, (in collaboration with Dr. Schreier) we have examined some of these clones using assay systems which look specifically at the nature of the AC compartment as inducer of T_H proliferation. Our data suggest that the DC can sometimes replace the classic macrophage but that this varies from clone to clone.

In view of this antigen presentation, mechanism an important question was whether or not there is genetic restriction at the level of the T-cell clone. We have already noted that the AC–T cell interface is the critical site of the restriction and that this holds true for the clonal derivation systems. I-A-compatible AC are a prerequisite and I-A-incompatible cells are ineffective (Schreier *et al.*, 1982). Further selection of F_1 T-cell lines on AC of one or other parental strain type will produce clones which only proliferate in the presence of the correct phenotypic AC. The fact that some parental-derived clone may proliferate more effectively when exposed to the F_1 AC may reflect differences in the genetics of the strain types rather than aberrant restriction (Klein *et al.*, 1981).

The T-cell clones themselves have a potential for developing their own "heterogeneity" *in vitro* (Schreier *et al.*, 1982). Thus, some may stop proliferating and die off. More relevant are those which survive but lose their helper activity. Sometimes this coincides with increased growth. With these clones I-A-compatible AC stimulation is the obvious maneuver used to try to restore help. In the presence of antigen and AC it is usually possible to continue the proliferation but not necessarily to restore help. This type of change illustrates the subtle effects involved. Further, preselection may be particularly important in our understanding of the RES–T cell interaction since clones selected upon peritoneal washout cells adhered to plastic will not proliferate in the presence of other types of AC.

Another variation of the clonal system is that some clones will act *in vivo* as effective T helpers, while others will not (Schreier *et al.*, 1982). This does not seem to be related to the proliferative capacity of the particular clone. Also not related to the proliferative capacity of the clone is the ability of these cells to respond in an allogeneic culture system and to act as cytotoxic T cells (Sredni *et al.*, 1980). Both these findings add emphasis to the postulate that more than one pathway of T-cell activation is present in the cloned T_H circuit and that the early stages of selection are those at which the specific RES role is important.

Accessory cells do not produce TCGF themselves (Smith, 1980). The pure supernatant of a peritoneal washout adherent cell or spleen adherent cell is inadequate for this function. However, the presence of AC in the systems which do produce this factor in one form or another is striking (Andersson *et al.*, 1979). For example, both the secondary allogeneic response and the Con A response (which are the most commonly used sources of supernatants for this type of assay) are AC dependent in their initial stage. The role of the AC in relation to TCGF effect on clones is illustrated by the fact that AC restore TCGF responsiveness to clones which have lost their responsiveness (Schreier *et al.*, 1980). This observation supports the notion that the AC activate a TCGF receptor on T cells even at the clonal level. This would also conform with the unquestioned role the different types of AC can play in the proliferation of T-cell lines before the clonal types.

5. ROLE OF ACCESSORY CELLS IN T_H INDUCTION *IN VIVO*

Methods of depleting animals of Ac are far from perfect, and so our concepts of AC function in cell interaction *in vivo* are based on extrapolations from cell separation work *in vitro*. However, there are a number of studies which are compatible with *in vitro* concepts and tend to confirm them. Thus, the use of antigens which kill macrophages *in vivo*, such as silica or carrageenan, has tended to diminish antibody responses (Sheagren *et al.*, 1975), which is compatible with inhibition of helper (and other cell) induction.

As anti-I-A antibodies block helper cell induction *in vitro* it would be expected that sufficient concentrations would also inhibit the response *in vivo*.

Such experiments have been performed, with the predicted results, by the repeated injection of monoclonal anti-I-A ascites *in vivo* (Sprent, 1980).

Another way to look at *in vivo* AC–T cell interactions is to test the *in vivo* response to selected AC populations prepared *in vitro*. Antigen-pulsed Mϕ are potent inducers of T-cell priming *in vivo* (Mitchison, 1969); likewise, dendritic cells can have the same function (S. C. Knight, personal communication). At the clonal level, optimal short-term delayed type hypersensitivity responses are generated by a mixture of T_H cells, antigen, and peritoneal cells (Schreier *et al.*, 1981).

6. MACROPHAGE-DERIVED Ia–ANTIGEN COMPLEXES (GRF) IN T_H INDUCTION

In 1975 we demonstrated that the induction of T_H cells *in vitro* with protein or polypeptide antigens requires the participation of Mϕ-like AC (Erb and Feldmann, 1975a). However, direct contact between AC and T lymphocytes was not found to be essential, and mediators produced by antigen-incubated AC were also capable of inducing T_H. The activity of these mediators, called genetically related Mϕ factor (GRF), strikingly parallels that of AC and antigen, suggesting that they are a major or active principle of AC function in helper cell induction.

To obtain GRF, either normal PEC or PEC stimulated nonspecifically (e.g., 2% starch injected intraperitoneally 3–4 days before harvest) are plated on petri dishes and after several hours of incubation the nonadherent cells are washed away. The residual adherent cells are then incubated with antigen (e.g., KLH) for up to 4 days in serum-free medium. The supernatants (S/N) harvested from these cells (GRF) are tested for helper cell-inducing activity. Mϕ-depleted T cells are incubated with various doses of GRF for 4 days using the mini-Marbrook culture system. To assess helper activity a small number of living cells are added to normal spleen cells or anti-Thy = 1 + C′-treated spleen cells (as a source of B cells) and incubated with a hapten–carrier conjugate. Four days later the anti-hapten response is measured in a Cunningham plaque assay using hapten-coated SRBC. The number of antibody-forming cells obtained is a measure of whether T_H cells have been generated or not.

GRF used in a low concentration (1–10%) induced T_H in an antigen-specific manner, but only if GRF was derived from Mϕ identical at the *I-A* subregion of the *H-2* complex with the T cells (Erb *et al.*, 1979a). Using immunoadsorbent columns prepared with the IgG fraction of various antisera and antigen, it was found that GRF is a complex of Ia antigen and immunogenic fragments (Erb *et al.*, 1976). Both components are noncovalently associated, since the complex can be split by lowering the pH to 2.4. However, the components reassociate after raising the pH to 7.

The molecular weight of GRF was determinationed by either Sephadex G-75 columns or SDS–polyacrylamide gel electrophoresis. With Sephadex the GRF was found to be between 50,000 and 60,000 daltons; with SDS–PAGE, 70,000 daltons. Treatment of GRF with proteolytic enzymes completely abolished the T_H-inducing capacity (Feldmann *et al.*, 1979).

Using ^{125}I-labeled antigen, only the 70,000-dalton material can be removed by repeated treatment with anti-I-A sera, suggesting the antibody precipitates an unlabeled cellular product that is associated with a KLH fragment. In one experiment the 70,000-dalton material eluted from the gel induced KLH-specific T_H. However, the biochemical characterization is not yet complete; there are many more experiments needed to determine the exact chemical nature of GRF.

Puri and Lonai (1980) described a molecule consisting of Ia products and antigenic fragments which they term IAC (Ia-associated antigen complex). The characteristics of IAC closely resemble those of GRF, and it is highly likely that IAC and GRF are the same moieties.

It is interesting that when investigating the kinetics of GRF production we found that adherent PEC incubated with antigen release GRF on day 1, with increasing amounts on day 2 and 3. This is followed by a progressive decline in GRF production. This is different from the kinetics of IAC production which is found in the maximal concentration in the S/N of Mϕ after a short period of incubation with antigen. It may be significant that splenic adherent cells were used for the production of IAC, while GRF is obtained from PEC. Splenic adherent cells bear much more Ia antigen than PEC (Cowing *et al.*, 1978). Thus the kinetics of production and/or release of these factors may be different.

At the T-cell level the induction of T_H *in vitro* requires the interaction of two T cells. One is a short-lived, Ly-$1^+2^+3^+$ cell which acts as a T amplifier, and the other is a long-lived, recirculating Ly-$1^+2^-3^-$ cell which is the helper cell precursor (Feldmann *et al.*, 1979). GRF binds to both T-cell subsets, which thus most likely express the same recognition repertoire. However, they differ in their response to GRF because the T_H precursors require an additional "signal" provided by the amplifier T cell in order to become a helper cell. While the GRF–T amplifier/T_H precursor interaction is genetically restricted, the mediator provided by the amplifier T cells is not. The physical and chemical nature of this mediator is unclear, but functionally, it resembles TCGF (interleukin-2) which is essential for the proliferation of T cells (see above).

The receptor for binding of GRF to T cells has been analyzed by blocking experiments (Erb *et al.*, 1980). Out of a large panel of various reagents which were tested, only a few blocked the binding of GRF to T cells. These were anti-*H-2D* or *K* subregion sera, anti-MTLA (Fab fragments of a rabbit anti-mouse T-lymphocyte antiserum), and an excess of soluble antigen. The blocking of the GRF receptor by anti-*H-2D/K* sera was surprising in view of the fact that anti-Ia (or anti-I-A) did not block the receptor but did block GRF activity. Thus, the GRF receptor does not contain Ia products but either contains *H-2* specificities or may be in close proximity to H-2 molecules and therefore be blocked by steric hindrance. Other alternatives can also not be excluded to account for the effects of anti-H-2. For example, "impurities" or antiviral activity could have been present within the anti-H-2 sera used, which were conventional in type and not monoclonal. The blocking of the GRF receptor by anti-MTLA is interesting since this antisera may be directed against the T-cell receptor(s) for MHC gene products

(Woody *et al.*, 1979). If this is correct, their anti-MTLA Fab might bind to the receptor for Ia on T cells and thus specifically inhibit the interaction with the Ia part of GRF.

Blocking of the GRF receptor by an excess of native antigen poses a puzzling problem as it contrasts with the fact that free antigen does not block T-cell responses. It is not clear in our system whether indeed a receptor for antigen is blocked or whether another mechanism is working. In this context, it is interesting that the binding of labeled IAC to T cells takes place within 1 to 4 min and could be blocked by unlabeled IAC, but not by soluble antigen (Puri and Lonai, 1980). This binding of soluble antigen followed slow kinetics, i.e., soluble antigen did not block at the beginning, but inhibited after 30 min of incubation. Puri and Lonai suggest that native antigen had to be "processed" by AC to become IAC which then replaced the labeled homologous IAC at the T-cell receptor. It is possible that a similar mechanism is operational in our GRF blocking experiments, in which T cells are preincubated with soluble antigen for at least 1 hr before GRF is added. As our T cells are purified from spleen, are Mϕ depleted but not Mϕ free, it could be that during the incubation period IAC/GRF is produced by the few residual Mϕ which then block the receptor.

GRF was also treated for the capacity to restimulate T_H memory cells *in vitro*. Unpurified GRF did not restimulate memory cells, but anti-Ia column-purified GRF did (Erb *et al.*, 1981). The results suggest that crude GRF might contain inhibitors that prevent the restimulation of primed T_H. These inhibitors are apparently not effective at blocking in the activation of unprimed T cells.

As GRF is a complex of Ia products and immunogenic framgnets of antigen, it is possible that the Ia antigens are the Ir gene products which mediate the Ir gene-like function of the complex. Though there is no direct evidence for such a correlation, the properties of GRF are very suggestive. The activity of GRF closely parallels that of Mϕ and antigen in that only GRF obtained from responder but not from nonresponder Mϕ activates T cells to become helper cells (Table 2) (Erb *et al.*, 1979b). Similarly, only IAC obtained from responder Mϕ bound to responder F_1 T cells (Puri and Lonai, 1980). However, we do not know how this relates to the "nonresponder Mϕ"; do they not produce GRF, do they produce a "defective" GRF, or do the T cells lack the appropriate receptor site?

To assess the biological significance of GRF, it was tested *in vivo* by injecting small amounts intraperitoneally without adjuvant. After one or two injections T_H were generated as demonstrated by our *in vitro* cooperation assay. After three or more injections, secondary responses were obtained that were sometimes as high as if the mice had been primed with antigen in adjuvant. The amount of GRF injected corresponds to 3–5 μg of native antigen, a dose which only induces a marginal response if injected without adjuvant. In fact, the amount of native antigen in GRF is much lower, as most of it is degraded. These data, though preliminary, demonstrate that GRF also has activity *in vivo*. Similar results have been obtained by Puri and Lonai (1980) who showed that IAC was 100 to 1000 times more immunogenic *in vivo* than the same amount of soluble antigen.

TABLE 2. GRF IS A STABLE IR GENE PRODUCT[a,b]

1st culture (helper cell induction)		2nd culture (cooperation)		Anti-DNP response (AFC/3 × 10^6 cells ± S.E.)	
T cells	Antigen/GRF (μg/ml)	Helper cells	B cells + DNP-TGAL (1 μg/ml)	Expt. I	Expt. II
F_1 (B10 × CBA)	TGAL1.0	+	F_1 (B10 × CBA)	0	120 ± 105
F_1 (B10 × CBA)	F_1 (B10 × CBA) GRF_{TGAL}	+	F_1 (B10 × CBA)	187 ± 14	1479 ± 93[c]
F_1 (B10 × CBA)	CBA GRF_{TGAL}	+	F_1 (B10 × CBA)	157 ± 24[d]	1629 ± 426[d]
F_1 (B10 × CBA)	B10 GRF_{TGAL}	+	F_1 (B10 × CBA)	257 ± 24[d]	1401 ± 9[illegible][d]
NIL	NIL	−	F_1 (B10 × CBA)	27 ± 17	257 ± 1[illegible]0
F_1 (B10 × B10.S)	TGAL1.0		F_1 (B10 × B10.S)	30 ± 20	99 ± 60
F_1 (B10 × B10.S)	F_1 (B10 × B10.S) GRF_{TGAL}	+	F_1 (B10 × B10.S)	220 ± 50[c]	1149 ± 156[c]
F_1 (B10 × B10.S)	B10.S GRF_{TGAL} (a)	+	F_1 (B10 × B10.S)	17 ± 12[c]	99 ± 27[c]
F_1 (B10 × B10.S)	B10 GRF_{TGAL} (b)	+	F_1 (B10 × B10.S)	123 ± 14[c]	831 ± 114[c]
		a + b	F_1 (B10 × B10.S)	n.d.	1041 ± 99[d]
NIL	NIL	−	F_1 (B10 × B10.S)	7 ± 7	150 ± 51
CBA	TGAL1.0	+	CBA	117 ± 18	690 ± 51
CBA	CBA GRF_{TGAL}	+	CBA	636 ± 39[c]	2439 ± 120[c]
NIL	NIL	−	CBA	63 ± 28	411 ± 174
B10	TGAL1.0	+	B10	47 ± 24	171 ± 96
B10	B10 GRF_{TGAL}	+	B10	210 ± 23[c]	921 ± 180[c]
NIL	NIL	−	B10	50 ± 12	9 ± 9
B10.S	TGAL1.0	+	B10.S	0	261 ± 138
B10.S	B10.S GRF_{TGAL}	+	B10.S	13 ± 9	171 ± 54[d]
B10.S	KLH 0.1	+	B10.S + TNP-KLH[e]	n.d.	129 ± 84
B10.S	B10.S GRF_{KLH}	+	B10.S + TNP-KLH[e]	n.d.	807 ± 18[d]
NIL	NIL	−	B10.S + TNP-KLH[e]	n.d.	171 ± 54
NIL	NIL	−	B10.S −	43 ± 21	60 ± 20

[a]Reprinted with permission from Erb *et al.* (1979a).
[b]Helper cells induced with GRF (20 μl in 200-μl volume with 3 × 10^6 T cells), washed, counted, and recultured in the presence of anti-O and C^1-treated F_1 spleen cells and either DNP-(T, G)-A-L or TNP-KLH for 4 days in Minimarbrooks. IgM responses are shown using unprimed B cells (Expt. 1) or DNP-CGG-primed B cells (Expt. II). 2 × 10^5 helper cells in Expt. I, 10^5 in Expt. II.
[c]$P < .05$. Refers to two groups on either side of symbol.
[d]$P > 0.05$. Refers to two groups on either side of symbol.
[e]Does not contain DNP-TGAL.

7. ROLE OF OTHER FACTORS IN HELPER CELL INDUCTION

7.1. NONSPECIFIC MACROPHAGE FACTOR (NMF)

During the studies in which peritoneal cells were incubated with antigen, we found that the supernatants from such cultures contained an activity different from the GRF described above. If peritoneal cells were incubated not with a small soluble protein but rather with particulate or insolubilized antigen such as SRBC, or KLH coupled to Sepharose, or just cultured *in vitro,* a factor could be found which did not have the properties of GRF (Erb and Feldmann, 1975b). Since this supernatant factor could induce helper function in T cells from strains of mice other than in those in which it was induced but only with particulate antigens such as KLH–Sepharose, it was termed nonspecific macrophage factor (NMF; Erb and Feldmann, 1975b). This factor has not been extensively characterized biochemically but has several features different from GRF such as molecular weight (< 20,000), kinetics of release, and dose–response. Interestingly, conditions which generate GRF in culture do not result in significant NMF formation, suggesting that distinct biosynthetic pathways are involved.

7.2. ROLE OF IL-1 IN T_H INDUCTION

A decade ago an Mϕ-derived factor was described that enhanced the proliferation of mouse thymocytes to low concentrations of mitogens (Gery *et al.*, 1972). Subsequent work showed that this factor [lymphocyte activation factor (LAF), more recently termed interleukin-1] could substitute for Mϕ when lymphocytes were stimulated by mitogens (Rosenstreich and Mizel, 1979). It is apparent that the factor works on T-cell populations to induce proliferation and differentiation and it has been suggested that this effect is mediated by the subsequent release of TCGF (IL-2) (Larsson *et al.*, 1980) from the T cells responding to IL-1 and other reagents. Interestingly, IL-1 has no effect on nude spleen cells, presumably because the T-cell precursors are unable to synthesize TCGF (Smith, 1980).

However, there is little data on IL-1 effects in antigen-specific helper systems. Many studies have used allogeneic responses where the involvement of T_H cells is less clear-cut. It has been suggested that the activation of responder T cells in response to alloantigen is mediated by the soluble factors IL-1 and IL-2 (Wagner *et al.*, 1980) and further that IL-1 may act in combination with alloantigen to induce the differentation of cytotoxic cells (Paetkau *et al.*, 1980) in AC-depleted populations, thus replacing the requirement for the Ia^+ RES stimulator cell. This has also been shown in a syngeneic antigen-specific proliferation system: IL-1 can replace the antigen and the presenting cell signal (Rosenwasser and Rosenthal, 1978). However, other evidence from both mouse and man suggests that when RES cells are rigorously depleted from the responder population either by antiserum treatment (Raff *et al.*, 1980) or by physical methods (Sunshine *et al.*, 1982) IL-1 and antigen is not an effective substitute for AC. This has led us to postulate that IL-1 may act as an amplifying rather than an inducing signal in T-cell proliferation. Nonetheless, several interesting questions may still be posed about the nature and role of IL-1. It is not known, for example, whether all types of RES cells are capable of inducing IL-1 synthesis in the presence or absence of antigen: it will be important to determine whether dendritic cells are synthesizers of this activity. While clearly distinct from GRF described above, its relation to NMF and its role in generating antigen-specific T helpers in *in vitro* systems are well worth exploring, and the known biochemical properties do not exclude the possibility that NMF is IL-1.

8. CONCLUSIONS

The studies described above have implied a major role for the RES system in T_H cell induction. There are, however, serious gaps in our knowledge. The extent of AC heterogeneity and the role of each of these AC in lymphocyte triggering and regulation is not clear. Neither is the relative contribution of AC versus AC-derived soluble mediatory function in controlling and coordinating lymphocyte responses.

It should also be clear from this review that while new technology has greatly advanced our knowledge of the cell biology of lymphocytes in tissue culture and also of the molecular biology of lymphocytes (reviewed in *Immunol. Rev.* **59,** 1981), we know relatively little about lymphocyte function *in vivo.* Immune physiology is a much neglected discipline.

It is known that all T cells recirculate at a rapid rate and B cells do also, although somewhat more slowly as judged by thoracic duct cannulation studies (Sprent, 1978a,b). Thus, there is a dilemma—how do rapidly trafficking lymphocytes find each other in order to interact in the increasingly complex manner that is being proposed (Feldmann *et al.*, 1979; Cantor and Gershon, 1979; Herzenberg *et al.*, 1980)?

A simplifying concept, which we have discussed elsewhere, is that the RES as the fixed elements of the lymphoid organs is the means of integrating the complex signals to which lymphocytes respond. Thus, we envisage that lymphocytes recirculate through their distinct areas of the lymphoid system (e.g., T-cell areas in the parafollicular region of lymph nodes, B-cell areas in the follicles and marginal zone) and search for the signals that would activate them. The signals accumulate on the surface of the RES, the "accessory cells" which we have discussed here. This concept is compatible with all the known data: that all forms of lymphocyte activation require AC and that interactions between lymphocytes often involve the intermediary role of AC. This concept would predict that different lymphocytes respond to different signals and recirculate through different areas to respond to different AC.

Our current interest is in testing this hypothesis using refined methods. For example, we now know that there is specialization within the AC pool: dendritic cells do not stimulate B cells, but can stimulate T cells to proliferate; and both dendritic cells and macrophages have a role in relationship to T-cell clones

(Feldmann *et al.*, 1984). Thus, interaction with RES AC is essential in the evolution of T-cell help and this rate limiting step has still not been defined completely either with respect to cellular interactions or with respect to the soluble mediatiors involved.

ACKNOWLEDGMENTS. Our studies described here were funded by the Imperial Cancer Research Fund and the National Institutes of Health. We thank our colleagues for their help and encouragement and Philippa Wells for typing the manuscript.

REFERENCES

Andersson, J. O., Gronvik, K. O., Larsson, E. L., and Coutinho, A., 1979, Studies on T lymphocyte activation. I. Requirements for an Ia bearing accessory cell in Con A induced T cell proliferation, *Eur. J. Immunol.* **9**:581.

Cantor, H., and Gershon, R. K., 1979, Immunological circuits: Cellular composition, *Fed. Proc.* **38**:2058.

Cowing, C., Schwartz, B. D., and Dickler, H. B., 1978, Macrophage Ia antigens. I. Macrophage populations differ in their expression of Ia antigens, *J. Immunol.* **120**:378.

Diener, E., Shortman, K., and Russel, P., 1970, Induction of immunity and tolerance *in vitro* in the absence of phagocytic cells, *Nature (London)* **225**:731.

Drexhage, H. A., Mulliuk, H., de Groot, J., Clarke, J., and Balfour, B. M., 1979, A study of cells present in peripheral lymph of pigs with special reference to a type of cell resembling the Langerhans cell, *Cell Tissue Res.* **202**:407.

Erb, P., 1980, Analysis of the *in vitro* immune response to insulin. 1. Primary induction of insulin specific T helper cells and characterization of the genetic control of the helper cell response to bovine and procine insulin, *Immunol.* **40**:385.

Erb, P., and Feldmann, M., 1975a, Role of macrophages in the *in vitro* induction of T helper cells, *Nature (London)* **254**:352.

Erb, P., and Feldmann, M., 1975b, The role of macrophages in the generation of T helper cells. II. The genetic control of macrophages–T cell interaction of helper cell induction with soluble antigens, *J. Exp. Med.* **142**:460.

Erb, P., Feldmann, M., and Hogg, N., 1976, Role of macrophages in the generation of T helper cells. IV. Nature of genetically related factor derived from macrophages incubated with soluble antigen, *Eur. J. Immunol.* **6**:365.

Erb, P., Meier, B., and Feldmann, M., 1979a, Is genetically related macrophage factor (GRF) a soluble immune response (Ir) gene product?, *J. Immunol.* **122**:1916.

Erb, P., Meier, B., Matsunaga, T., and Feldmann, M., 1979b, Nature of T cell macrophage interaction in helper cell induction *in vitro*. II. Two stages of T helper cell differentiation analyzed in irradiation and allophenic chimeras, *J. Exp. Med.* **149**:686.

Erb, P., Vogt, P., Matsunaga, T., Rosenthal, A., and Feldmann, M., 1980, Nature of T cell–macrophage interaction in helper cell induction *in vitro*. III. Responsiveness of T cells differentiating in irradiation or allophenic chimeras depends on the genotype of the host, *J. Immunol.* **124**:2656.

Erb, P., Vogt, P., Cecka, M., and Feldmann, M., 1981, Activation of T cells by I region products released by macrophages, in: *Lymphokine Reports* (E. Pick, ed.), p. 125, Vol. 2, Academic Press, New York.

Feldmann, M., and Palmer, J., 1971, The requirement for macrophages in the secondary immune response to antigens of small and large size *in vitro*, *Immunology* **21**:685.

Feldmann, M., Erb, P., and Kontiainen, S., 1975, Cell collaboration between T and B lymphocytes and macrophages in antibody production, in: *Lymphocytes and Cell Interactions* (R. C. Williams, ed.), pp. 1–22, Raven Press, New York.

Feldmann, M., Rosenthal, A. S., and Erb, P., 1979, Macrophage–lymphocyte interactions in immune induction, *Int. Rev. Cytol.* **60:**149.

Feldmann, M., Sunshine, G. H., and Katz, D. R., 1984, RES-Leucocyte Interactions, in: *The Reticuloendothelial System, Vol. 7A: Physiology* (S. M. Reichard and J. P. Filkins, eds.), pp. 267–288. Plenum Press.

Gery, I., Gershon, R. K., and Waksman, B. M., 1972, Potentiation of T lymphocyte responses to mitogens, *J. Exp. Med.* **136:**128.

Gorczynski, R. M., 1977, Role of macrophage-derived factors in the generation of cytotoxic and antibody responses, *Scand. J. Immunol.* **6:**665–674.

Greineder, D. K., and Rosenthal, A. S., 1975, Macrophage activation of allogeneic lymphocyte proliferation in the guinea pig mixed leukocyte culture, *J. Immunol.* **114:**154.

Herzenberg, L. A., Black, S. J., and Herzenberg, L. A., 1980, Regulatory circuits and antibody responses, *Eur. J. Immunol.* **10:**1.

Humphrey, J. H., and Grennan, D., 1981, Different macrophage populations distinguished by means of fluorescent polysaccharides: Recognition and properties of marginal zone macrophages, *Eur. J. Immunol.* **11:**221.

Inaba, K., Nabane, K., and Muramatsu, S., 1981, Cellular synergy in the manifestation of accessory cell activity for *in vitro* antibody responses, *J. Immunol.* **127:**452.

Klaus, G. G. B., Humphrey, H. J., Kunkl, A., and Dongworth, D. W., 1980, The follicular dendritic cell: Its role in antigen presentation and in the generation of immunological memory, *Immunol. Rev.* **53:**3.

Klein, J., Juretic, A., Baxevanis, C. N., and Nagy, Z. A., 1981, The traditional and a new version of the mouse H-2 complex, *Nature (London)* **291:**455.

Larsson, E. L., Coutinhu, A., and Carlos-Martinez, A., 1980, A suggested mechanism for T lymphocyte activation: Implications of the acquisition of functional reactivities, *Immunol. Rev.* **51:**61.

Mitchison, N. A., 1969, The immunogenic capacity of antigen taken up by peritoneal exudate cells, *Immunology* **16:**1.

Mosier, D. E., 1969, Cell interactions in the primary immune response *in vitro:* A requirement for specific cell clusters, *J. Exp. Med.* **129:**351.

Nossal, G. J. V., and Ada, G. L., 1971, *Antigens, Lymphoid Cells, and the Immune Response,* Academic Press, New York.

Paetkau, V., Shaw, J., Mills, G., and Caplan, B., 1980, Cellular origins and targets of co-stimulator (IL2), *Immunol. Rev.* **51:**157.

Pierce, C. W., Kapp, J., and Benacerraf, B., 1976, Regulation by the H-2 gene complex of macrophage lymphoid cell interactions in secondary antibody responses *in vitro, J. Exp. Med.* **144:**371.

Puri, J., and Lonai, P., 1980, Mechanism of antigen binding by T cells: H-2 (IA) restricted binding of antigen plus Ia by helper cells, *Eur. J. Immunol.* **10:**273.

Raff, H. Y., Picher, L. J., and Stobo, J. D., 1980, Macrophage heterogeneity in man, *J. Exp. Med.* **152:**581

Rosenstreich, D. L., and Mizel, S. B., 1979, Signal requirements for T lymphocyte activation, *J. Immunol.* **22:**1749.

Rosenthal, A. S., and Shevach, E. M., 1973, Function of macrophages in antigen recognition by guinea pig T lymphocytes, *J. Exp. Med.* **138:**1194.

Rosenwasser, L. J., and Rosenthal, A. S., 1978, Adherent cell function in murine T lymphocyte recognition, I. Macrophage-dependent T cell proliferative assay in the mouse, *J. Immunol.* **120:**1991.

Scher, M. G., Beller, D. I., and Unanue, E. R., 1980, Demonstration of a soluble mediator that induces exudates rich in Ia-positive macrophages, *J. Exp. Med.* **152:**1684.

Schreier, M. H., and Tees, R., 1980, Clonal induction of helper T cells: Conversion of specific signals into non-specific signals, *Int. Arch. Allergy Appl. Immunol.* **61:**227.

Schreier, M. H., Iscove, N. N., Tees, R., Awden, L., and von Boehmer, H., 1980, Clones of killer and helper T cells: Growth requirements, specificity and relation of function in long term culture, *Immunol Rev.* **51:**315.

Schreier, M. H., Tees, R., and Nordin, A., 1982, Establishment and characterization of helper T cell clones: Their function, heterogeneity and effect on the B cell responses to particulate, soluble and T independent antigens, in *Lymphokines,* Vol. 5 (M. Feldmann and M. H. Schreir, eds.), pp. 443–465, Academic Press, New York.

Sheagren, J. N., Simon, H. B., Tuazon, C. U., and Mehrotra, P. P., 1975, Cell mediated immunity *in vitro,* in: *Monoclonal Phagocytes* (R. van Furth, ed.), Blackwell, Oxford.

Smith, K. A., 1980, T cell growth factor, *Immunol. Rev.* **51:**337.

Sprent, J., 1978, Role of H-2 gene products in the function of T helper cells from normal and chimeric mice measured *in vivo, Immunol. Rev.* **42:**108.

Sprent, J., 1978, Restricted helper function of F_1–parent bone marrow chimeras controlled by K end of H-2 complex, *J. Exp. Med.* **147:**1838.

Sprent, J., 1980, Blocking T cell function *in vivo* with anti Ia antibody, *J. Exp. Med.* **152:**996.

Sredni, B., Tse, H. Y., and Schwartz, R. H., 1980, Alloreactivity of an antigen specific T cell clone, *Nature (London)* **283:**581.

Steinman, R. M., and Cohn, Z. A., 1973, Identification of a novel cell type in the peripheral lymphoid organs of mice, *J. Exp. Med.* **137:**1142.

Stingl, G., Tamaki, K., and Katz, S. I., 1980, Origin and function of epidermal Langerhans cells, *Immunol. Rev.* **53:**149.

Sunshine, G. H., Katz, D. R., and Feldmann, M., 1980, Dendritic cells induce T cell proliferation to synthetic antigens under Ir gene control, *J. Exp. Med.* **152:**1817.

Sunshine, G. H., Katz, D. R., and Czitrom, A. A., 1982, Heterogeneity of accessory cells in the murine mixed leucocyte response, *Eur. J. Immunol.* **12:**9.

Veerman, A. J., 1974, On the interdigitating cells in the thymus dependent use of the rat spleen: A relation between the mononuclear phagocyte system and T lymphocytes, *Cell Tissue Res.* **148:**247.

Vogt, P., Erb, P., Keller, B., and Feldmann, M., 1980, Nature of macrophage T cell interaction in secondary helper cell generation *in vitro:* Genetic restriction of macrophage–T cell interaction which also determines T–B genetic restriction, *Eur. J. Immunol.* **11:**377.

Von Boehmer, H., Hans, W., and Jerne, N. K., 1978, MHC linked immune responsiveness is acquired by lymphocykes of low responder mice differentiating in the thymus of high responder mice, *Proc. Natl. Acad. Sci. USA* **75:**2439.

Wagner, H., Feldman, M., Boyle, W., and Scrader, J. W., 1972, Cell mediated immune responses *in vitro.* III. The requirement for macrophages in cytotoxic reactions against cell bound and subcellular alloantigens, *J. Exp. Med.* **136:**33.

Wagner, H., Hardt, C., Heeg, K., Pfizenmaier, K., Solbach, W., Bartlett, R., Stockingher, H., and Rollinghoff, M., 1980, T–T interactions during cytotoxic T lymphocyte responses: T cell derived helper factor (interleukin-2) as a probe to analyse CTL responsiveness and thymic maturation of CTL progenitors, *Immunol. Rev.* **51:**215.

Watson, J. D., 1979, Continuous proliferation of murine antigen specific helper T lymphocytes in culture, *J. Exp. Med.* **150:**1510.

Woody, J., Zvaifler, N., Rees, A., Ahmed, A., Hartzman, R., Strong, M., Howie, S., Kantor, F., and Feldmann, M., 1979, Human and mouse specific T cell helper factors assayed *in vivo* and *in vitro:* Implications for human Ir genes, *Transplant Proc.* **11:**382.

Zinkernagel, R. M., Althage, A., Waterfield, E., Kindred, B., Welsh, R. M., Callahan, G., and Pincett, P., 1980, Restriction specificities, alloreactivity and allotolerance expressed by T cells from nude mice reconstituted with H-2 compatible or incompatible thymus grafts, *J. Exp. Med.* **151:**376.

9

The Role of Macrophages in the Processing and Presentation of Protein Antigens to T Lymphocytes

THOMAS R. MALEK and ETHAN M. SHEVACH

1. INTRODUCTION

It is clear that macrophages serve as antigen-presenting cells for a variety of specific immune responses and that many antigens are presented by macrophages to T lymphocytes in the context of the products of the *I* region of the major histocompatibility gene complex (MHC) of a species. For example, *I*-region-controlled genetic restrictions have been described for the development and expression of helper T cells (Erb and Feldmann, 1975a; Marrack and Kappler, 1978), for T-lymphocyte proliferation (Rosenthal and Shevach, 1976; Schwartz *et al.*, 1978), and for delayed-type hypersensitivity (Miller, 1978). The use of recombinant and congenic mice and inbred guinea pigs has been an invaluable tool in establishing the role of the *I* region in antigen presentation. Furthermore, alloantisera to *I*-region gene products have demonstrated the necessity for the expression of Ia antigens on the surface of macrophages (Yamashita and Shevach, 1977; Cowing *et al.*, 1978). The ability of multispecific anti-Ia sera to produce marked inhibition of *in vitro* antigen-specific T-lymphocyte proliferation to conventional and immune response (Ir) gene-controlled antigens (Shevach, 1978) indicated that a complex of Ia antigens and the nominal antigen was seen by the T lymphocyte. The use of monoclonal anti-Ia antibodies in antigen-specific T-lymphocyte DNA synthetic responses of bulk cultured (Burger and Shevach, 1980; Lerner *et al.*, 1980) or cloned T cells (Clark *et al.*,1982) has demonstrated that the observed inhibition is most likely due to direct blocking of

THOMAS R. MALEK and ETHAN M. SHEVACH • Laboratory of Immunology, National Institute of Allergy and Infectious Diseases, National Institutes of Health, Bethesda, Maryland 20205.

Ia on the antigen-presenting macrophage and suggests that discrete epitopes on Ia are seen by an individual clone of antigen-specific T cells.

However, besides displaying antigen in the context of MHC gene products, it is believed that macrophages may be required to "process" or alter antigen prior to presentation to T cells. In this review we will concentrate on the problem of macrophage antigen handling. We will present the experimental evidence which has led to the concept of "processing" of antigen by macrophages and our most recent functional and biochemical data addressing this question. In addition, the relationships between macrophage antigen "processing" and the possible role of macrophages as the site of Ir gene expression will also be discussed.

2. EVIDENCE FOR ANTIGEN "PROCESSING" BY MACROPHAGES

The term antigen "processing" has been coined not to describe a discrete biological mechanism but to account for a series of functional experiments which suggest that native determinants of the nominal antigen are not presented by macrophages to the appropriate T lymphocytes. These studies, therefore, imply that the macrophage has altered the antigen before presentation to T cells.

2.1. THE EFFECT OF ANTIANTIGEN ANTIBODY ON T-CELL ANTIGEN RECOGNITION

In contrast to the success of anti-Ia antibody in defining the requirement for Ia in antigen presentation, antibodies to protein antigens have not been successfully employed to determine the nature of the nominal antigen displayed by macrophages. The early studies of Uhr and Pappenheimer (1958) which demonstrated that immunization with antigen–antibody complexes formed in antibody excess were potent inducers of delayed hypersensitivity, yet simultaneously caused marked suppression of antibody formation, suggested that antibody to antigen was incapable of inhibiting what we now know to be a T-cell-mediated phenomenon. Ellner and Rosenthal (1975) demonstrated that both guinea pig and rabbit antibodies to 2,4-dinitrophenyl (DNP)-guinea pig albumin present continuously in culture did not affect the degree of guinea pig T-cell proliferation induced by DNP-guinea pig albumin-bearing macrophages. Similarly, Ben-Sasson *et al.* (1977) were unable to inhibit the binding of antigen-specific T cells to autologous antigen-pulsed macrophages with antibody to antigen; even when a second layer of antibody to the heterologous antibody was used no inhibition was observed. These studies, therefore, suggest that immunologically relevant antigen is either in a site inaccessible to antibody or that the antigen-specific receptor on T cells is reactive with a moiety not present on the native protein antigen, e.g., a macrophage-"processed" antigen fragment or an antigen-induced alteration of the Ia molecule on the cell surface.

A possible exception to the general observation that antiantigen antibody has no effect on T-lymphocyte function was seen in the studies of Thomas *et al.* (1978) using trinitrophenyl (TNP)-modified macrophages as antigen-presenting cells. These studies demonstrated that high-titer guinea pig anti-TNP sera added either to the primary or secondary culture could substantially inhibit the TNP-specific T-cell proliferative response. However, the stimulatory capacity of macrophages which had been TNP-modified but cultured at 37°C for 24 hr (aged) prior to addition to primed T cells was unaffected by similar treatment. This result was consistent with the view that the macrophage must process membrane-conjugated TNP in a manner so that it was inaccessible to anti-TNP antibody to create the relevant immunogen recognized by the T cell.

Further analysis of the guinea pig T-cell response to hapten-modified macrophages, however, has suggested that the failure of antihapten antibody to inhibit responses when aged hapten-modified macrophages were the source of presenting cells was simply due to too low a density of hapten to allow for efficient binding of antihapten antibody (Shevach *et al.*, 1979; Shevach, 1980). These studies demonstrated that the available density of TNP groups on the aged, TNP-modified macrophage was 2% of that on freshly modified cells and that when the density of haptenic groups on the surface of the aged, TNP-modified macrophage was increased by subsequent treatment with the non-cross-reactive (at the T cell level, but not antibody level) DNP hapten, the TNP-specific proliferative response induced by these doubly haptenated cells could be inhibited when the cultures were performed in the presence of anti-TNP antibody.

The results in the TNP system, therefore, suggested that the failure of others to demonstrate an effect of antiantigen antibody on T-cell activation was simply secondary to the low density of antigenic determinants on the macrophage membrane with resultant low-affinity binding of antibody to antigen. We have recently directly tested this hypothesis by using the TNP hapten as a probe for the soluble antigen rather than as the antigenic moiety itself. The basic experimental protocol was to assess the effect of anti-TNP antibodies present continuously in culture on the antigen-specific (not TNP-specific) T-cell proliferative response to macrophages pulsed with soluble protein antigens when the macrophages had been treated with TNP following the pulse exposure to the protein antigen. A summary of a series of such experiments is presented in Table 1. When macrophages which were pulsed with soluble protein antigen and then TNP-modified were cultured with the appropriate primed T cells in the presence of anti-TNP antibodies, a marked inhibition of the T-cell proliferative response to the soluble protein antigen under study was observed. However, in order for inhibition to be seen, a lag period (aging) of at least 1–3 hr was required following pulse exposure to the protein antigen and prior to TNP modification of the macrophage surface (Groups 3, 4, 5). For inhibition to be observed the protein antigen must contain a sufficient number of free amino groups assessible to TNP modification. Thus, the antigen-specific T-cell proliferative response to L-glutamic acid, L-Tyrosine (GT) which only contains one free amino group (the N-terminal amino acid) was not inhibited by anti-TNP antibodies in these experiments (Group 6). Therefore, this result and the observation that inhibition by

TABLE 1. INHIBITION OF THE T-CELL PROLIFERATIVE RESPONSE INDUCED BY MACROPHAGES WHICH WERE BOTH PULSED WITH ANTIGEN AND TNP-MODIFIED BY ANTI-TNP ANTIBODIES[a]

Group	Immune T cells[b]	Macrophage treatment	% inhibition
1	OVA	TNP/OVA	0
2	OVA	OVA/TNP	0
3	OVA	OVA/21 hr aged per TNP	64 ± 5
4	GL	GL/21 hr aged per TNP	91 ± 7
5	PPD	PPD/21 hr aged per TNP	51 ± 8
6	GT	GT/21 hr aged per TNP	8 ± 4

[a]Macrophages were pulsed with the indicated antigen and either immediately TNP-modified (Group 2) or aged for 21 hr prior to TNP modification (Groups 3–6). Some macrophages were TNP-modified prior to pulse exposure to antigen (Group 1). These macrophages (1×10^5) were cultured for 3 days with the indicated primed T cells (1×10^5) in 5% NGPS or 5% anti-TNP serum. The data are calculated as % inhibition as follows: 1 − (Δcpm in anti-TNP serum/Δcpm in NGPS)100. The Δcpm reflect the responses generated to antigen-pulsed macrophages minus the response to unpulsed macrophages. Each value represents the mean inhibition of 4–6 experiments ± S.E.
[b]OVA, Ovalbumin; GL, L-glutamic acid, L-lysine; GT, L-glutamic acid, L-tyrosine.

anti-TNP did not occur when the macrophages were TNP-modified before pulse exposure to antigen (Group 1) demonstrated the necessity of directly modifying the nominal antigen with TNP. Since pulse exposure of the macrophages with TNP-derivatized proteins without TNP modification of the macrophage membrane failed to lead to inhibition of proliferation, TNP modification of macrophage membrane molecules also appeared to be required.

Only intact IgG and $F(ab')_2$, but not monomeric Fab, fractions of anti-TNP antibodies were effective inhibitors of the proliferative response (Table 2). The necessity for bivalent binding raised the possibility that capping and shedding of TNP-modified nominal antigen along with TNP-modified membrane glycoproteins from the surface of the macrophage might account for the inhibition by anti-TNP antibodies. Data in support of this possibility were obtained from

TABLE 2. THE REQUIREMENT FOR BIVALENT BINDING OF ANTI-TNP ANTIBODY FOR INHIBITION OF PROLIFERATION TO AGED ANTIGEN-PULSED TNP-MODIFIED MACROPHAGES[a]

Immune T cells	Macrophage treatment	Anti-TNP	% inhibition
OVA	OVA/24 hr per TNP	IgG	65 ± 5
		$F(ab')_2$	54 ± 4
		Fab	12 ± 6
PPD	PPD/24 hr per TNP	IgG	55 ± 7
		$F(ab')_2$	48 ± 2
		Fab	3 ± 1
GL	GL/24 hr per TNP	IgG	95 ± 6
		$F(ab')_2$	73 ± 11

[a]Macrophages were pulsed with the indicated antigen and aged for 24 hr before TNP modification. These macrophages (1×10^5) were cultured for 3 days with the indicated primed T cells (1×10^5) in 5% NGPS or the indicated fraction of anti-TNP antibodies. Data are calculated as shown in Table 1.

pretreatment studies in which pulsed-aged TNP-modified macrophages were briefly cultured in anti-TNP serum, washed extensively, and then used as antigen-presenting cells with the appropriate immune T cells in cultures containing normal guinea pig serum. Marked inhibition of the proliferative response was detected when the macrophages were precultured with anti-TNP antibodies (Table 3). This result, therefore, supports a capping and shedding mechanism as responsible for the observed functional inhibition.

Thus, our studies in the TNP system strongly suggest that the failure of antibodies to nominal antigen to inhibit T-cell function was not due to the nominal antigen being sequestered in a site where it was inaccessible to the antibody. These studies suggest that the density of antigen on the macrophage cell surface is critical in order for antiantigen antibody to produce inhibition of T-cell function. These experiments, however, do not directly assess the biochemical nature of the nominal antigen associated with the macrophage membrane. Thus, the failure of others to block T-cell function with antiantigen antibodies may still reflect a macrophage-induced alteration of the nominal antigen. Furthermore, the requirement in our studies that the antigen-pulsed macrophages be cultured for several hours prior to TNP modification in order for inhibition to be seen is also consistent with the view that a macrophage processing event may occur.

2.2. T-CELL REACTIVITY TO DENATURED PROTEIN ANTIGENS

Studies employing denatured protein antigens have demonstrated that some T-cell responses do not require recognition of native antigen. Gell and Benacerraf (1959) demonstrated that delayed-type hypersensitivity could be elicited in animals primed with native bovine serum albumin (BSA) when challenged with either native or urea-denatured BSA. Subsequently, several additional studies have demonstrated that T-cell responses could be generated with native and either denatured or chemically modified antigens regardless of the form of antigen used for priming the T lymphocytes; however, secondary anti-

TABLE 3. INHIBITION OF MACROPHAGE PRESENTATION BY BRIEF EXPOSURE TO ANTI-TNP ANTIBODY[a]

Immune T cells	Macrophage treatment	Preculture	cpm
OVA	OVA/21 hr per TNP	NGPS	60,877
		anti-TNP	16,474
GL	GL/21 hr per TNP	NGPS	22,275
		anti-TNP	4,155

[a]Macrophages were pulsed with the indicated antigen and cultured for 21 hr before TNP modification. Treated macrophages were then incubated for an additional 3 hr at 37°C in 20% NGPS or anti-TNP serum and then washed. These macrophages (1×10^5) were cultured for 3 days with the indicated immune T cells in 5% NGPS. The results are exposed as Δcpm/culture of [^{3}H]-TdR incorporation which represents the cpm obtained from cultures with antigen-pulsed macrophages minus the cpm from cultures with unpulsed macrophages.

body responses were detected only when the same form of the antigen was used to prime and challenge the animals (Ishizaka *et al.*, 1975; Takatsu and Ishizaka, 1975; Schirrmacher and Wigzell, 1972).

In several recent studies Grey and his colleagues (Endres and Grey, 1980b; Chesnut *et al.*, 1980) extended these observations by demonstrating that the T-cell proliferative response and tolerance induction to native and denatured forms of ovalbumin are highly cross-reactive and that the same set of T cells may be responding to both forms of the antigen. In contrast, a similar cross-reactivity between these forms of ovalbumin was not observed for the development of suppressor T-cell activity (Endres and Grey, 1980a). These authors argue that the observed cross-reaction between native and denatured forms of antigen can be best explained by a macrophage "processing" step in which the same "sequential" determinants are generated from both forms of the antigen. Yet in experiments which examined the ability of antibodies to denatured ovalbumin to inhibit T-cell proliferation to both forms of the antigen, no inhibition was detected.

The studies with denatured and native protein antigens deserve further comment. Clearly these studies illustrate that the T cell may react with antigenic determinants not seen by antibodies. With the exception of the study by Chesnut *et al.* (1980), no one has addressed the question of whether the same clone of T cells is reactive to both forms of the antigen. Nevertheless, data demonstrating this point do not prove that macrophages must "process" antigen. Macrophages are phagocytic cells and through the action of proteolytic enzymes may break down an antigen to its component fragments. Similar fragments may be derived from native and denatured forms of a given antigen. These fragments may then be released into the surrounding environment only to later become associated with the macrophage cell surface. If a particular fragment is recognized as foreign, a T-cell response is generated with the resulting observation that either the native or the denatured form of the antigen is presented effectively to a clone of antigen-specific T cells. Physiologically, this breakdown of antigen by the macrophage may be crucial for presentation of a particulate antigen such as *Listeria* as suggested by Unanue (1981). The question, however, which remains is whether this type of degradation of an antigen is in fact equivalent to "processing" and is it an obligate requirement for antigen presentation.

2.3. IMMUNOGENIC MATERIAL FROM SUPERNATANTS OF ANTIGEN-PULSED MACROPHAGES

Additional functional experiments which have supported the notion of macrophage "processing" of antigen are the observations that supernatant fluids from cell cultures containing macrophages and antigen are capable of inducing T-helper cells *in vitro* (Erb and Feldmann, 1975b) or binding to T-helper cells (Puri and Lonai, 1980). Each study has demonstrated that the biologically active material is restricted by the *I* region of the MHC in its action and that the biological activity can be removed by immunosorbent coated with anti-Ia antibodies. The nature of the antigen associated with these factors is unknown. Erb *et al.* (1976) indicated that antiantigen immunosorbent was not able to remove biological activity. Puri and Lonai (1980) have suggested that their factor contains determinants derived from the nominal antigen because radioactive antigen could be retained on anti-Ia immunosorbent columns.

3. Ir GENE DEFECT AT THE LEVEL OF THE MACROPHAGE

The ability of an animal to respond to a variety of synthetic polypeptide antigens and some conventional antigens, e.g., insulin and cytochrome *c*, is controlled by genes mapping within the *I* region of the MHC of the species under study. The cellular level of expression of the genetic defect which leads to nonresponsiveness to these antigens has still not been definitively established. Nevertheless, one candidate for the expression of the Ir gene defect is the antigen-presenting macrophage. This possibility has been suggested by a number of investigators using a variety of experimental models either *in vitro* or *in vivo* including radiation chimeras. Although it is beyond the scope of this chapter to review these experiments (for a recent review see Longo *et al.*, 1981) the critical observation in these studies is the failure of macrophages from the nonresponder parental strain to present antigen to primed (nonresponder × responder) F_1 T cells.

Here again we are confronted with the situation in which a series of functional experiments suggest that the macrophage must actively do something to the antigen prior to presentation. Thus, an Ir gene defect in the macrophage may be due to ineffective "processing" of the antigen and/or inappropriate association of the nominal antigen on the macrophage surface with Ia in forming the immunogenic moiety seen by T cells. Benacerraf (1978) has suggested that the Ia molecule on macrophages interacts specifically with a unique amino acid sequence on the native antigen. The determinant selection model of Rosenthal (1978) suggests that the macrophage plays a fundamental role in displaying the determinants to be seen by the T cell.

An alternative explanation for these experiments, however, is that the observed Ir gene defect is expressed at the level of the T cell, not the macrophage. Certainly, experiments which demonstrated that nonresponder macrophages are effective antigen-presenting cells would favor this view. The experiments of Pierce *et al.* (1976) which successfully primed responder mice with antigen-pulsed nonresponder macrophages support this notion although the potential for allogeneic effects and suppressor T-cell activity in this system raises the possibility that other factors may account for their results. Recently, Ishii *et al.* (1981) have reported experiments in which following deletion of alloreactive T cells, nonresponder macrophages presented several Ir gene-controlled antigens to responder T cells using a sensitive T-cell proliferation assay. Studies in our laboratory have resulted in the detection of T-cell clones from responder guinea pigs which recognized L-glutamic acid, L-lysine (GL) in association with nonresponder Ia (Clark and Shevach, 1982). In this system the alloreactive T cells could be completely separated from the antigen-specific T cells by cloning in soft agar and expanding the appropriate colonies with antigen in the presence of nonresponder macrophages. Similar results have also been noted with insulin as the antigen under study (Drs. G. Dos Reis and E. M. Shevach, unpublished data). Collectively these data question whether an Ir gene defect is expressed at the level of the macrophage. Therefore, although macrophages may "process" antigen prior to presentation, this phenomenon may not be related to Ir gene expression.

4. DIRECT ANALYSIS OF MACROPHAGE-ASSOCIATED NOMINAL ANTIGEN

An approach to the question of whether macrophages "process" antigen and an analysis of the nature of the stimulatory moiety on this cell population requires experiments which directly examine macrophage-associated nominal antigen. Unfortunately, the few experiments reported in the literature along these lines have not been particularly revealing with regard to these questions and have in some instances led to contradictory conclusions.

The experiments which follow the fate of antigen in macrophages involve the pulse exposure of macrophages to radiolabeled antigen, the determination of the amount of antigen taken up by these cells, and an estimate of the persistence and cellular compartmentalization (cell surface versus intracellular) of the retained antigen. In general, these studies demonstrated that 0.2–0.6% of the antigen was cell-associated after pulse exposure and of this material 10–20% resisted early destruction depending on the molecular species of antigen under study (Unanue and Cerottini, 1970; Ellner and Rosenthal, 1975). Five hours after pulse exposure, very little of the remaining macrophage-retained antigen was lost upon further culture. Studies in both the mouse (Unanue and Cerottini, 1970) and the guinea pig (Ellner and Rosenthal, 1975) have shown that after 1 day of culture, 15–20% of the residual cell-bound antigen remained trypsin-sensitive and was presumably located on the cell surface. Attempts to directly demonstrate antigen on the cell surface, however, using electron microscopy have been unsuccessful (Steinman and Cohn, 1973).

Considerable controversy exists concerning the significance of the cell surface-associated trypsin-sensitive component. Unanue and Cerottini (1970) evaluated in an *in vivo* model the immunogenicity of antigen-pulsed trypsin-treated macrophages and demonstrated that two-thirds of the immune response was abrogated by trypsinization of the macrophages after uptake of antigen. In contrast, Ellner and Rosenthal (1975) in an *in vitro* assay which measured T-cell proliferation and Ben-Sasson *et al.* (1977) in an *in vitro* assay which assessed specific binding of immune T cells to antigen-pulsed macrophages could detect no effect after trypsin treatment of the pulsed cells. However, Ben-Sasson *et al.* (1977) did note that the enzyme Pronase was capable of diminishing the capacity of macrophages previously pulsed with antigen to bind specific T lymphocytes.

Therefore, the failure of trypsin may be related to its restricted sites of proteolytic activity.

Our demonstration that the stimulatory capacity of antigen-pulsed macrophages which had been modified with TNP was markedly reduced in the presence of anti-TNP antibodies suggested that the determinants of the nominal antigen required for the induction of a T-cell proliferative response were modified by the TNP hapten. Furthermore, since the conjugation of the TNP hapten to the macrophage is predominantly a cell surface phenomena (Bonsall and Hunt, 1971; Arrotti and Garvin, 1972; Comoglio *et al.*, 1978; Kaplan *et al.*, 1979), this result also suggested that the immunologically relevant antigen was located on the macrophage cell surface.

We have also used the TNP hapten as a cell surface-specific probe to immunochemically reassess the cellular compartmentalization of antigen in macrophages. Our first experiments on the fate of antigen in the macrophage sought to measure the uptake of antigen in macrophages and to attempt to directly demonstrate TNP-modified antigen on the macrophage cell surface. All these experiments were performed using the terpolymer L-glutamic acid, L-lysine, L-tyrosine (GLT) as the antigen. GLT was chosen since it may be radioiodinated as well as modified with TNP and since the response to it is under the control of MHC-linked Ir genes in guinea pigs.

Our antigen uptake studies with GLT demonstrated results very similar to those seen with other antigens in either the mouse or the guinea pig (Table 4). Immediately after antigen pulsing, 0.32% of the ^{125}I-labeled GLT was associated with the macrophages and 19 and 7% of the initial ^{125}I-labeled GLT remained cell-associated after a 3- and 24-hr culture, respectively.

Our approach for the detection of nominal antigen on the cell surface of macrophages was to first pulse macrophages with ^{125}I-labeled GLT and then TNP-modify these cells at various times after the pulse exposure. We predicted that GLT on the cell surface would contain the ^{125}I label as well as the TNP-haptenic group while intracellular GLT would contain only the ^{125}I label. These molecular species of antigen could be distinguished by quantitative radioprecipitation analysis of detergent extracts from fresh and aged GLT-pulsed TNP-modified macrophages with anti-GLT and anti-TNP antisera.

A summary of several experiments is shown in Table 5. Fresh and aged GLT-pulsed TNP-modified macrophages always contained [^{125}I]-GLT which

TABLE 4. UPTAKE OF GLT BY MACROPHAGES[a]

	% GLT cell associated
Fresh	0.320
3 hr aged	0.061
24 hr aged	0.022

[a]Macrophages were pulsed with [^{125}I]-GLT for 1 hr at 37°C and the amount of cell-associated cpm was determined immediately after the pulse exposure (fresh) or after a 3- and 24-hr culture period (aged).

TABLE 5. EXPRESSION OF GLT ON THE SURFACE OF FRESH AND AGED MACROPHAGES[a]

		NP-40 extract % ^{125}I cpm precipitated	
Group	Macrophage treatment	Anti-GLT	Anti-TNP
1	GLT/TNP	35	17
2	GLT/3 hr aged per TNP	34	28
3	GLT/24 hr aged per TNP	22	20
4	TNP/GLT	37	4
5	GLT	36	3

[a]Macrophages were pulsed with [^{125}I]-GLT and then modified with TNP immediately (Group 1), after a 3- or 24-hr aging culture (Groups 2 and 3), or were not subject to TNP modification (Group 5). Macrophages were also TNP-modified before the pulse exposure to GLT (Group 4). After treatment, the cell-associated radioactive GLT was extracted with 0.5% NP-40 and radioprecipitation assays with anti-TNP and anti-GLT sera were performed on these extracts. Data are expressed as percentage of radioactivity precipitated with the indicated antisera minus the percentage precipitated with NGPS. This NGPS value ranged from 4 to 10%.

was precipitable with anti-TNP (Groups 1, 2, 3). Therefore, this result demonstrated the presence of cell surface-associated nominal antigen on macrophages. A consistent observation was that the amount of GLT precipitated with anti-GLT from extracts of fresh-pulsed cells was always substantially greater than that precipitated with anti-TNP (Group 1), suggesting that a pool of GLT escaped TNP modification and was presumably intracellular. In contrast, a similar percentage of radioactivity was precipitated by anti-GLT and anti-TNP when extracts of aged-pulsed TNP-modified macrophages were analyzed (Groups 2, 3). Sequential radioprecipitation studies (data not shown) demonstrated that most of the cell surface-associated GLT of the fresh and aged macrophages (anti-TNP precipitable) also contained determinants of the native antigen (anti-GLT precipitable).

Control experiments demonstrated that detergent extracts from macrophages which had been TNP-modified prior to GLT-pulsing or from macrophages which had been GLT-pulsed but not TNP-modified contained [^{125}I]-GLT precipitable with anti-GLT but not anti-TNP antisera (Groups 4, 5). Therefore, precipitation of GLT with anti-TNP was due to covalent association of TNP with GLT and not secondary to the association of TNP-modified membrane molecules and unmodified GLT.

One intriguing observation in these experiments was the demonstration of a pool of intracellular GLT in the fresh-pulsed cells and its absence in the aged-pulsed macrophages. These results suggested that internalized antigen may have been recompartmentalized to the macrophage cell surface during the aging culture and, therefore, may represent macrophage-"processed" antigen. A series of experiments which directly test this possibility are summarized in Table 6. Macrophages were pulsed with GLT and then TNP-modified; detergent extracts were prepared from some cells immediately after the TNP modification while other aliquots of these pulsed-haptenated cells were aged for various times (1–24 hr) before detergent extraction. We hypothesized that if the cell surface antigen

TABLE 6. TNP-MODIFIED GLT FROM FRESH-PULSED MACROPHAGES IS RETAINED BY AGED ANTIGEN-PULSED MACROPHAGES[a]

	NP-40 extract % ^{125}I cpm precipitated	
Macrophage treatment	Anti-GLT	Anti-TNP
GLT/TNP	28	17
GLT/TNP per 2 hr aged	27	17
GLT/TNP per 4 hr aged	21	12
GLT/TNP per 20 hr aged	21	15

[a]Macrophages were pulsed with [^{125}I]-GLT and then immediately treated with TNP. Some macrophages were immediately extracted with NP-40 while others were aged for 2, 4, or 20 hr, as indicated, before detergent extraction. Assay and data were analyzed as indicated in Table 5.

of the aged macrophage was comprised of GLT that was first internalized, these antigen molecules should have escaped TNP modification when the cells were haptenated immediately after the pulse, and, therefore, the amount of [^{125}I]-GLT precipitable with anti-TNP from these cells should significantly decrease with aging these macrophages. Surprisingly, the percentage of anti-TNP-precipitable material was similar at each time point during the culture. These results suggest that the GLT molecules present in the intracellular compartment of the macrophage immediately following pulse exposure are not expressed on the cell surface of the macrophage at a later time.

One difficulty encountered in the interpretation of this experiment is that a lag period of 1–24 hr elapsed between the time of TNP modification and the time of detergent extraction. Thus, we have no direct proof that the TNP-modified GLT extracted from these cells was in fact present on the cell surface at the time

TABLE 7. THE CELL SURFACE RETENTION OF GLT FROM ANTIGEN-PULSED MACROPHAGES[a]

		NP-40 extract % ^{125}I cpm precipitated	
Group	Macrophage treatment	Anti-GLT	Anti-TNP
1	GLT/16 hr aged per TNP	24	22
2	GLT/TNP per 16 hr aged	24	23
3	GLT/TNP/16 hr aged per TNP	24	29

[a]Macrophages were pulsed with [^{125}I]-GLT and some were modified with TNP after a 16-hr aging culture (Group 1). Other aliquots were immediately modified with TNP after the pulse exposure to GLT and aged for 16 hr (Group 2); the macrophages in Group 3 received a second TNP treatment after the aging culture. NP-40 extracts were prepared from each group and the assay and data were analyzed as in Table 5.

of detergent extraction. In fact, the TNP-modified GLT may have been recompartmentalized from the cell surface to some intracellular site during the aging culture. In order to rule out this possibility, we TNP-modified the cells immediately after pulse exposure and again 16 hr later just prior to detergent extraction (Table 7). We reasoned that if the TNP-modified GLT present after a 16-hr aging culture from cells that were haptenated only after pulse exposure was in an intracellular site, then the amount of anti-TNP-precipitable material should be significantly greater in aliquots of cells that were haptenated twice, immediately after pulse exposure and again prior to extraction. However, it is clear from Table 7 (compare Group 3 to Group 2) that the percentage of [^{125}I]-GLT reactive with anti-TNP is independent of the time of TNP modification and is similar in all groups. A slight increase (~ 3–5%) for the doubly haptenated cells (Group 3) was observed in several experiments. These data indicate that essentially all the cell surface GLT of the fresh-pulsed macrophages is retained on the cell surface after aging and that very little of the intracellular GLT bound by the fresh-pulsed cells has been recompartmentalized to the surface of the macrophage during the aging culture.

Our functional studies indicated that the immunologically revelant antigen resides in the pool of antigen which is located on the cell surface of the aged-pulsed macrophage. The companion experiments which examined the fate of GLT in macrophages demonstrated that the cell surface pool of GLT of the aged-pulsed cells was predominately derived from GLT which was initially cell surface associated. The antigen associated with the aged macrophage represents approximately 10% of the GLT associated with the fresh-pulsed macrophage. Furthermore, during the aging culture it appears that cell surface and intracellular GLT are degraded at similar rates (T. R. Malek, L. T. Clement, and E. M. Shevach, unpublished data).

In evaluating these data it is necessary to consider the level at which macrophage "processing" of GLT may have occurred. First, macrophage "processing" of a soluble antigen may be a rapid event which takes place during the pulse-exposure period (generally 45–60 min in our studies) with resulting cell surface expression of the immunogenic moiety. Second, all "processing" of GLT might be mediated by ectoenzymes on the macrophage cell surface without a requirement for internalization of the antigen. Third, it is conceivable that the very small pool of GLT which has apparently been recompartmentalized from the interior to the cell surface of the macrophage may represent "processed" antigen and the entire pool of immunologically relevant antigen resides here. Our failure to inhibit the T-cell proliferative response with anti-TNP antibodies when fresh-pulsed TNP-modified macrophages were the source of antigen-presenting cells is consistent with this view; however, it is also likely that other factors, such as incomplete capping and shedding of the nominal antigen, may be operative in the failure to inhibit the response generated to the fresh-pulsed cell. Lastly, it seems equally possible as originally suggested by Unanue and Cerottini (1970) that the immunogenic moiety is not a "processed" fragment and that the membrane of the macrophage contains a site(s) where some molecules of antigen escape degradation and retain their original structure.

5. CONCLUSION

At this point we believe that the experimental data accumulated do not decisively prove that macrophages actively "process" antigen prior to presentation. Although the failure of antiantigen antibody to block T-cell proliferation, the cross-reactivity at the T-cell level between native and denatured forms of antigen, and the apparent inability of nonresponder macrophages to serve as antigen-presenting cells have often been interpreted to favor macrophage "processing" models to explain these phenomena, other models, not requiring macrophages to "process" antigens, may also explain these observations. Therefore, the failure of antiantigen antibody to inhibit T-cell proliferation may simply be due to the low concentration of antigen on the macrophage cell surface as our experiments employing TNP as an antigen itself or a probe for soluble protein antigens have suggested. Furthermore, recent experiments in our laboratory (Clark and Shevach, 1982) and by Ishii *et al.* (1981) seriously question whether the Ir gene defect is in fact expressed at the level of the antigen-presenting cell.

Clearly, biochemical studies of macrophage-associated nominal antigen are necessary for precisely establishing the nature of the immunogenic moiety on macrophages. The difficulties in performing such studies thus far have been due not only to the heterogeneous nature of the cell populations used but also to the small amounts of antigen associated with these cells. The recent demonstration of antigen-presenting function of several cloned B-cell tumor lines (McKean *et al.*, 1981; Glimcher *et al.*, 1982) and a dendritic cell-like clone isolated from the P388 cell line (Cohen and Kaplan, 1981) may now provide a homogeneous population of cells to overcome the former obstacle for biochemical studies of nominal antigen associated with a presenting cell.

REFERENCES

Arrotti, J. J., and Garvin, J. E., 1972, Reaction of human serum albumin and human erythrocytes with tritiated 2,4,6-trinitrobenzene sulfonic acid and tritiated picryl chloride, *Biochim. Biophys. Acta* **225**:79.

Benacerraf, B., 1978, A hypothesis to relate the specificity of T lymphocytes and the activity of I region-specific Ir genes in macrophages and B lymphocytes, *J. Immunol.* **120**:1809.

Ben-Sasson, S. Z., Lipscomb, M. F., Tucker, T. F., and Uhr, J. W., 1977, The specific binding of T lymphocytes to macrophages. II. Role of macrophage-associated antigen, *J. Immunol.* **119**:1493.

Bonsall, R. W., and Hunt, S., 1971, The reactivity of the human erythrocyte membrane to sodium trinitrobenzenesulphonate, *Biochim. Biophys. Acta* **249**:281.

Burger, R., and Shevach, E. M., 1980, Monoclonal antibodies to guinea pig Ia antigens. II. Effect on alloantigen, antigen, and mitogen induced T lymphocyte proliferation in vitro, *J. Exp. Med.* **152**:1011.

Chesnut, R. W., Endres, R. O., and Grey, H. M., 1980, Antigen recognition by T cells and B cells: Recognition of cross-reactivity between native and denatured forms of globular antigens, *Clin. Immunol. Immunopathol.* **15**:397.

Clark, R. B., and Shevach, E. M., 1982, Generation of T cell colonies from responder strain 2 guinea pigs that recognize the copolymer L-glutamic acid, L-lysine in association with nonresponder strain 13 Ia antigens, *J. Exp. Med.* **155**:635.

Clark, R. B., Chiba, J., Zweig, S. E., and Shevach, E. M., 1982, T cell colonies recognize antigen in association with specific epitopes on Ia molecules, *Nature (London)* **294**:412.

Cohen, D. A., and Kaplan, A. M., 1981, Adherent Ia$^+$ murine tumor lines with characteristics of dendritic cells. I. Morphology, surface phenotype, and induction of syngeneic mixed lymphocyte reaction, *J. Exp. Med.* **154**:1881.

Comoglio, P. M., Tarone, G., and Bertini, M., 1978, Immunochemical purification of probe-labeled plasma membrane proteins: An approach to the molecular anatomy of the cell surface, *J. Supramol. Struct.* **8**:301.

Cowing, C., Pincus, S. H., Sachs, D. H., and Dickler, H. B., 1978, A subpopulation of adherent accessory cells bearing both I-A and I-E or C subregion antigens is required for antigen-specific murine T lymphocyte proliferation, *J. Immunol.* **121**:1680.

Ellner, J. J., and Rosenthal, A. S., 1975, Quantitative and immunologic aspects of the handling of 2,4-dinitrophenyl guinea pig albumin by macrophages, *J. Immunol.* **114**:1563.

Endres, R. O., and Grey, H. M., 1980a, Antigen recognition by T cells. I. Suppressor T cells fail to recognize cross-reactivity between native and denatured ovalbumin, *J. Immunol.* **125**:1515.

Endres, R. O., and Grey, H. M., 1980b, Antigen recognition by T cells. II. Intravenous administration of native or denatured ovalbumin results in tolerance to both forms of the antigen, *J. Immunol.* **125**:1521.

Erb, P., and Feldmann, M., 1975a, The role of macrophages in the generation of T-helper cells. II. The genetic control of the macrophage–T-cell interaction for helper cell induction with soluble antigens, *J. Exp. Med.* **142**:460.

Erb, P., and Feldmann, M., 1975b, The role of macrophages in the generation of T helper cells. III. Influence of macrophage-derived factor in helper cell induction, *Eur. J. Immunol.* **5**:759.

Erb, P., Feldmann, M., and Hogg, N., 1976, Role of macrophages in the generation of T helper cells. IV. Nature of genetically related factor derived from macrophages incubated with soluble antigen, *Eur. J. Immunol.* **6**:365.

Gell, P. G. H., and Benacerraf, B., 1959, Studies on hypersensitivity. II. Delayed hypersensitivity to denatured proteins in guinea pigs, *Immunology* **2**:64.

Glimcher, L. H., Kim, K.-J., Green, I., and Paul, W. E., 1982, Ia antigen-bearing B cell tumor lines can present protein antigen and alloantigen in a major histocompatibility complex-restricted fashion to antigen-reactive T cells, *J. Exp. Med.* **155**:445.

Ishii, N., Baxevanis, C. N., Nagy, Z. A., and Klein, J., 1981, Responder T cells depleted of alloreactive cells react to antigen presented on allogeneic macrophages from nonresponder strains, *J. Exp. Med.* **154**:978.

Ishizaka, K., Okudaira, H., and King, T. P., 1975, Immunogenic properties of modified antigen E. II. Ability of urea-denatured antigen and α-polypeptide chain to prime T cells specific for antigen E, *J. Immunol.* **114**:110.

Kaplan, G., Unkeless, J. C., and Cohn, Z. A., 1979, Insertion and turnover of macrophage plasma membrane proteins, *Proc. Natl. Acad. Sci. USA* **76**:3824.

Lerner, E. A., Matis, L. A., Janeway, C. A., Jones, P. P., Schwartz, R. H., and Murphy, D. B., 1980, Monoclonal antibody against an Ir gene product, *J. Exp. Med.* **152**:1085.

Longo, D. L., Matis, L. A., and Schwartz, R. H., 1981, Insights into immune response gene function from experiments with chimeric animals, *CRC Crit. Rev. Immunol.* **2**:83.

McKean, D. J., Infante, A. F., Nilson, A., Kimoto, M., Fathman, C. G., Walker, E., and Warner, N., 1981, Major histocompatibility complex-restricted antigen presentation to antigen reactive T cells by B lymphocyte tumor cells, *J. Exp. Med.* **154**:1419.

Marrack, P., and Kappler, J., 1978, The role of H-2 linked genes in helper T cell function. III. Expression of immune response genes for trinitrophenyl conjugates of poly-L(Tyr, Glu)-poly D,L-Ala-poly-L-Lys in B cells and macrophages, *J. Exp. Med.* **147**:1596.

Miller, J. F. A. P., 1978, Restrictions imposed on T lymphocyte reactivities by the major histocompatibility complex: Implications for T cell repertoire selection, *Immunol. Rev.* **42**:76.

Pierce, C. W., Kapp, J. A., and Benacerraf, B., 1976, Regulation by the H-2 gene complex of macrophage–lymphoid cell interactions in secondary antibody responses *in vitro*, *J. Exp. Med.* **144**:371.

Puri, J., and Lonai, P., 1980, Mechanism of antigen-binding by T cells: H-2 (I-A)-restricted binding of antigen plus Ia by helper cell, *Eur. J. Immunol.* **10**:273.
Rosenthal, A. S., 1978, Determinant selection and macrophage function in genetic control of the immune response, *Immunol. Rev.* **40**:136.
Rosenthal, A. S., and Shevach, E. M., 1976, The function of macrophages in T-lymphocyte antigen recognition, *Contemp. Top. Immunobiol.* **5**:47.
Schirrmacher, V., and Wigzell, H., 1972, Immune responses against native and chemically modified albumins in mice. I. Analysis of non-thymus-processed (B) and thymus-processed (T) cell responses against methylated bovine serum albumin, *J. Exp. Med.* **136**:1616.
Schwartz, R. H., Yano, A., and Paul, W. E., 1978, Interaction between antigen-presenting cells and primed T lymphocytes, *Immunol. Rev.* **40**:153.
Shevach, E. M., 1978, The guinea pig I-region: A functional analysis of Ia–Ir associations, *Springer Semin. Immunopathol.* **1**:207.
Shevach, E. M., 1980, The role of antigenic determinants in macrophage–T lymphocyte interaction, in: *Macrophage Regulation of Immunity* (E. R. Unanue and A. S. Rosenthal, eds.), p. 59, Academic Press, New York.
Shevach, E. M., Chan, C., Thomas, D. W., and Clement, L. T., 1979, What is the nature of the antigenic complex recognized by T lymphocytes?, in: *T and B Lymphocytes: Recognition and Function* (F. H. Bach, B. Bonavida, E. S. Vitetta, and G. F. Fox, eds.), p. 405, Academic Press, New York.
Steinman, R. M., and Cohn, Z. A., 1973, The interaction of soluble horseradish peroxidase with mouse peritoneal macrophages *in vitro*, *J. Cell Biol.* **55**:186.
Takatsu, K., and Ishizaka, K., 1975, Reagenic antibody formation in the mouse. VI. Suppression of IgE and IgG antibody responses to ovalbumin following the administration of high dose urea-denatured antigen, *Cell. Immunol.* **20**:276.
Thomas, D. W., Clement, L. T., and Shevach, E. M., 1978, T lymphocyte stimulation by hapten-conjugated macrophages: A model system for the study of immunocompetent cell interactions, *Immunol. Rev.* **40**:181.
Uhr, J. W., and Pappenheimer, H. M., Jr., 1958, Delayed hypersensitivity. II. Induction of hypersensitivity in guinea pigs by means of antigen–antibody complexes, *J. Exp. Med.* **108**:891.
Unanue, E. R., 1981, The regulatory role of macrophages in antigenic stimulation. Part two. Symbiotic relationship between lymphocytes and macrophages, *Adv. Immunol.* **31**:1.
Unanue, E. R., and Cerottini, J. C., 1970, The immunogenicity of antigen bound to the plasma membrane of macrophages, *J. Exp. Med.* **131**:711.
Yamashita, U., and Shevach, E. M., 1977, The expression of Ia antigens on immunocompetent cells in the guinea pig. II. Ia antigens on macrophages, *J. Immunol.* **119**:1584.

10

Requirement for Macrophages in Primary and Secondary Humoral Responses

CARL W. PIERCE

1. INTRODUCTION

The involvement of macrophages in the initiation and regulation of humoral and cellular immune responses and the functions of macrophages as nonspecific effector cells of the immune system have become better understood during the past 20 years. This began with the demonstration that antigens localized and were retained in lymphoid tissues in areas rich in macrophages and dendritic cells. Further, evidence was presented that macrophages, after ingestion and degradation of antigen, presented antigenic fragments which were highly immunogenic and critical for initiation of immune responses by lymphocytes. Later, several investigators demonstrated that antigen associated with macrophages was the important immunogen both *in vivo* and *in vitro*. The development of tissue culture systems capable of supporting development of both antibody and cellular immune responses and procedures to separate macrophages from complex cell mixtures has permitted more detailed and definitive investigations of functions of macrophages in immune responses.

Macrophages are important in the uptake, catabolism, and presentation of antigen to responding T cells and B cells which results in the activation of the immune system and the development of antibody and/or cell-mediated responses, such as lymphokine production and delayed hypersensitivity and rejection phenomena (Nelson, 1976; Pierce, 1980; Unanue, 1972, 1981). In this capacity, macrophages present relevant antigenic determinants in highly immunogenic configurations and may function to convert an antigen from a tolerogen to an immunogen. Macrophages may also serve important immunoregulatory

CARL W. PIERCE • Department of Pathology and Laboratory Medicine, The Jewish Hospital of St. Louis, and Department of Pathology and of Microbiology and Immunology, Washington University School of Medicine, St. Louis, Missouri 63110.

functions by presenting antigen in a manner to influence the balance between cell-mediated and antibody responses. Moreover, the manner in which macrophages present antigen in the context of Ia molecules may be important in determining the balance between stimulation of helper or amplifier T cells and stimulation of suppressor T cells both of which are important in the regulation of immune responses (Pierce, 1980; Unanue, 1981). A second broad area in which macrophages are more active than previously realized is the secretion of a variety of biologically active substances. These include not only enzymes and complement components, but products active in the inflammatory process and nonspecific regulation of T- and B-lymphocyte functions, such as interleukin-1 (Nelson, 1976; Unanue, 1981). Other functions of macrophages may be classified as nonspecific accessory effector cell functions, where macrophages are activated by products of T and B cells to protect the host against invasion by infectious organisms or neoplastic cells. Other chapters in this treatise deal with the multitude of functions of macrophages in immune and inflammatory responses. This chapter will review briefly the functions of macrophages in primary and secondary antibody responses as assessed for the most part in tissue culture systems.

2. ANTIBODY RESPONSES TO T-CELL-DEPENDENT ANTIGENS

The first demonstration that macrophages were required for the development of antibody responses *in vitro* was by Mosier (1967), who separated spleen cells from nonimmune mice into adherent (macrophages) and nonadherent (lymphoid) cells by allowing macrophages to adhere to a series of plastic culture dishes. Neither population alone developed a primary IgM plaque-forming cell (PFC) response to sheep red blood cells (SRBC), whereas cultures of the recombined macrophages and lymphoid cells responded as well as unmanipulated spleen cells. These types of experiments were confirmed by several laboratories for responses to SRBC (Pierce, 1969; Roseman, 1969; Pierce and Benacerraf, 1969; Talmage *et al.*, 1969; Hartmann *et al.*, 1970; Haskill *et al.*, 1970; Shortman *et al.*, 1970; Shortman and Palmer, 1971; Cosenza and Leserman, 1972; Unanue, 1972; Claman and Mosier, 1972; Feldmann, 1972; Sjoberg *et al.*, 1972; Chen and Hirsch, 1972; Lee *et al.*, 1976; Niederhuber, 1978; Niederhuber and Allen, 1980; Wong and Herscowitz, 1979), and have been extended to responses to other T-cell-dependent antigens, such as hapten conjugates of proteins (Katz and Unanue, 1973; Feldmann and Nossal, 1972), erythrocytes (Kettman and Dutton, 1971), viruses (Bluestein and Pierce, 1973), synthetic polypeptide antigens (GAT) (Kapp *et al.*, 1973b; Pierce *et al.*, 1974, 1976; Pierce, 1980), and TNP conjugates of polypeptides such as (TG)-AL or (HG)-AL (Hodes and Singer, 1978; Singer *et al.*, 1978; Hodes *et al.*, 1978). The T-cell-dependent nature of all these antigens has been established using several experimental methods for T-cell deprivation both *in vivo* and *in vitro*. I am unaware of any T-cell-dependent antigen that will stimulate primary antibody responses in cultures of macrophage-depleted T and B lymphocytes.

Further studies demonstrated that macrophages from T-cell-deprived mice (Mosier *et al.*, 1970; Munro and Hunter, 1970) or mice tolerant to SRBC (Forbes, 1969) were capable of supporting antibody responses *in vitro* to SRBC by normal lymphoid cells. Macrophages from normal or proteose peptone-induced periotoneal exudate, bone marrow, or lymph node support primary responses to T-cell-dependent antigens *in vitro* as efficiently, on a per cell basis, as splenic adherent cells (Hoffmann, 1970; Pierce *et al.*, 1974).

When spleen cells were fractionated by velocity sedimentation (Miller and Phillips, 1970; Osoba, 1970; Gorczynski *et al.*, 1971) or density gradient centrifugation (Haskill *et al.*, 1970; Mishell *et al.*, 1970), those cells recovered in fractions known to contain macrophages were also able to support PFC responses in cultures of lymphoid cells, but failed to develop significant responses alone. Macrophages separated from spleen cells from immune and virgin mice support primary responses to SRBC by separated lymphoid cells from virgin mice with equal efficiency, showing that immunization does not lead to an augmentation of macrophage function (Cosenza *et al.*, 1971). However, recent studies (Johnson *et al.*, 1982; C. M. Johnson, V. Hauptfeld, J. R. Little, and C. W. Pierce, unpublished observations) with cloned macrophages derived from murine bone marrow have shown these macrophages to be very efficient at the function of antigen presentation; optimal responses by splenic lymphoid cells (5×10^6/culture) require 5×10^4 splenic adherent or proteose peptone-induced peritoneal exudate macrophages, whereas 100–500 cloned macrophages stimulate comparable responses. These cloned macrophages will be useful for future experiments on macrophage function in antibody responses.

The requirement for macrophages for antibody responses *in vitro* by lymphoid cells from the spleens of previously immunized mice may now be resolved. Early experiments showed that after priming with antigen, lymphoid cells became less dependent on macrophages for the development of secondary antibody responses. This phenomenon was not manifested by lymphoid cells until 7 to 10 days after priming, but persisted for at least 1 year after a single injection of antigen (Pierce, 1969). Other investigators have confirmed these results in part using spleen cells from mice immune to DNP-hemocyanin (Katz and Unanue, 1973) and TNP-ϕx virus (Bluestein and Pierce, 1973). Other investigators have stressed the importance of cell density and the shape of the culture vessel in this phenomenon (Theis and Thorbecke, 1970). Thus, in cultures with high cell density, either in dishes or tubes, this phenomenon is easier to observe. Other studies in which macrophages were rigorously depleted by glass bead columns followed by antimacrophage serum and complement, showed that macrophages were required for the development of secondary antibody responses by lymphoid cells from primed mice (Feldmann and Palmer, 1971). Additional studies using iron carbonyl (Sjoberg *et al.*, 1972) or Sephadex G-10 (Ly and Mishell, 1974) to deplete macrophages have shown that primed lymphoid cells require macrophages to develop secondary antibody responses. Further studies using antigen-pulsed macrophages have also shown that virgin and immune lymphoid cells are strictly dependent on macrophages for development of antibody responses (Pierce *et al.*, 1974, 1976; Pierce, 1980).

3. ANTIGEN-PRESENTATION FUNCTIONS OF MACROPHAGES

The involvement of macrophages in the presentation of antigen to lymphocytes for the initiation of antibody responses *in vivo* and *in vitro* has been appreciated for many years; excellent review articles on this subject are available (Nelson, 1976; Cohn, 1968; Unanue, 1972, 1981). It will be useful for later sections of this treatise to review antigen-presentation functions of macrophages in the GAT system, where the development of antibody responses is controlled by *H-2*-linked immune response genes. The primary antibody response to GAT in cultures of spleen cells from responder strains of mice (all *H-2* haplotypes except $H\text{-}2^{p,q,s}$) is comparable in terms of GAT dose requirements, magnitude, kinetics, and Ig class to responses in the spleen after *in vivo* immunization. This antigen stimulates only IgG GAT-specific PFC responses; IgM PFC have not been detected either *in vivo* or *in vitro* by the assay methods employed (Kapp *et al.*, 1973a). Furthermore, primary antibody responses to GAT are strictly dependent on the presence of macrophages and T cells in the cultures (Kapp *et al.*, 1973b). This antigen has been extremely useful in exploring antigen-presentation functions of macrophages in the development of primary antibody responses *in vitro*.

To probe this question directly, we compared the primary responses stimulated by the optimal dose of soluble GAT (10 μg/culture) and macrophage-bound GAT in cultures of splenic lymphoid cells from responder strains of mice, e.g., C57BL/10 (Pierce *et al.*, 1974). GAT, trace-labeled with ^{125}I, was reacted with extensively washed peritoneal exudate macrophages in the cold for 30 min (100 μg GAT/2 × 10^6 cells/ml). After further extensive washing, the amount of GAT bound per 7 × 10^4 macrophages was determined and a known amount of GAT bound to a known number of macrophages was added to the lymphoid cell cultures. In numerous experiments, these reaction conditions resulted in approximately 1.5 ng GAT per 7 × 10^4 macrophages. The amount of GAT bound by 7 × 10^4 macrophages is directly related to the concentration of GAT per 10^6 macrophages in the reaction mixture up to 50 μg GAT per 10^6 macrophages; greater than 50 μg GAT per 10^6 macrophages does not result in significantly greater uptake of GAT. The binding of GAT by macrophages at 4 and 37°C is equivalent, and the absence of serum in the reaction mixture does not affect the uptake of GAT (Pierce and Kapp, 1976a).

Experiments using GAT bound to macrophages clearly demonstrated an antigen-presentation function for macrophages in the development of primary and secondary antibody responses *in vitro* (Pierce *et al.*, 1974, 1976). Macrophage-bound GAT was a significantly more efficient immunogen than soluble GAT; 10 μg of soluble GAT stimulated optimal PFC responses *in vitro*, whereas comparable responses were stimulated by 1.5 ng GAT bound to 7 × 10^4 macrophages. The detailed analyses performed by Katz and Unanue (1973) of secondary antibody responses were not repeated for primary and secondary responses to GAT, but where such experiments were done the results are comparable. Thus, the efficiency of macrophage-bound antigen in stimulating primary and secondary antibody responses *in vitro* is similar.

4. ROLE OF MACROPHAGES IN ANTIBODY RESPONSES TO ANTIGENS UNDER THE CONTROL OF *H-2*-LINKED Ir GENES

Antibody responses to certain antigens, such as GAT, are controlled by autosomal dominant Ir genes which map in the *I* region of the *H-2* complex of mice. Antibody responses to GAT by spleen cells *in vitro* follow the same genetic restrictions as serological responses in immunized mice. Spleen cells from responder strains of mice (all strains of mice except those of $H\text{-}2^{p,q,s}$ haplotypes) develop IgG GAT-specific PFC responses *in vitro* to both GAT and GAT-MBSA, whereas spleen cells from nonresponder strains of mice develop responses only to GAT-MBSA (Kapp *et al.*, 1973a). Thus, B cells are not the site of expression of the genetic defect, since GAT-specific PFC responses develop in cultures of nonresponder spleen cells stimulated with GAT-MBSA (Kapp *et al.*, 1973b).

When macrophages and lymphoid cells from responder and nonresponder mice were cultured in syngeneic combinations, all cultures responded to SRBC and GAT-MBSA, but only cultures of responder cells responded to GAT. When allogeneic combinations of macrophages and lymphoid cells were used, all cultures developed responses to SRBC and GAT-MBSA, which were comparable to responses in cultures of syngeneic combinations. Macrophages from responder mice do not confer the ability to develop PFC responses to GAT on lymphoid cells from nonresponder mice, whereas macrophages from nonresponder mice support development of normal responses to GAT by responder lymphoid cells (Kapp *et al.*, 1973b; Pierce and Kapp, 1976a,b; Pierce, 1980).

However, since lymphoid cell preparations were not entirely free of macrophages (approximately 1% contaminating macrophages), it could be argued that the nonresponder macrophages support the viability of the responder lymphoid cells (Pierce *et al.*, 1974), but the few contaminating responder macrophages actually present GAT in a manner that stimulates development of antibody responses by the responder lymphoid cells. Macrophages from nonresponder and responder mice were pulsed with GAT; responder and nonresponder macrophages bearing approximately 1.5 ng GAT per 7×10^4 macrophages stimulated comparable PFC responses by responder lymphoid cells. Neither GAT-bearing macrophage stimulates responses by nonresponder lymphoid cells, making it highly unlikely that relevant GAT is transferred from nonresponder macrophages to macrophages contaminating the responder lymphoid cells to stimulate the antibody response. All of these data strongly indicated that macrophage function with regard to GAT in responder and nonresponder mice is the same and that the macrophage is not the site of the genetic defect in nonresponder spleen cells (Kapp *et al.*, 1973b). Thus, responsiveness to GAT is determined by the genotype of the lymphoid cells, and more specifically, by the genotype of the T cells (Kapp *et al.*, 1975; Pierce and Kapp, 1976b).

The defect in genetic nonresponder spleen cells appears to be the failure of GAT-specific T cells to provide effective helper function for responses to GAT by B cells (Kapp *et al.*, 1974, 1975). However, GAT bound to macrophages can, in some instances, circumvent this defect; GAT macrophages stimulate development of GAT-specific helper T cells *in vivo* in nonresponder mice, which mediate "normal helper functions" in antibody responses to GAT-MBSA by B cells *in vitro* (Kapp *et al.*, 1975). Further experiments demonstrated that expression of the Ir gene in nonresponder mice resulted in preferential stimulation of suppressor T cells, which appear to act by preempting the stimulation and/or function of helper T cells (Kapp *et al.*, 1974; Pierce and Kapp, 1976b). The major conclusions from these studies were: (1) macrophages were not the site of expression of Ir genes in nonresponder mice; and (2) the Ir gene most probably was expressed in a regulatory T-cell subset. The observation that syngeneic and allogeneic macrophages could support comparable primary responses to GAT led to another series of studies.

5. ABILITY OF SYNGENEIC AND ALLOGENEIC MACROPHAGES TO SUPPORT PRIMARY AND SECONDARY ANTIBODY RESPONSES *IN VITRO*

Efficient physiologic interactions among macrophages, T cells, and B cells are controlled or restricted by products encoded by the *I* region of the MHC of the species (Katz, 1977; Pierce *et al.*, 1976; Pierce, 1980; Unanue, 1981). These restrictions control interactions between T cells and B cells in secondary IgG antibody responses (Katz *et al.*, 1975; Pierce and Klinman, 1975; Sprent and Von Boehmer, 1976) and between macrophages and T cells in: (1) generation and functional expression of carrier-specific murine helper T cells *in vitro* (Erb and Feldmann, 1975); (2) primary antibody responses to certain antigens such as TNP-(TG)-AL and TNP-hemocyanin (Hodes *et al.*, 1978; Singer *et al.*, 1977, 1978); (3) secondary antibody responses (Pierce *et al.*, 1976; Kappler and Marrack, 1976; Swierkosz *et al.*, 1979); (4) DNA synthetic responses to antigen by immune guinea pig (Rosenthal and Shevach, 1976) and murine T lymphocytes (Schwartz *et al.*, 1978); and (5) expression of delayed hypersensitivity reactions in mice (Miller, 1978).

The nature of macrophage–lymphocyte (T cell) interactions in antibody responses, especially the apparent lack of restrictions on these interactions in primary antibody response to GAT and the strict control of these interactions by *I*-region products in secondary antibody responses, was investigated further. First, lymphoid cells (spleen cells depleted of macrophages) from virgin mice (strain A) stimulated with GAT-Mϕ from syngeneic A mice or allogeneic B mice (bearing 1–2 ng GAT/10^5 Mϕ) developed comparable primary IgG GAT-specific PFC responses (Table 1). If these GAT-Mϕ were cultured for 24 hr, approximately 90% of the GAT originally associated with the macrophages was shed into the medium as small nonimmunogenic GAT; further culturing resulted in little subsequent shedding of GAT. Cultured syngeneic A and allogeneic B GAT-Mϕ also stimulated comparable primary PFC responses, suggesting that the ability of allogeneic B GAT-Mϕ to stimulate primary responses was not due to

TABLE 1. PRIMARY AND SECONDARY ANTIBODY RESPONSES TO GAT STIMULATED BY SYNGENEIC AND ALLOGENEIC MACROPHAGES

Lymphoid cells from A mice primed with[a]	PFC responses to GAT[b]	
	A GAT-Mϕ	B GAT-Mϕ
Virgin	Response	Response
A GAT-Mϕ	Response	No response
B GAT-Mϕ	No response	Response
A GAT-Mϕ + B GAT-Mϕ	Response	Response

[a]A mice were immunized 21 days previously by intraperitoneal injection of 4×10^6 of the indicated Mϕ bearing 20 ng GAT/10^6 cells. At culture initiation, spleen cells from these animals had < 25 IgG GAT-specific PFC/10^7 cells.
[b]Data from representative published experiments are presented as response or no response to illustrate the phenomenon of the genetic restrictions in secondary PFC responses.

transfer of GAT from these B macrophages to syngeneic A macrophages contaminating the lymphoid cell population which actually stimulate the response (Pierce *et al.*, 1976; Pierce, 1980).

A ready explanation for the ability of allogeneic macrophages to support development of a primary response as well as syngeneic macrophages was that these macrophages stimulated a positive allogeneic effect which augmented the response (Pierce *et al.*, 1976). Direct evidence supporting this explanation was not found; mixed lymphocyte response or enhancing factors in culture supernatant fluids were never detected. More recently, the explanation has been found in experiments designed for another reason. Nude mice (strain A) were engrafted with (A × B)F_1 thymus glands; T cells from these mice were tolerant to B alloantigens by several criteria. Moreover, the spleen cells from these mice failed to develop primary responses to B GAT-Mϕ; responses to A GAT-Mϕ were intact. This failure to respond to B GAT-Mϕ was absolute and did not involve suppressive mechanisms. However, if the macrophages differed from B macrophages in any fashion (e.g., *H-2K* or *D; I* region or non-MHC antigens), these macrophages stimulated responses comparable to A GAT-Mϕ. Addition of supernatant fluids from cultures of strain B lymphocytes and MHC or non-MHC genetically disparate macrophages to the lymphoid cells from nude A mice engrafted with (A × B)F_1 thymus permitted B GAT-Mϕ to stimulate primary antibody responses comparable to A GAT-Mϕ. Collectively, these data suggest that allogeneic macrophages support primary antibody responses by presenting the relevant antigen and by stimulating production of a factor(s) which enhances the responses of lymphocytes to antigen presented on allogeneic macrophages. In the absence of this factor, allogeneic macrophages apparently cannot stimulate a primary response (Lake and Pierce, 1984).

By contrast, immune A lymphoid cells preferentially developed secondary

PFC responses to GAT when stimulated with GAT-Mϕ syngeneic to the macrophages which presented GAT to the lymphoid cells during the *in vivo* immunization process. Thus, A lymphoid cells from mice immunized with A GAT-Mϕ responded to A GAT-Mϕ, but not to allogeneic B GAT-Mϕ (Table 1). Conversely, A lymphoid cells from mice immunized with allogeneic B GAT-Mϕ developed secondary responses to B GAT-Mϕ but failed to respond to syngeneic A GAT-Mϕ. Lymphoid cells from A mice immunized with both A and B GAT-Mϕ responded equally well *in vitro* to either GAT-Mϕ (Table 1, Pierce *et al.*, 1976; Pierce, 1980). Other experiments have suggested that the observed response patterns were not due to allogeneic effects, but this is difficult to rule out completely. The genetic restrictions in secondary PFC responses were antigen-specific, demonstrable only for a limited period of time, after a single immunization with GAT-Mϕ and are controlled by products encoded by the *I-A* subregion of the complex (Pierce and Kapp, 1978a; Pierce, 1980). Recombination cultures of virgin and/or immune T cells and B cells or immune T cells and B cells from mice immunized with syngeneic and allogeneic GAT-Mϕ clearly demonstrated that the genetic restrictions operated at the level of interactions between the GAT-Mϕ and the immune T cell. The mode of immunization of the B cells did not influence the genetic restriction or the responses observed (Pierce *et al.*, 1976; Pierce and Kapp, 1978a; Pierce, 1980).

Similar restrictions on macrophage–T cell interactions have been made in secondary antibody responses to fowl gamma globulin. However, in this system, lymphoid cells rigorously depleted of macrophages must be used, because antigen-transfer and/or release of immunogenic fowl gamma globulin can readily be detected. Consequently, in the presence of contaminating syngeneic macrophages, allogeneic macrophages pulsed with fowl gamma globulin appear to present antigen as effectively as syngeneic macrophages (Pierce and Malek, 1980).

These experiments using GAT showed that lymphoid cells from mice immune to GAT developed secondary PFC responses to GAT-Mϕ syngeneic with the macrophages used for *in vivo* immunization; minimal PFC responses developed when these immune lymphoid cells were stimulated with GAT-M′ϕ allogeneic to those used for immunization. This phenomenon was most apparent when A mice were immunized with allogeneic B GAT-Mϕ and developed secondary PFC responses *in vitro* when stimulated with B GAT-Mϕ, but failed to develop a significant response when stimulated with syngeneic A GAT-Mϕ (Table 1). The possibility that suppressor cells in the immune T-cell populations accounted for the failure of the immune lymphoid cells to develop primary responses to GAT-Mϕ allogeneic to those used for immunization *in vivo* was examined. It was shown that immune spleen cells that responded only to the GAT-Mϕ syngeneic to those used for priming also had suppressor T cells capable of suppressing primary responses by virgin spleen cells stimulated by GAT-Mϕ allogeneic to the macrophages used for the *in vivo* primary of the restricted immune T-helper cells (Pierce and Kapp, 1978b; Pierce, 1980).

6. FUNCTIONS OF RESPONDER AND NONRESPONDER MACROPHAGES IN RESPONSES TO GAT BY (RESPONDER × NONRESPONDER)F_1 SPLEEN CELLS

The preceding experiments are complicated by potential allogeneic effects influencing the restrictions on macrophage–immune T cell interactions in secondary responses and more pointedly on the ability of allogeneic macrophages to support primary antibody responses. Further, at the time the experiments were done, the notion that Ir gene functions were expressed at the level of the macrophage was in vogue. Consequently, the ability of macrophages from mice which are responders and nonresponders to GAT was examined to determine their ability to stimulate antibody responses by (responder × nonresponder)F_1 lymphoid cells. The use of F_1 lymphocytes eliminates potential allogeneic effect problems. The salient features of the Ir gene control of responses to GAT will be reviewed. First, the failure of nonresponder mice to develop antibody responses to soluble GAT appears to be due to a preferential stimulation of GAT-specific suppressor T cells, which inhibit the activation of helper T cells and thus the development of an antibody response (Kapp *et al.*, 1974; Pierce and Kapp, 1976b). However, GAT-specific helper T cells can be demonstrated in nonresponder mice immunized with GAT-MBSA or GAT-Mϕ (Kapp *et al.*, 1975; Pierce and Kapp, 1976b). The Ir gene defect is not expressed in macrophages in responses to GAT, since allogeneic nonresponder and syngeneic responder GAT-Mϕ stimulate comparable primary PFC responses by responder lymphoid cells *in vitro* (Kapp *et al.*, 1973b; Pierce *et al.*, 1976; Pierce 1980) and nonresponder GAT-Mϕ stimulate GAT-specific helper T cells in responder mice *in vivo* that function *in vitro* only when stimulated with nonresponder GAT-Mϕ (Pierce *et al.*, 1976; Pierce, 1980).

However, experiments in other systems indicated that Ir gene functions are expressed in Mϕ and were involved in mediating genetic restrictions in Mϕ–T cell interactions (Benacerraf and Germain, 1978; Rosenthal and Shevach, 1976; Singer *et al.*, 1978; Marrack and Kappler, 1978; Kappler and Marrack, 1978; Rosenthal, 1978). In the GAT system, virgin (responder A × nonresponder B)F_1 spleen cells developed comparable primary responses to both parental, A and B, and F_1 GAT-Mϕ (Table 2). F_1 spleen cells from mice immunized with either responder A or nonresponder B parental GAT-Mϕ developed secondary responses only when stimulated with the parental GAT-Mϕ used for immunization or F_1 GAT-Mϕ. These results were entirely consistent with the restrictions on macrophage–immune helper T cell interactions in the allogeneic situations described above. However, spleen cells from F_1 mice immunized with soluble GAT developed secondary responses only when stimulated with responder A parental or F_1 GAT-Mϕ (Table 2).

Thus, a contradiction exists between the ability of nonresponder GAT-Mϕ to stimulate primary responses by (responder A × nonresponder B)F_1 spleen cells and to prime these mice in such a way that the development of secondary

TABLE 2. PRIMARY AND SECONDARY RESPONSES TO GAT STIMULATED BY PARENTAL RESPONDER (A), NONRESPONDER (B), AND (A × B)F_1 MACROPHAGES IN RESPONDER × NONRESPONDER (A × B)F_1 SPLEEN CELLS

(A × B)F_1 spleen cells primed with[a]	PFC responses to GAT[b] A GAT-Mϕ	B GAT-Mϕ	(A × B)F_1 GAT-Mϕ
Virgin	Response	Response	Response
A GAT-Mϕ[b]	Response	No response	Response
B GAT-Mϕ[b]	No response	Response	Response
(A × B)F_1 GAT-Mϕ[b]	Response	Response	Response
Soluble GAT[c]	Response	No response	Response

[a](A × B)F_1 mice were immunized 21 days previously by intraperitoneal injection of 4 × 10^6 A, B, or (A × B)F_1 GAT-Mϕ bearing 30 ng GAT/10^6 cells.
[b]Data from representative published experiments are presented as response or no response to illustrate responses to responder parental (A), nonresponder parental (B), and (A × B)F_1 macrophages by (A × B)F_1 lymphoid cells.
[c](A × B)F_1 mice were immunized 28 days previously by intraperitoneal injection of 10 μg GAT in Maalox-pertussis.

responses is restricted to stimulation by nonresponder B GAT-Mϕ, and the failure of spleen cells from F_1 mice primed with soluble GAT to develop secondary responses to nonresponder B GAT-Mϕ. This latter observation is compatible with the concept that Ir gene function may be expressed in macrophages in the GAT system under some circumstances. Alternatively, the physical state of GAT used for immunization, soluble GAT versus GAT-Mϕ, may be crucial in the priming process and the subsequent response patterns of immune F_1 spleen cells to parental GAT-Mϕ *in vitro*. The simultaneous administration of soluble GAT with parental A or B GAT-Mϕ or F_1 GAT-Mϕ to (responder A × nonresponder B)F_1 mice converted the response patterns normally produced by a parental or F_1 GAT-Mϕ to the response pattern normally induced by soluble GAT alone (Pierce and Kapp, 1978b).

Thus, the physical state of the GAT used for immunization was critical in determining the subsequent response patterns of the primed F_1 spleen cells. Soluble GAT can alter the response patterns normally induced by priming with parental or F_1 GAT-Mϕ such that these immune spleen cells responded as if immunized with soluble GAT alone. Since these F_1 mice can develop secondary PFC responses to nonresponder GAT-Mϕ after immunization with these GAT-Mϕ, but soluble GAT reverses this response pattern, the possibility of suppressor cell activity preferentially induced by soluble GAT in these (responder × nonresponder)F_1 mice was investigated. F_1 spleen cells from mice primed with soluble GAT had a population of radiosensitive T cells which suppressed the responses of virgin F_1 spleen cells stimulated by nonresponder parental B GAT-Mϕ (Pierce and Kapp, 1978b). Moreover, F_1 spleen cells from mice immunized with F_1 GAT-Mϕ lacked suppressor T cells able to suppress responses of virgin F_1 spleen cells stimulated with responder A or nonresponder B parental GAT-Mϕ. The possibility that these suppressor T cells induced by soluble GAT in (responder A × nonresponder B)F_1 mice represent the analog of the suppressor

T cells induced in nonresponder mice by soluble GAT is currently being investigated.

7. CONCLUSIONS

These experiments demonstrate several salient points concerning modulation of immune responses by macrophages and restrictions regulating macrophage–T cell interactions in antibody responses. First, restrictions governing interactions between macrophages and virgin helper T cells in the generation of primary antibody responses may not be stringent; syngeneic and allogeneic macrophages appear to stimulate comparable responses by activating appropriate virgin helper T cells. Exceptions to this generality have been noted by Singer *et al.* (1977, 1978). Moreover, the importance of allogeneic effects stimulated by minimal genetic differences on allogeneic macrophages need to be explored further (Lake and Pierce, 1984). Second, immune helper T cells are stimulated to provide restricted helper function for B cells only by macrophages syngeneic with macrophages which "primed" the helper T cells. Third, the lymphoid cells from (responder × nonresponder)F_1 mice immunized with F_1 GAT-Mϕ developed secondary responses when stimulated with either responder or nonresponder parental GAT-Mϕ or F_1 GAT-Mϕ. By contrast, lymphoid cells from F_1 mice primed with soluble GAT (which should be presented on F_1 macrophages for priming T and B cells) responded to F_1 and responder parental GAT-Mϕ but not to nonresponder GAT-Mϕ. However, lymphoid cells from F_1 mice primed with nonresponder parental GAT-Mϕ subsequently responded to nonresponder parental GAT-Mϕ. Moreover, both responder and nonresponder macrophages stimulate comparable primary responses by virgin (responder × nonresponder)F_1 lymphoid cells. Collectively, these observations provide incontravertible evidence against functional expression of Ir genes controlling the response to GAT in macrophages. Fourth, the responses of F_1 lymphoid cells immunized simultaneously with soluble GAT and nonresponder parental GAT-Mϕ were clearly different from responses of F_1 lymphoid cells immunized with nonresponder parental GAT-Mϕ. The former F_1 lymphoid cells no longer respond to nonresponder parental GAT-Mϕ and appear to respond as if immunized with soluble GAT alone. These observations demonstrated the critical importance of the physical state of the GAT used for immunization and that soluble GAT can block priming of helper T cells that are normally primed by and respond to subsequent stimulation with nonresponder parental GAT-Mϕ. Lastly, F_1 lymphoid cells, after priming with soluble GAT, have sorcsuppressor T cells that can inhibit primary responses of virgin F_1 spleen cells stimulated with nonresponder parental GAT-Mϕ. Soluble GAT, therefore, stimulated at least two populations of T cells in F_1 mice: helper T cells for responses stimulated by responder parental GAT-Mϕ, and suppressor T cells, which act in primary responses of virgin F_1 spleen cells stimulated by nonresponder parental GAT-Mϕ.

ACKNOWLEDGMENTS. The investigations of the author have been supported by USPHS Grants AI-09897 and AI-13915 and Research Career Development Award AI-70173. I thank Paula Ryan for patient secretarial assistance.

REFERENCES

Benacerraf, B., and Germain, R. N., 1978, The immune response genes, of the major histocompatibility complex, *Immunol. Rev.* **38:**70.

Bluestein, H. G., and Pierce, C. W., 1973, Development of primary γM, γG, and γA anti-TNP plaque-forming cell responses *in vitro, J. Immunol.* **111:**130.

Chen, C., and Hirsch, J. G., 1972, The effects of mercaptoethanol and of peritoneal macrophages on the antibody forming capacity of non-adherent mouse spleen cells *in vitro, J. Exp. Med.* **136:**604.

Claman, H. N., and Mosier, D. E., 1972, Cell–cell interactions in antibody production, *Prog. Allergy* **16:**40.

Cohn, Z., 1968, The structure and function of monocytes and macrophages, *Adv. Immunol.* **9:**163.

Cosenza, H., and Leserman, L. D., 1972, Cell interactions *in vitro*. I. Role of the third cell in the *in vitro* response of spleen cells to erythrocyte antigens, *J. Immunol.* **108:**418.

Cosenza, H., Leserman, L. D., and Rowley, D. R., 1971, The third cell type required for the immune response by spleen cells *in vitro, J. Immunol.* **107:**414.

Erb, P., and Feldmann, M., 1975, The role of macrophages in the generation of T-helper cells. II. The genetic control of the macrophage–T-cell interaction for helper cell induction with soluble antigens, *J. Exp. Med.* **142:**460.

Feldmann, M., 1972, Cell interactions in immune responses *in vitro*. II. The requirements for macrophages in lymphoid cell collaboration, *J. Exp. Med.* **135:**1049.

Feldmann, M., and Nossal, G. J. V., 1972, Tolerance, enhancement and the regulation of interactions between T cells, B cells, and macrophages, *Transplant. Rev.* **13:**3.

Feldmann, M., and Palmer, J., 1971, The requirement for macrophages in the secondary immune response to antigens of small and large size, *Immunology* **21:**685.

Forbes, I. J., 1969, Analysis *in vitro* of tolerance, *Immunology* **16:**699.

Gorczynski, R. M., Miller, R. G., and Phillips, R. A., 1971, *In vivo* requirement for a radiation resistant cell in the immune response to sheep erythrocytes, *J. Exp. Med.* **134:**1201.

Hartmann, K.-U., Dutton, R. W., McCarthy, M. M., and Mishell, R. I., 1970, Cell components in the immune response. II. Cell attachment separation of immune cells, *Cell. Immunol.* **1:**182.

Haskill, J. S., Byrt, P., and Marbrook, J., 1970, *In vitro* and *in vivo* studies of the immune response to sheep erythrocytes using partially purified cell preparations, *J. Exp. Med.* **131:**57.

Hodes, R. J., and Singer, A., 1978, Cellular and genetic control of antibody responses *in vitro*. I. Cellular requirements for the generation of genetically controlled primary IgM responses to soluble antigens, *Eur. J. Immunol.* **7:**892.

Hodes, R. J., Ahmann, G. B., Hathcock, K. S., Dickler, H. B., and Singer, A., 1978, Cellular and genetic control of antibody responses *in vitro*. IV. Expression of Ia antigens on accessory cells required for responses to soluble antigens including those under Ir gene control, *J. Immunol.* **121:**1501.

Hoffmann, M., 1970, Peritoneal macrophages in the immune response to SRBC *in vitro, Immunology* **18:**791.

Johnson, C., Little, J. R., Hauptfeld, V., and Pierce, C. W., 1982, Functional and phenotypic heterogeneity among clones of bone marrow macrophages derived from a single mouse, *Fed. Proc.* **41:**380.

Kapp, J. A., Pierce, C. W., and Benacerraf, B., 1973a, Genetic control of immune responses *in vitro*. I. Development of primary and secondary plaque-forming cell responses to the random terpolymer L-glutamic acid^{60}-L-alanine^{30}-L-tyrosine^{10} (GAT) by mouse spleen cells *in vitro, J. Exp. Med.* **138:**1107.

Kapp, J. A., Pierce, C. W., and Benacerraf, B., 1973b, Genetic control of immune responses *in vitro*.

II. Cellular requirements for the development of primary plaque-forming cell responses to the random terpolymer L-glutamic acid^{60}-L-alanine^{30}-L-tyrosine^{10} (GAT) by mouse spleen cells *in vitro*, *J. Exp. Med.* **138:**1121.

Kapp, J. A., Pierce, C. W., Schlossman, S., and Benacerraf, B., 1974, Genetic control of immune responses *in vitro.* V. Stimulation of suppressor T cells in nonresponder mice by the terpolymer L-glutamic acid^{60}-L-alanine^{30}-L-tyrosine^{10} (GAT), *J. Exp. Med.* **140:**648.

Kapp, J. A., Pierce, C. W., and Benacerraf, B., 1975, Genetic control of immune responses *in vitro.* VI. Experimental conditions for the development of helper T cell activity specific for the terpolymer L-glutamic acid^{60}-L-alanine^{30}-L-tyrosine^{10} (GAT) in nonresponder mice, *J. Exp. Med.* **142:**40.

Kappler, J. W., and Marrack, P. C., 1976, Helper T cells recognize antigen and macrophage surface components simultaneously, *Nature (London)* **262:**297.

Kappler, J. W., and Marrack, P. C., 1978, The role of H-2 linked genes in helper T cell function. I. *In vitro* expression in B cells of immune responses controlling helper T cell activation, *J. Exp. Med.* **146:**1748.

Katz, D. H., 1977, *Lymphocyte Differentiation, Recognition and Regulation,* Academic Press, New York.

Katz, D. H., and Unanue, E. R., 1973, Critical role of determinant presentation in the induction of specific responses in immunocompetent lymphocytes, *J. Exp. Med.* **137:**967.

Katz, D. W., Graves, M., Dorf, M. E., Dimuzio, H., and Benacerraf, B., 1975, Cell interactions between histoincompatible T and B lymphocytes. VII. Cooperative responses between lymphocytes are controlled by genes in the I region of the H-2 complex, *J. Exp. Med.* **141:**263.

Kettman, J. R., and Dutton, R. W., 1971, Radioresistance of the enhancing effect of cells from carrier-immunized mice in an *in vitro* primary immune response, *Proc. Natl. Acad. Sci. USA* **68:**699.

Lake, J. P., and Pierce, C. W., 1984, Immune responses by thymus gland grafted nude mice, *J. Immunol.*, in press.

Lee, K. C., Shiozara, C., Shaw, C., and Diener, E., 1976, Requirement for accessory cells in the antibody response to T cell-independent antigens *in vitro, Eur. J. Immunol.* **6:**63.

Ly, I. A., and Mishell, R. I., 1974, Separation of mouse spleen cells by passage through columns of Sephadex G-10, *J. Immunol. Methods* **5:**239.

Marrack, P., and Kappler, J. W., 1978, The role of H-2 linked genes in helper T cell function: III. Expression of immune response genes for trinitrophenyl conjugates of poly L(Tyr, Glu)-poly-D,L-Ala-poly-L-Lys in B cells and macrophages, *J. Exp. Med.* **147:**1596.

Miller, J. F. A. P., 1978, Restrictions imposed on T lymphocyte reactivities by the major histocompatibility complex: Implications for T cell repertoire selection, *Immunol. Rev.* **42:**76.

Miller, R. G., and Phillips, R. A., 1970, Separation of cells by velocity sedimentation, *J. Cell. Physiol.* **73:**191.

Mishell, R. I., Dutton, R. W., and Raidt, D. J., 1970, Cell components in the immune response. I. Gradient separation of immune cells, *Cell. Immunol.* **1:**175.

Mosier, D E., 1967, A requirement for two cell types for antibody formation *in vitro, Science* **158:**1575.

Mosier, D. E., Fitch, F. W., Rowley, D. A., and Davies, A. J. S., 1970, Cellular deficit in thymectomized mice, *Nature (London)* **225:**276.

Munro, A , and Hunter, P., 1970, *In vitro* reconstitution of the immune response of thymus-deprived mice to sheep red blood cells, *Nature (London)* **225:**277.

Nelson, D. S. (ed.), *Immunobiology of the Macrophage,* Academic Press, New York.

Niederhuber, J. E., 1978, Macrophage–T cell interaction in a primary antibody response dependent on an I-J subregion macrophage determinant, in: *Macrophage Regulation of Immunity* (E. R. Unanue and A. S. Rosenthal, eds.), pp. 197–212, Academic Press, New York.

Niederhuber, J. E., and Allen, P., 1980, Role of I region gene products in macrophage induction of an antibody response. II. Restriction at the level of the T cell recognition of I-J subregion macrophage determinants, *J. Exp. Med.* **151:**1103.

Osoba, P., 1970, Some physical and radiobiological properties of immunologically reactive mouse spleen cells, *J. Exp. Med.* **132:**369.

Pierce, C. W., 1969, Immune response *in vitro.* I. Cellular requirements for the immune response by non-primed and primed spleen cells *in vitro, J. Exp. Med.* **130:**345.

Pierce, C. W., 1980, Macrophages: Modulators of immunity, *Am. J. Pathol.* **98:**10.

Pierce, C. W., and Benacerraf, B., 1969, Independence of "activated" lymphoid cells in the immune response *in vitro, Science* **166:**1002.

Pierce, C. W., and Kapp, J. A., 1976a, The role of macrophages in antibody responses *in vitro,* in: *Immunobiology of the Macrophage* (D. S. Nelson, ed.), Academic Press, New York.

Pierce, C. W., and Kapp, J. A., 1976b, Regulation of immune responses by suppressor T cells, *Contemp. Top. Immunobiol.* **5:**91.

Pierce, C. W., and Kapp, J. A., 1978a, Functions of macrophages in antibody responses *in vitro, Fed. Proc.* **37:**86.

Pierce, C. W., and Kapp, J. A., 1978b, Antigen-specific suppressor T-cell activity in genetically restricted immune spleen cells, *J. Exp. Med.* **148:**1271.

Pierce, C. W., and Kapp, J. A., 1978c, Suppressor T-cell activity in responder × nonresponder (C57BL/10 × DBA/1)F_1 spleen cells responsive to L-glutamic acid^{60}-L-alanine^{30}-L-tyrosine^{10}, *J. Exp. Med.* **148:**1282.

Pierce, C. W., and Malek, T. R., 1980, Restrictions on macrophage–lymphoid cell interactions in secondary antibody responses to fowl gamma globulin *in vitro,* in: *Macrophage Regulation of Immunity* (E. R. Unanue and A. S. Rosenthal, eds.), pp. 35–46, Academic Press, New York.

Pierce, C. W., Kapp, J. A., Wood, D. C., and Benacerraf, B., 1974, Immune responses *in vitro.* X. Functions of macrophages, *J. Immunol.* **112:**1181.

Pierce, C. W., Kapp, J. A., and Benacerraf, B., 1976, Regulation by the H-2 gene complex of macrophage–lymphoid cell interactions in secondary antibody responses *in vitro, J. Exp. Med.* **144:**371.

Pierce, S. K., and Klinman, N. R., 1975, The allogeneic bisection of carrier-specific enhancement of monoclonal B-cell responses, *J. Exp. Med.* **142:**1165.

Roseman, J., 1969, X-ray resistant cell required for the induction of *in vitro* antibody formation, *Science* **165:**1125.

Rosenthal, A. S., 1978, Determinant selection and macrophage function in genetic control of the immune response, *Immunol. Rev.* **40:**135.

Rosenthal, A. S., and Shevach, E. M., 1976, The function of macrophages in T-lymphocyte antigen recognition, *Contemp. Top. Immunobiol.* **5:**47.

Schwartz, R. H., Yano, A., and Paul, W., 1978, Interactions between antigen-presenting cells and primed T lymphocytes: An assessment of Ir gene expression in the antigen-presenting cell, *Immunol. Rev.* **40:**153.

Shortman, K., and Palmer, J., 1971, The requirement for macrophages in the *in vitro* immune responses, *Cell. Immunol.* **2:**399.

Shortman, K., Diener, E., Russell, P., and Armstrong, W. D., 1970, The role of nonlymphoid accessory cells in the immune response, *J. Exp. Med.* **131:**461.

Singer, A., Dickler, H. B., and Hodes, R. J., 1977, Cellular and genetic control of antibody responses *in vitro.* II. Ir gene control of primary IgM responses to trinitrophenyl conjugates of poly-L-(Tyr,Glu)-poly-D,L-Ala-poly-L-Lys and poly-L-(His,Glu)-poly-D,L-Ala-poly-L-Lys, *J. Exp. Med.* **146:**1096.

Singer, A., Cowing, C., Hathcock, K. S., Dickler, H. B., and Hodes, R. J., 1978, Cellular and genetic control of antibody response *in vitro.* III. Immune response gene regulation of accessory cell function, *J. Exp. Med.* **147:**1611.

Singer, A., Hathcock, K. S., and Hodes, R. J., 1979, Cellular and genetic control of antibody responses *in vitro.* V. Helper T cell recognition of determinants on accessory cells but not B cells, *J. Exp. Med.* **149:**1208.

Sjoberg, O., Andersson, J., and Moller, 1972, Requirement for adherent cells in the primary and secondary immune response *in vitro, Eur. J. Immunol.* **2:**123.

Sprent, J., and Von Boehmer, H., 1976, Helper function of T cells depleted of alloantigen-reactive lymphocytes by filtration through irradiated F_1 hybrid recipients. I. Failure to collaborate with allogeneic B cells in a secondary response to sheep erythrocytes measured *in vivo, J. Exp. Med.* **144:**617.

Swierkosz, J. E., Marrack, P. C., and Kappler, J. W., 1979, The role of H-2 linked genes in helper T cell function. V. I-region control of helper T cell interactions with antigen presenting macrophages, *J. Immunol.* **123**:654.

Talmage, D. W., Radovich, J., and Hemmingsen, H., 1969, Cell interaction in antibody synthesis, *Adv. Immunol.* **12**:271.

Theis, G. A., and Thorbecke, G. J., 1970, The proliferative and anamnestic antibody response of rabbit lymphoid cells *in vitro*: Requirement for adherent and nonadherent cells for the responses to particulate antigens in spleen cell cultures, *J. Exp. Med.* **131**:970.

Unanue, E. R., 1972, The regulatory role of macrophages in antigenic stimulation, *Adv. Immunol.* **15**:95.

Unanue, E. R., 1981, The regulatory role of macrophages in antigenic stimulation. Part two. Symbiotic relationship between lymphocytes and macrophages, *Adv. Immunol.* **31**:1.

Wong, D. M., and Herscowitz, H. B., 1979, Immune activation by T independent antigens: Lack of effect of macrophage depletion on theimmune response to TNP-LPS, PVP and dextran, *Immunology* **27**:765.

11

Regulation of Macrophage Functions by Complement, Complement Receptors, and IgG-Fc Receptors

GORDON D. ROSS and SIMON L. NEWMAN

1. INTRODUCTION

Membrane receptors provide the essential recognition function required for control of macrophage responses to changes in their cellular environment. Considering the complexity and number of different functions performed by macrophages, it is likely that only a small proportion of the total number of different types of receptors are presently known. Among these various receptors there are at least six distinct types of complement (C) receptors and three different types of IgG-Fc receptors (Table 1). Of these nine types of receptors, only four have been characterized structurally. Although a function has been described for six of these receptors, it is possible that each of these receptors may control several other additional functions that are presently unknown.

Macrophages have a complex interaction with the C system that goes beyond the expression of C receptors. Macrophages have been shown to synthesize many different C components in an active form, but functions have been proposed for only a few of these different intrinsic C components. For example, C5 molecules synthesized by macrophages are expressed on outer membrane surfaces, and are believed to be responsible for triggering macrophage differentiation in response to C-activating substances. Activated macrophages may also release factor B in an activated form known as Bb, a serine protease that has the ability to convert plasminogen into plasmin (Sundsmo and Wood, 1981). The generation of such a plasminogen activator has long been recognized to be a

GORDON D. ROSS and SIMON L. NEWMAN • Division of Rheumatology–Immunology, Department of Medicine, and Department of Microbiology–Immunology, University of North Carolina, Chapel Hill, North Carolina 27514.

TABLE 1. TYPES OF COMPLEMENT RECEPTORS AND IgG-Fc RECEPTORS EXPRESSED BY MONOCYTE-MACROPHAGES AND NEUTROPHILS

Receptor type	Specificity	Molecular weight	Expression on other cell types
CR_1	C4b, C3b, C5b, iC3b, C3c	205,000	Lymphocytes, renal epithelial cells, eosinophils, erythrocytes
CR_3	iC3b	155,000 and 94,000	Large granular lymphocytes (NK cells)
C1q-R	C1q	?	Lymphocytes
H-R	Factor H	50,000 and 100,000	Lymphocytes
C5a-R	C5a, C5a des Arg-cochemotaxin	?	Eosinophils, lymphocytes, mast cells
C3a-R	C3a, C4a	?	Eosinophils, lymphocytes, mast cells
FcR I (mouse and rat)	IgG2a	67,000	?
FcR II (mouse and rat)	IgG1, IgG2b	52,000	Lymphocytes
FcR III (mouse)	IgG3	?	?
FcR (human)	IgG1, IgG3	?	Lymphocytes, eosinophils, platelets

marker of macrophage activation. Furthermore, brief treatment of lymphocytes with Bb triggers blastogenesis (Sundsmo, 1983). Finally, preliminary evidence has been obtained that macrophage endogenous factor H and factor I may participate in phagocytosis and the respiratory burst response to C3b-coated particles.

2. STRUCTURE AND FUNCTION OF MACROPHAGE C RECEPTORS

2.1. RECEPTOR TYPE 1 (CR_1)

CR_1, the classic immune adherence receptor, was first described in 1953 by Nelson, who demonstrated that primate erythrocytes bound to C3-bearing immune complexes. Subsequently, the same CR_1 was shown to be present on monocytes, macrophages, neutrophils, lymphocytes, eosinophils, and renal epithelial cells. CR_1 is specific for a site in the C3c region of C3b (Fig. 1) that is not exposed in native C3, but is exposed in denatured native C3 (C3i) (Berger *et al.*, 1981), iC3b (Ross *et al.*, 1983), and C3c (Ross and Polley, 1975; Ross *et al.*, 1983a). In addition, CR_1 also binds to C4b (Cooper, 1969; Ross and Polley, 1975; Dobson *et al.*, 1981a) and C5b (Dierich and Landen, 1978). Based on studies with sheep erythrocytes containing limited amounts of bound C3 or C4 (EC3 or EAC14) and rosette formation with human erythrocytes that have only 360–2000 CR_1/cell,

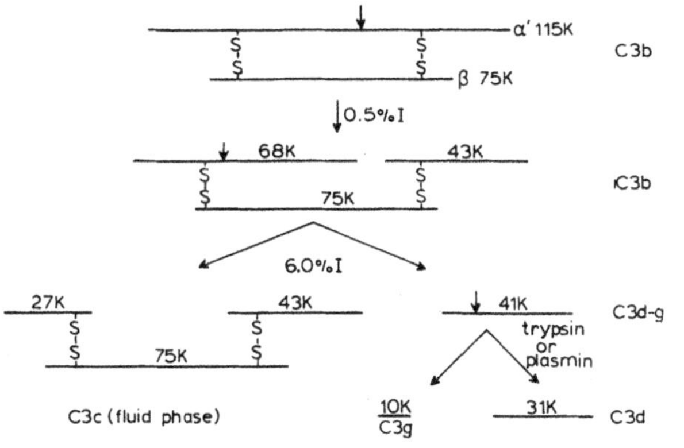

FIGURE 1. Cleavage of bound C3b by factor I. C3b is bound or fixed to microbial cells or immune complexes by way of a covalent ester or amide bond formed by a glutamate residue that is near the N-terminal of the d region of C3b (Tack *et al.*, 1980). After proteolytic digestion of bound C3b by factor I and other enzymes, the small C3d fragment and all larger fragments containing C3d (iC3B and C3d-g) remain bound because of this covalent attachment. The cofactor for factor I cleavage of C3b is factor H, whereas the cofactor for factor I cleavage of iC3b is erythrocyte CR_1 (Ross *et al.*, 1982; Medof *et al.*, 1982). After bound iC3b is converted to bound C3d-g, the C3c fragment is released into the fluid phase. The binding site for CR_1 is exposed in C3b, iC3b, and C3c, whereas the binding site for CR_2 is exposed in iC3b, C3d-g, and C3d. The binding site for CR_3 is exposed only in iC3b.

CR_1 has been shown to have the highest affinity for bound C3b, and less affinity for bound C4b (Cooper, 1969) and iC3b (Ross *et al.*, 1983a). Because fluid-phase monomeric C3b, C4b, C3c, and iC3b have a much lower affinity for CR_1 than do C3b dimers or bound C3b (Arnaout *et al.*, 1981), it is likely that *in vivo* unbound C3 fragments do not compete for CR_1 with bound C3 fragments. In plasma it is known that C3b is rapidly degraded to iC3b and then more slowly into C3d-g (Fig. 1). Thus, iC3b rather than C3b may be the major ligand that binds to CR_1.

Initial studies with anti-human erythrocyte sera indicated that the CR_1 expressed on erythrocytes was antigenically similar to the CR_1 expressed on macrophages, lymphocytes, and neutrophils (Ross *et al.*, 1973; Ross and Polley, 1975). This was later confirmed when CR_1 was isolated from erythrocytes (Fearon, 1979), and the specific anti-CR_1 elicited with the pure receptor was shown inhibit both C3b (Fearon, 1980) and C4b (Dobson *et al.*, 1981a) rosetting, and to immunoprecipitate a similar molecular weight CR_1 from various different cell types (Fearon, 1980). On each cell type examined, CR_1 was shown to be a single-chain glycoprotein of 205,000 daltons. Immunofluorescent studies with anti-CR_1 demonstrated that the CR_1 antigen was also present on renal epithelial cells that previously had been shown to bind C3b complexes (Kazatchkine *et al.*, 1982; M. Papamichael, J. D. Lambris, and G. D. Ross, unpublished observation, 1981). Using [^{125}I]-Fab'-anti-CR_1, the number of CR_1 antigens per cell was quantitated with different cell types (Fearon, 1980; Dobson *et al.*, 1981a; Iida *et al.*, 1982; Wilson *et al.*, 1982), and the numbers obtained were in good agreement with those obtained in previous direct binding studies with [^{125}I]-C3b (Tack *et al.*,

1978; Arnaout *et al.*, 1981). Erythrocytes express only 360–2000 CR_1/cell, whereas monocytes and neutrophils express 30,000–60,000 and B lymphocytes 20,000–30,000 (Fearon, 1980; Arnaout *et al.*, 1981).

Anti-CR_1 $F(ab')_2$ and Fab′ fragments have proven to be useful reagents to explore CR_1 functions. Because C3b complexes added to phagocytic cells are converted subsequently to iC3b complexes, C3d-g complexes, and finally C3d complexes by intrinsic factor H, factor I, and elastase or other proteases (Lambris *et al.*, 1980; Ross and Lambris, 1982), it cannot be assumed that functions induced by added C3b are CR_1-dependent. Furthermore, some C3b-mediated functions may require cell-associated factor H, and be less dependent upon CR_1. For example, Fab′-anti-CR_1 produced only 10 to 50% inhibition of the neutrophil superoxide burst triggered by pure C3b-coated zymosan particles (Dobson *et al.*, 1981b). By contrast, nearly complete inhibition of superoxide release was demonstrated with either affinity-purified Fab-anti-C3c or Fab′-anti-H. In addition, no respiratory burst was triggered by $F(ab')_2$ anti-CR_1 alone. The inhibition by anti-C3c demonstrated that the C3b on the zymosan was required for a respiratory burst. However, the complete inhibition by anti-H and only partial inhibition by anti-CR_1, suggested that intrinsic factor H, rather than CR_1, might be responsible for triggering the respiratory burst. CR_1 probably contributes to the respiratory burst by promoting the binding of C3b-zymosan to neutrophils as suggested by Newman and Johnston (1979). Recent studies have demonstrated that CR_3 binds to zymosan directly, and is the zymosan-recognition receptor of neutrophils and monocyte-macrophages (Ross and Lachmann, 1983).

Monocyte-macrophage CR_1, as well as neutrophil CR_1, play a major role in the phagocytosis of C4b-, C3b, and iC3b-coated bacteria and soluble complexes. Phagocytosis proceeds in two distinct steps: binding and ingestion. With monocytes, neutrophils, and resting macrophages, CR_1 functions only to bind C4b- and C3b-coated particles to the phagocytic cells, and ingestion is triggered synergistically by particle-bound IgG antibody and phagocyte Fc receptors (Ehlenberger and Nussenzweig, 1977; Newman and Johnston, 1979). Fc receptors on neutrophils and monocytes have a lower affinity for IgG than do CR_1 for C3b, so that bacteria coated only with small amounts of IgG are not bound to phagocytes in the absence of C. CR_1 has been shown to acquire the ability to induce ingestion independently of Fc receptors when either human blood monocytes are cultured for 7 to 10 days in autologous serum (Newman *et al.*, 1980) or mouse peritoneal macrophages are elicited *in vivo* with thioglycollate (Bianco *et al.*, 1975) or activated *in vitro* with T lymphokines (Griffin and Griffin, 1979). The mechanism of this change in CR_1 function is unknown. Possibly, differentiated macrophages express greater numbers of CR_1 per cell. However, the CR_1 on thioglycollate-elicited or T lymphokine-activated macrophages have been shown to have the ability to migrate across the membrane surface to the site of particle attachment, whereas the CR_1 on resident macrophages have a relatively fixed membrane distribution (Griffin and Mullinax, 1981). This suggests that macrophage CR_1 may have transmembrane linkages to microtubules or microfilaments that are responsible for mobilizing receptors. Particle size may also be important for controlling CR_1 function. Some types of small bacteria that are coated only with C3b are ingested by neutrophils, whereas larger C3b-coated particles such as erythrocytes are not ingested (Schreiber *et al.*, 1982). However, the mechanism of C3b-mediated ingestion of small particles and soluble complexes by neutrophil CR_1 appears to be absorptive endocytosis or pinocytosis rather than phagocytosis (Fearon *et al.*, 1981). This latter finding suggests that CR_1 on blood neutrophils may have an important function in the clearance of circulating immune complexes coated with C3b, iC3b, or C4b.

2.2. C RECEPTOR TYPE 3 (CR_3)

Phagocytic cells and natural killer cells express CR_3 (Perlmann *et al.*, 1981; Ross and Lambris, 1982; Ross and Lachmann, 1983). In several studies in the past (Reynolds *et al.*, 1975; Ehlenberger and Nussenzweig, 1977; Ross *et al.*, 1978), CR_3 was not distinguished from CR_2 (the C3d receptor) that is expressed primarily on B lymphocytes. CR_3 is a lectin that binds to a carbohydrate expressed only in iC3b, and does not bind to other types of C3 fragments (Ross *et al.*, 1983a; Ross and Lachmann, 1983). CR_2 binds to the d region of C3d-g, as well as to C3d fragments and the d region of iC3b (Fig. 1). When fixed iC3b binds to erythrocyte CR_1, the CR_1 functions as the essential cofactor for factor I cleavage of the fixed iC3b into fixed C3d-g and fluid-phase C3c (Ross *et al.*, 1982; Medof *et al.*, 1982). Although it has a similar molecular weight, the C3g fragment is distinct from the C3e fragment (Ghebrehiwet and Muller-Eberhard, 1979), because anti-C3e is unreactive with C3d-g (M. K. Pangburn and Ghebrehiwet, 1981). According to Lachmann (1981), bound C3b *in vivo* is degraded into iC3b and then into C3d-g, but little if any of the bound C3d-g is degraded fully into C3d. We have found that CR_3 activity is only detectable when C3b is converted into iC3b. However, because the fixed iC3b also binds to both CR_1 and CR_2, all three C3 receptor types are actually iC3b receptors (Ross *et al.*, 1983a). Subsequently, when the bound iC3b is converted into C3d-g, the bound C3d-g reacts only with CR_2, and the loss of CR_1 activity can be traced to the C3c fragment that is released from the bound iC3b during formation of the C3d-g (Fig. 1). When purified C3c fragments were attached to fluorescent microspheres, the microspheres rosetted with CR_1-bearing cells, and the C3c-microsphere rosettes could be inhibited completely by anti-CR_1 (Ross *et al.*, 1983a).

Structural characterization of CR_3 came from two different observations. First, two anti-macrophage monoclonal antibodies were identified that selectively inhibited CR_3 activity. Anti-Mac-1, a rat anti-mouse macrophage antibody was found to inhibit both mouse and human CR_3 (Beller *et al.*, 1982; Ross *et al.*, 1983a) and to immunoprecipitate a mouse macrophage antigen of 190,000 and 105,000 daltons (Ault and Springer, 1981). MN-41, a mouse anti-human CR_3, was also found to inhibit human CR_3 and to react with a human cell antigen of 155,000 and 94,000 daltons (Eddy *et al.*, 1983). Confirmation that these two antibodies were CR_3-specific (and did not inhibit CR_3 by reaction with a nearby unrelated antigen), came from the finding of three different patients with a genetic deficiency of both CR_3 activity and the antigens detected by anti-Mac-1 and MN-41. Because these CR_3-deficient patients were also unreactive with OKMI and Mo-1, it was also established that these two other "macrophage-specific" antibodies were also anti-CR_3. All four monoclonal anti-CR_3 antibodies were shown to react with a human cell surface antigen containing two chains of 155,000 and 94,000 daltons that was absent in the CR_3-deficient patients (Ross *et al.*, 1983b).

CR_3 has an important role in host defense because all three patients with CR_3 deficiency had a history of repeated bacterial skin infections (Ross *et al.*, 1983b). In addition to being an iC3b receptor, CR_3 also binds directly to unopsonized yeast (zymosan) lacking fixed C3, and functions as the zymosan recognition receptor of neutrophils and monocytes. Inhibition of CR3 activity by EDTA and by N-acetyl-D-glucosamine suggests that CR_3 is a lectin that is analogous to bovine serum conglutinin (Ross and Lachmann, 1983). Because the CR_3-deficient patients had repeated bacterial (but not yeast) infections, it is possible that CR_3 also binds to bacterial sugars. Even though both EC3bi and zymosan bind to neutrophil and monocyte CR_3, it is unclear why only zymosan and not EC3bi is readily ingested and induces a superoxide burst. Macrophage CR_3 does trigger phagocytosis of EC3bi, and appears to be much more efficient in phagocytosis than is CR_1 (Newman *et al.*, 1983). Perhaps the difference with neutrophils and monocytes is that zymosan (but not EC3bi) binds to the mannose-fucose receptor in addition to CR_3, and that triggering this other receptor in addition to CR_3 is necessary for inducing phagocytosis. This hypothesis is supported by the finding that isolated yeast mannan did not bind to CR_3, and that anti-CR_3 inhibited neutrophil yeast ingestion by a maximum of 81% (Ross and Lachmann, 1983). Also, CR_3-deficient neutrophils and monocytes did ingest 5%–10% as many yeast particles as did normal neutrophils and monocytes (Ross *et al.*, 1983b). These two findings suggest a CR_3-independent mechanism for yeast binding and ingestion that may involve the mannose-fucose receptor that is known to be able to bind isolated yeast mannan. Monocytes and neurophils may require this secondary binding of zymosan to the mannose-fucose receptor, whereas macrophage CR_3 may function independently of the mannose-fucose receptor.

2.3. FACTOR H RECEPTORS (H-R)

H-R have been demonstrated on B lymphocytes and neutrophils, and preliminary data suggest that the same receptor may also be present on monocyte-macrophages (Lambris *et al.*, 1980; Dobson *et al.*, 1981b; Newman *et al.*, 1981; Schopf *et al.*, 1982). B-lymphocyte H-R bind H aggregates or H that is complexed with C3b, and trigger the immediate release of B-cell endogenous factor I. This released factor I was shown to convert EC3b into EC3bi which then bound to lymphocyte CR_2 (Lambris *et al.*, 1980). The B-lymphocyte H-R was found to have a binding site for H that resembled both C3b and the binding site (idiotype) of goat anti-H antibody. A rabbit antibody specific for the idiotype of goat anti-H was found to block lymphocyte H-R and to bind to EC3b (Lambris and Ross, 1982). This anti-idiotypic antibody ($\alpha\alpha$H) also triggered B cells to release endogenous factor I in a manner similar to factor H complexes. Thus, the ααH appeared to recognize a common binding site structure for factor H that was shared with B-cell H-R and C3b. Immunoprecipitation and SDS–PAGE analysis of the B-cell antigen reactive with ααH indicated that the H-R contained two protein components of 100,000 and 50,000 daltons, with the 100,000-dalton component made up of two 50,000-dalton disulfide-linked subunits.

Current data suggest that the normal ligand for H-R is probably a C3b,H complex present on either a microbial cell or an immune complex. It appears possible that H and H-R may serve as alternative C3b receptors having a distinct function from CR_1. This was suggested by the finding that the neutrophil superoxide burst response to C3b-zymosan was blocked completely by anti-H, but only partially by anti-CR_1 (Dobson *et al.*, 1981b).

H-R seem to have a similar activation function on the various cell types that express the receptor. For example, monocyte-macrophages, B lymphocytes, and neutrophils each release intracellular stores of factor I when exposed to aggregated H or C3b,H complexes (Lambris *et al.*, 1980; Dobson *et al.*, 1981b; Newman *et al.*, 1981). In addition, lymphocyte blastogenesis is triggered by aggregated H (Hammann *et al.*, 1981), and, as mentioned above, factor H and H-R may also have a role in stimulating the neutrophil respiratory response to C3b-zymosan. However, the neutrophil response to C3b-zymosan may involve multiple triggering signals in addition to H and H-R, as attempts to trigger a neutrophil superoxide burst with either aggregated H or EC3b,H have so far been unsuccessful. Recently, however, Schopf *et al.* (1982) have reported that purified H alone would trigger a human monocyte respiratory burst.

2.4. C5a RECEPTORS (C5a-R)

Monocyte-macrophage and neutrophil receptors for C5a have long been recognized because of the potent chemotactic activity induced by C5a. Similar C5a-R are also present on mast cells and possibly a low proportion of lymphocytes. With lymphocytes, C5a has been shown to trigger lymphocyte activation and may have an important function in regulation of the immune response (Weigle *et al.*, 1982). However, this lymphocyte response to C5a may be indirect, involving first C5a binding to C5a-R on macrophages, and then followed by macrophage stimulation of lymphocytes. Mast cells release histamine in response to C5a "anaphylatoxin," and this produces both smooth muscle contraction and an increase in capillary vasculature permeability.

C5a is a 16,000-dalton peptide derived from the N-terminus of the α-chain of C5 by cleavage with either the C4b2a3b convertase of the classical pathway or the C3bBbP convertase of the alternative pathway. C5a-R are specific for C5a and have a 30-fold lower affinity for C5a from which the C-terminal arginine has been removed by serum carboxypeptidase (C5a-des Arg) (Chenoweth and Hugli, 1980). Since the conversion of C5a to C5a-des Arg occurs very rapidly in serum, it was at first unclear how C5a could be chemotactic *in vivo*. Later, when it was shown that C5a was indeed chemotactic in serum, further studies demonstrated a normal serum protein that bound to C5a-des Arg and restored its chemotactic activity (Perez *et al.*, 1981). Other studies have also suggested that noncomplement enzymes such as trypsin or thrombin might cleave C5 and produce chemotactic fragments much larger than C5a (Wetsel and Kolb, 1982). At this time it is unknown whether these other chemotactic C5 fragments react with the C5a-R or with some other macrophage receptor. Likewise, it is unknown which macrophage receptor is responsible for the chemotactic activity that has been described for the fluid-phase C567 complex (Ward *et al.*, 1966).

The finding that C5a produces measurable chemotaxis at concentrations as low as 4×10^{-10} M (Chenoweth and Hugli, 1980) implies that the C5a-R have a relatively high binding affinity. Binding studies with human neutrophils have indicated that C5a-R have an affinity in the range of $3\text{–}7 \times 10^{-9}$ M (Chenoweth and Hugli, 1978). However, in these studies competitive dissociation of [^{125}I]-C5a from the cells with unlabeled C5a was only 5–10% after 1 hr, precluding an exact determination of the C5a-R binding affinity constant. Later studies have suggested that C5a binding to C5a-R was irreversible, and that bound C5a was degraded antigenically (Gerard *et al.*, 1979). The differential morphology of the blood cells binding [^{125}I]-C5a, as well as [^{125}I]-C3a, was investigated by examining cell smears by simultaneous autoradiography and Wright-Giemsa staining (Glovsky *et al.*, 1979). C5a-R were expressed on 35% of monocytes, 98% of neutrophils, 65% of eosinophils, and 2% of lymphocytes.

C5a-R have an important function in attracting macrophages and neutrophils to the site of C activation. Various types of *in vitro* and *in vivo* experiments with C5-deficient or C5-depleted sera have demonstrated a striking absence of neutrophil infiltration into sites of extravascular C activation (Rosenfeld *et al.*, 1976a,b; Snyderman *et al.*, 1979). Also, C5-deficient mice are known to be more susceptible to pneumococcal infection than are normal mice (Shin *et al.*, 1969).

2.5. C3a–C4a RECEPTORS (C3a-R)

Receptors for C3a that are distinct from C5a-R have been demonstrated on several leukocyte types and mast cells. Cross-inhibition studies have demonstrated that C4a binds to the same receptor as C3a, but with lower affinity than C3a (Gorski *et al.*, 1979). The mast cell C3a-R, though distinct from the C5a-R, also triggers histamine release with resultant smooth muscle contraction and increased vascular permeability. However, it now appears that C3a and C3a-R do not trigger chemotaxis (Fernandez *et al.*, 1978). Previous findings of C3a-mediated chemotaxis were probably due to trace contamination of C3a with C5a. Despite this absence of chemotactic activity, studies using [^{125}I]-C3a and autoradiography in combination with Wright–Giemsa staining have demonstrated C3a-R on neutrophils, monocytes, and eosinophils. When neutrophils are exposed to highly purified C3a, the cells are triggered to release histamine (Glovsky *et al.*, 1979). Control of this C3a-induced histamine release may come from C3b, which is generated simultaneously with C3a, and which has been shown to trigger neutrophil release of histaminase (Herman *et al.*, 1981). Highly purified C3a has also been shown to suppress lymphocyte blastogenic responses, suggesting the presence of critical C3a-R on either lymphocytes or macrophages (Hobbs *et al.*, 1982; Weigle *et al.*, 1982).

Similar to C5a, the activity of C3a with C3a-R depends on the presence of a C-terminal arginine that is removed rapidly by serum carboxypeptidase. However, no serum factor that restores the activity of C3a-des Arg has yet been described. Considerable data about the essential amino acids that make up the active site structure of C3a have been gained by synthesis of various octapeptides and pentapeptides that resemble the C-terminus of C3a (Hugli and Erickson, 1977). These data also provided some clues about the active site of the C3a-R, whose structure is expected to complement the shape, charge, and hydrophobicity of the C3a-binding site.

3. ROLE OF INTRINSIC C COMPONENTS IN MACROPHAGE FUNCTIONS

3.1. SYNTHESIS OF C BY MACROPHAGES

The synthesis of various C components by macrophages has been recognized for many years (Stecher *et al.*, 1967; Einstein *et al.*, 1976), but little is known about the role of intrinsic C in macrophage functions. It is probably significant that most macrophage-synthesized C components are secreted in either a native or an active form. These include C2 (Einstein *et al.*, 1976), Clq, Clr, Cls (Muller *et al.*, 1978), C3 (Strunk *et al.*, 1982), C5, and factors B, D, P, H, and I (Whaley, 1980). Synthesis has been demonstrated in three different ways. First, cultured macrophage supernatants have been tested by specific hemolytic assays for the individual components, and a cycloheximide-inhibitable increase in C activity during the cultivation period has been taken as evidence for synthesis. Since non-C proteins might be able to mimic the activity of certain C proteins, other more specific assays are preferable. In particular, leukocyte elastase and other proteolytic enzymes are known to have factor D-like activity (Brade *et al.*, 1974), CR_1 is known to have factor H-like activity (Fearon, 1979), and other unknown macrophage proteases may be able to mimic the proteolytic activities of C2, Clr, Cls, B, or I. As a second method, macrophage C synthesis has been characterized by cultivation of cells in radiolabeled amino acids followed by either immunoprecipitation or immunodiffusion and autoradiographic analysis of macrophage proteins reactive with specific anti-C component antibodies. This type of test has demonstrated components not readily detectable by functional assay, including C4, C3, C5, and factor H (Stecher *et al.*, 1967; Whaley, 1980). However, several different potential artifacts may contribute to false-positive results in immunoprecipitation of cellular antigens. Also, an antibody that is specific for a particular C component among serum proteins, may have unrecognized additional specificities among cellular proteins. This problem can be somewhat overcome by analysis of intrinsically labeled immune precipitates by

SDS–PAGE. In this way, the human monocyte antigen detected with anti-C5 was shown to have the same molecular weight and subunit structure as plasma C5 (Sundsmo and Götze, 1981). In addition, intrinsic C5 was demonstrated on the outer membrane surfaces of cultured human monocytes by immunofluorescence with $F(ab')_2$-anti-C5. This indicated that monocyte intrinsic C5 was firmly bound to exposed external membrane surfaces. Macrophage intrinsic C3 was not detectable by similar membrane surface immunofluorescence staining techniques.

3.2. FUNCTION OF INTRINSIC C IN PHAGOCYTOSIS

As mentioned previously, C receptor-triggered phagocytosis occurs only with activated or differentiated macrophages, and not with human blood monocytes and neutrophils or with murine resting peritoneal macrophages. Elicitation of murine peritoneal macrophages with thioglycollate is known to be C-dependent (Bianco *et al.*, 1976), and is possibly triggered by cleavage of membrane surface C5 by factor Bb that is generated as a product of C activation (Götze *et al.*, 1979; Sundsmo and Götze, 1981). Macrophage intrinsic factors H and I may convert particle-bound C3b into iC3b, allowing opsonized particles to be bound by CR_3, as well as by CR_1. This results in more bound particles per macrophage, and two- or threefold more ingested particles per macrophage than when particles are coated with C3b alone (Newman *et al.*, 1981).

Even though monocytes usually do not ingest unopsonized cells, cells that are activators of the alternative pathway may be ingested by human monocytes due to recognition by a trypsin-sensitive monocyte surface protein (Czop *et al.*, 1978). Zymosan, rabbit erythrocytes, and desialated sheep erythrocytes (but not normal sheep erythrocytes) are ingested to some degree. As mentioned previously, CR_3 is the primary recognition receptor for zymosan. It is unknown if CR_3 can also bind to other C-activating particles such as rabbit erythrocytes. Only a small percentage of blood monocytes have the ability to ingest rabbit erythrocytes, and this percentage varies greatly among different individuals. The recognition system appears to be independent of C3b and CR_1, as a C3b coating on the particles is not required (Czop and Austen, 1980). Also, low concentrations of trypsin abrogate particle ingestion without affecting the ability of the cells to form C3b-dependent rosettes. Since cultured monocytes synthesize all of the recognition components of the alternative pathway (C3, B, D, P, H, and I), and are activated by Bb that is a product of alternative pathway activation, it is possible that the recognition system may involve these intrinsic C components. The functional activities of several of these C proteins is known to be trypsin-sensitive (C3, B, and H).

Recent data have suggested that macrophage endogenous Clq may function as one type of macrophage Fc receptor (Loos *et al.*, 1980). Similarly with lymphocytes, extrinsic Clq has been shown to promote the binding of aggregated IgG to cells bearing Clq-R (Tenner and Cooper, 1980). Since some monocytes express Clq-R (Tenner and Cooper, 1980), it may be possible that macrophage Clq-R function with intrinsic Clq to bind IgG to macrophage surfaces. If this were the case, intrinsic Clq and Clq-R might be able to trigger ingestion of IgG-coated particles, since this is a known function of macrophage Fc receptors.

3.3. ROLE OF MACROPHAGE INTRINSIC C IN PROMOTING CELL DIFFERENTIATION

When macrophage surface C5 is either cleaved by factor Bb or aggregated by $F(ab')_2$-anti-C5 (Sundsmo and Götze, 1979), macrophages adhere to a surface and spread, rapidly acquiring many properties that are characteristic of activated cells. The fate of the macrophage surface C5 following Bb cleavage is unknown. It is presumed that Bb cleavage of exposed C5 would produce C5a, and then this intrinsic C5a might react with C5a-R and act as a negative feedback control mechanism for macrophage activation (Sundsmo and Götze, 1981). This is because C5a alone causes the reverse of adherence and spreading, that is, macrophages stay small and rounded, do not attach, and instead move rapidly toward a C5a gradient (chemotaxis). It appears possible that endogenous factors B, D, P, and C3 might also participate in this reaction by forming an intrinsic C5-convertase. Future studies with monoclonal antibodies directed to these intrinsic C components may be able to confirm this hypothesis.

4. STRUCTURE AND FUNCTION OF IgG-Fc RECEPTORS

4.1. CLASS SPECIFICITY AND CELL POPULATION

The Fc receptor is a distinct and specific site on a cell membrane which is capable of recognizing and binding the Fc portion of the immunoglobulin molecule. Although Fc receptors specific for IgM (Uher *et al.*, 1981; Haesert, 1979), IgA (Fanger *et al.*, 1980, 1981), and IgE (Joseph *et al.*, 1978; Spiegelberg and Melewicz, 1980; Anderson and Spiegelberg, 1981; Boltz-Nitulescu and Spiegelberg, 1981) have been described, the majority of studies have focused on the biology and biochemistry of the Fc receptor for IgG. Fc receptors for IgG are ubiquitous in nature and have been found on a myriad of cell types in addition to those of phagocytic lineage. Fc receptors have been demonstrated to be on B lymphocytes, T-lymphocyte subpopulations, T-cell lymphomas, K cells, placental cells and fetal yolk sac membranes, on herpes simplex- or cytomegalovirus-infected fibroblasts, and on the surface of several neoplastic tissues (Zuckerman and Douglas, 1979). The fact that Fc receptors appear on such a variety of cell types suggests that their functional importance goes beyond their ability to trigger phagocytosis, and that they may play several vital roles, depending on the cell type and stage of cellular differentiation.

All phagocytic cells that have been examined have been found to possess membrane Fc receptors for IgG. Cells and species studied include human monocytes and neutrophils (Huber and Fudenberg, 1968; Henson, 1969; Messner and

Jelinek, 1970), alveolar macrophages (Reynolds *et al.*, 1975), and *in vitro* cultured monocyte-derived macrophages (Newman *et al.*, 1980); guinea pig neutrophils (Henson, 1969), peritoneal macrophages (Sugiyama *et al.*, 1981), and spleen and liver macrophages (Huber *et al.*, 1969); rabbit neutrophils (Henson, 1969) and alveolar macrophages (Reynolds *et al.*, 1975); rat peritoneal and alveolar macrophages (Boltz-Nitulescu *et al.*, 1981), and Kupffer cells (Munthe-Kaas, 1976); mouse neutrophils (Lay and Nussenzweig, 1968) and peritoneal macrophages (Rabinovitch, 1967; Holland *et al.*, 1972); canine monocytes (Lucas *et al.*, 1980); and swine alveolar macrophages (Charley and Frenove, 1980). Fc receptors have also been studied on macrophage-like cell lines such as the mouse cell lines P388D1 and J774 and their variants (Unkeless, 1980), and the human cell line U937 (Anderson and Abraham, 1980).

4.2. ASSAYS FOR THE DETECTION OF Fc RECEPTOR-BEARING CELLS

As with the C3 receptor, the most popular technique for assaying Fc receptor activity has been rosette formation. Heterologous erythrocytes (E) from sheep or oxen are coated with IgG anti-E antibody prepared in rabbits or mice (EA or EIgG), and the percentage of cells that bind EA to their surface is enumerated. A positive rosette is usually defined as a cell with three or more EA bound to its membrane. When neutrophils, monocytes, or macrophages are studied, binding of EA is usually followed by erythrophagocytosis, thus allowing ingestion to be quantitated with the same EA reagent. Although this assay has been used extensively, several laboratories may have used assay conditions that were not optimal for the cells under study. Zuckerman and Douglas (1978) demonstrated that EA rosette formation was both time and temperature dependent, with maximal values attained after 1 hr at 37°C. However, if the cell mixture was centrifuged prior to incubation, maximal values were reached after only 10 min at 37°C. EA rosette formation also requires metabolically active cells, an intact cytostructure, and magnesium and calcium (Passwell *et al.*, 1978). Using thin-section transmission electron microscopy, Douglas (1978) has shown that there is a broad zone of close interaction between the erythrocyte membrane and the receptor-bearing cell, with the distance between the membranes being approximately 100 Å. A freeze-fracture analysis of the receptor–ligand interaction has revealed a redistribution of intramembranous particles (IMP) from a random distribution into clusters or patches. This redistribution of IMPs has been seen with both lymphoid and macrophage cell types.

A second technique for identifying Fc receptor-bearing cells has involved the use of soluble immune complexes or aggregated IgG, the binding of which is detected by incorporation of either a fluorescent or ^{125}I label (Ishizaka and Ishizaka, 1960). The binding of these soluble aggregates to individual cells can thus be detected microscopically by immunofluorescence and autoradiography, or by quantitation of counts bound using a gamma counter. Since different preparations of aggregated IgG are heterogeneous in size and binding affinity, quantitation of receptors with this reagent tends to vary considerably. In some cell systems, radiolabeled monomeric IgG has been used successfully to quantitate receptor number and binding affinity (Unkeless and Eisen, 1975).

4.3 QUANTITATIVE ANALYSIS OF Fc RECEPTORS

The number and/or affinity of Fc receptors for IgG depends on the particular phagocytic cell, species, and the manner in which the cells are obtained. Fc receptors on phagocytic cells exhibit high-affinity binding and a finite number of receptors per cell as evidenced by saturation binding kinetics at high ligand concentration (Dorrington, 1976). True quantitative analysis of Fc receptors has been limited to macrophages and macrophage-like cell lines, since only these cells have been demonstrated to bind monomeric immunoglobulin (Arend and Mannik, 1973; Unkeless and Eisen, 1975; Leslie and Cohen, 1976; Unkeless, 1977; Segal and Hurwitz, 1977). These studies have suggested that the number of Fc receptors ranged from 10^5 to 10^6 sites per cell. Observed receptor numbers and binding affinities depended on which ligands were used, and whether or not the macrophages were "activated."

Although not truly quantitative, some differences in Fc receptor activity among various phagocytic cells have been detected using the EA rosette assay. For example, the majority of mouse peritoneal macrophages avidly phagocytized EIgG, whereas less than 10% of mouse neutrophils were even able to bind the EIgG under the same experimental conditions (Lay and Nussenzweig, 1968, 1969). In other studies, EA ingestion by human neutrophils was found to require 50 to 100 times more molecules of IgG per EA than did ingestion by human monocytes (Ehlenberger and Nussenzweig, 1977). The binding avidity of EA to guinea pig peritoneal macrophages was found to be three times greater than the binding avidity to alveolar macrophages. However, the alveolar cells were heterogeneous and contained cells with a broader range of binding avidities than did the peritoneal cells. Furthermore, comparison of normal unstimulated peritoneal macrophages with mineral oil-induced inflammatory exudate macrophages revealed a sixfold increase in the proportion of high-avidity cells in the latter population (Rhodes, 1975). Finally, mouse alveolar macrophages have shown greater Fc receptor activity than resident peritoneal macrophages both in their ability to form IgG rosettes, and in their phagocytic capacity (Hearst *et al.*, 1980).

4.4. SUBCLASS SPECIFICITY OF Fc RECEPTORS

It is well known that human and murine IgG immunoglobulin is further subdivided into discrete subclasses based on the amino acid composition of the constant regions of their heavy and light chains (Spiegelberg, 1974). Using the binding assays described above and competitive inhibition experiments with different IgG subclasses, some animal macrophages have been found to possess discrete Fc receptors for IgG which exhibit distinct subclass specificity (Unkeless,

1980; Diamond and Yelton, 1981). Further evidence for the existence of these discrete Fc receptors has come from their differential protease sensitivity, the isolation and characterization of Fc receptor variants from macrophage-like cell lines, the preparation of monoclonal anti-Fc receptor antibody, and the isolation of the Fc receptors from solubilized macrophage membranes. The most well-characterized Fc receptors are those that are found on mouse peritoneal macrophages and mouse macrophage-like cell lines. Mouse macrophages have been shown to possess three distinct Fc receptors (Table 1): FcR I, specific for IgG2a (Unkeless, 1977); FcR II, specific for IgG1 and IgG2b (Unkeless, 1977; Diamond and Scharff, 1980); and FcR III, specific for IgG3 (Diamond and Yelton, 1981). FcR I binds monomeric and aggregated mouse IgG2a, is sensitive to trypsin, and shows decreased binding at 4°C and in the presence of cytochalasin B. FcR II binds aggregated or immune-complexed mouse IgG1 and IgG2b, is resistant to trypsin and cytochalasin B, and functions at 4°C (Diamond *et al.*, 1978; Diamond and Scharff, 1980). The recently described FcR III (Diamond and Yelton, 1981) binds aggregated mouse IgG3, is also resistant to trypsin and cytochalasin B, and functions at both 4 and 37°C. These three distinct types of Fc receptors are also present on thioglycollate-elicited macrophages and the macrophage-like cell lines P388D1, J774, J774.2, and FC-1 (Unkeless, 1977; Diamond *et al.*, 1978; Haeffner-Cavaillon *et al.*, 1979a; Diamond and Scharff, 1980; Diamond and Yelton, 1981). Species specificity studies have indicated that the Fc receptors of mouse, rabbit, and human macrophages are structurally related (Haeffner-Cavaillon *et al.*, 1979a,b).

Despite the fact that these receptors show subclass specificity, all three types of Fc receptors have been found to be capable of mediating phagocytosis and antibody-dependent cellular cytotoxicity (ADCC) (Ralph *et al.*, 1980). This is in contrast to the earlier studies of Walker (1977) who reported that in the macrophage-like cell line IC-21, the Fc receptor for IgG2a mediated phagocytosis, whereas the Fc receptor for IgG2b mediated ADCC. Although the reason for this discrepancy is unknown, there remains a possibility that the differences resides in the use of different macrophage cell lines for the two studies.

Structural evidence for the existence of at least two Fc receptors on mouse perioneal macrophages has been provided by Lane *et al.*, (1980). Macrophage Fc receptors from radiolabeled thioglycollate-elicited macrophages were solubilized in Nonidet P-40, and separated on affinity columns containing aggregated mouse myeloma proteins of different IgG subclasses. They found that a trypsin-sensitive peptide of 67,000 daltons bound IgG2a, whereas a trypsin-resistant 52,000-dalton peptide bound IgG1 and IgG2b.

Rat peritoneal and alveolar macrophages and guinea pig peritoneal macrophages also appear to have two distinct Fc receptors based on IgG subclass specificity. Like mouse macrophages, rat macrophages possess one membrane Fc receptor specific for rat IgG2a, and a second receptor specific for rat IgG1 and IgG2b (Boltz-Nitulescu *et al.*, 1981). In the guinea pig, one Fc receptor binds to homologous IgG2 antibody alone, and the other receptor binds both IgG2 and IgG1 antibodies (Sugiyama *et al.*, 1981).

Sulica *et al.* (1979a,b,c) have described two separate and distinct Fc receptors on mouse macrophages based on their ability to bind either monomeric IgG or polymeric IgG contained in either heat aggregates or immune complexes. The "cytophilic" Fc receptor, which bound monomeric IgG, was sensitive to phospholipase C and resistant to Pronase. The "opsonic" Fc receptor, which bound polymeric IgG, was sensitive to Pronase but resistant to phospholipase C. Both receptors could be modulated with anti-IgG independently of one another. At 37°C, the "cytophilic" Fc receptor migrated across the membrane slowly, forming small patches but not capping. In contrast, the "opsonic" Fc receptor capped rapidly. Macrophages that had capped their "opsonic" Fc receptors were capable of regenerating them within 8 hr at 37°C. The relationship of these Fc receptors to the previously described IgG subclass-specific receptors remains to be investigated.

In the human system, studies with myeloma proteins have established that IgG1 and IgG3 immunoglobulin subclasses, but not IgG2 and IgG4, are preferentially bound to Fc receptors on neutrophils, monocytes, and the human macrophage cell line U937 (Abramson *et al.*, 1970; Hay *et al.*, 1972; Alexander, 1980; Anderson and Abraham, 1980). Fc receptor binding through IgG1 and IgG3 appeared to take place through the same binding site on the immunoglobulin molecule (Huber *et al.*, 1971). Coincidentally, the IgG1 and IgG3 subclasses were also the most efficient subclasses in activating the classical pathway (Spiegelberg, 1974).

4.5. BIOCHEMISTRY OF THE Fc RECEPTOR

Experiments attempting to define the specific domain of the Fc fragment that binds to the Fc receptor have given conflicting results. Studies performed using human IgG have suggested that the CH_3 region is the site recognized by the Fc receptor (Yasmeen *et al.*, 1973; Okafor *et al.*, 1974; Ciccimarra *et al.*, 1975), whereas other experiments performed with rabbit IgG have suggested that the CH_2 region contained the cytophilic binding site (Ovary *et al.*, 1976; Ganczankowski and Leslie, 1979). Diamond *et al.* (1979) used homogeneous myeloma immunoglobulins with either specific deletions of portions of the heavy chain or different heavy chain region recombinations produced by variants of MPC 11, an IgG2b-producing mouse myeloma cell line, to determine the portion of the Fc region of IgG2b that bound to mouse macrophage Fc receptors. They too reported that the CH_2 region was the site of binding for the Fc receptor. Recently, experiments studying the binding of human immunoglobulin fragments to human monocytes (Foster *et al.*, 1980) or the mouse macrophage-like cell line P388D1 (Haeffner-Cavaillon *et al.*, 1979a) have confirmed a role for the CH_3 region in Fc receptor recognition. However, these studies also suggested some requirement, either direct or indirect, for the CH_2 domain. The authors further suggested that the cytophilic site might be formed cooperatively by interactions between the two different heavy chain domains. The integrity of the hinge region appeared to be essential for full expression of cytophilic activity, since reduction of hinge region disulfides in both human IgG and its Fc fragment markedly decreased their binding affinity for Fc receptors. In addition, a mutant IgG1 molecule lacking the hinge region was found to be significantly less cytophilic than its normal counterpart. The N-acetylglucosamine and mannose carbohydrate moieties of IgG have also been found to be required for the cytophilic activity of the IgG molecule (Koide *et al.*, 1977).

The effect of various enzymes on Fc receptor function has been explored in an attempt to relate the enzymatic sensitivity of the receptor to an understanding of the composition and active moieties required for receptor expression. Unfortunately, results from studies of this type have been contradictory, perhaps due to biochemical heterogeneity in receptor composition. Furthermore, individual enzymes have been found to have both receptor enhancing and inhibiting properties, depending on the concentration of the enzyme. Finally, since it cannot be determined whether an enzyme effect on Fc receptor function was due to either direct modification of the receptor or some other membrane component, experiments of this type have not been very informative.

4.6. ACQUISITION OF Fc RECEPTORS DURING CELL DIFFERENTIATION

Although much information has been obtained concerning the biochemical and biological aspects of Fc receptors on phagocytic cells, comparatively little is known about the appearance of Fc receptors during hematopoiesis, or the fate of Fc receptors during differentiation of monocytes into macrophages. Rabellino and Metcalf (1975) cultured mouse marrow in semisolid medium and used the rosette assay to determine the proportions of cells with Fc receptors in individual colonies. They found that newly developed macrophage colonies showed 28, 35, 85, and 83% of Fc receptor-positive cells on days 3, 4, 6, and 8, respectively. The corresponding figures for neutrophil colonies were 14, 18, 21, and 55%, indicating more rapid development of Fc receptors in macrophage colonies than in neutrophil colonies. In a study of human bone marrow cells (Herborn *et al.*, 1979), Fc receptors were demonstrated on 46% of neutrophil promyelocytes, and greater than 90% of myelocytes and metamyelocytes. Cells that appeared to be promonocytes by morphological criteria also expressed Fc receptors. In the mouse system, Rabellino *et al.* (1978) reported expression of Fc receptors on metamyelocytes and myelocytes, but not on promyelocytes or myeloblasts. In addition, the ability of the cells to ingest particles bound to Fc receptors was not expressed in immature myeloid cells and was only acquired at later stages of maturation. Thus, as with macrophage C receptors, there are two separate maturation steps required for development of functional neutrophil Fc receptors. In a study of the M_1 myeloid leukemia cell line of the SL mouse strain, it has been shown that Fc receptor-negative blast cells (M_1^-) can be induced to differentiate into mature Fc receptor-positive macrophages (M_1^+) within 48 hr, when cultured in conditioned medium from murine embryonic fibroblasts (Yodoi *et al.*, 1978). The newly acquired Fc receptors mediated phagocytosis and were resistant to trypsin and Pronase.

In a study by Newman *et al.* (1980), the Fc receptor function of human monocytes was evaluated during *in vitro* differentiation into monocyte-derived macrophages. On day 0, approximately 65% of plastic-adherent monocytes exhibited Fc-mediated phagocytosis. During the first 3 days in culture in M199 containing 5% autologous serum, monocyte Fc receptor activity declined. Thereafter, the percentage of maturing macrophages capable of ingesting EIgG increased with time in culture until day 7. At this point, and on day 10, 65% of macrophages phagocytized EIgG. However, Fc receptor activity was markedly enhanced in the macrophages (day 7 and 10) in that they ingested two to three times as many EIgG than did day 0 monocytes. A recent report by Kay and Douglas (1981) has suggested that the loss of Fc receptor function during the first few days in culture is due to shedding of the Fc receptors into the culture medium.

4.7. TOPOLOGY OF Fc RECEPTORS

Although there have been only a few studies that examined the topology of Fc receptors on phagocytic cells, they have been very informative. First, Fc receptors on macrophages do not appear to be related to membrane antigens encoded by the major histocompatibility complex (MHC). Treatment of mouse peritoneal macrophages with anti-H-2 antibody did not diminish the binding of EA to membrane Fc receptors (Schlesinger and Chaouat, 1975; Kerbel, 1976). Furthermore, a rat monoclonal antibody specific for the mouse macrophage IgG1/IgG2b Fc receptor (FcR II) inhibited EA rosette formation regardless of the H-2 haplotype from which the macrophages were obtained (Unkeless, 1979).

The distribution of Fc receptors on human neutrophils was examined by electron microscopy using ferritin antiferritin immune complexes (An, 1980). The complexes were prepared in antigen excess so that they were composed of one antiferritin antibody molecule and one or two ferritin molecules, and acted as a monovalent ligand. Neutrophil Fc receptors were then labeled at 0°C in the presence of sodium azide. The receptors were found to be clustered as discontinuous patches of varying length over the cell surface. Preincubation of neutrophils at 37°C did not alter this pattern, nor did cross-linking of the soluble complexes with $F(ab')_2$ antiferritin. A similar clustered distribution pattern has also been reported for the CR_1 expressed on both human monocytes and neutrophils (Petty *et al.*, 1980a). Furthermore, this natural clustering of Fc receptors and CR_1 is apparently not mediated by either microfilaments or microtubules (An *et al.*, 1981; Fearon *et al.*, 1981). Clustering of receptors into patches over the cell surface may relate to their functional ability to trigger neutrophil cellular responses (Newman and Johnston, 1979). This arrangement would be more effective than individual receptor molecules scattered diffusely in the neutrophil membrane. Interestingly, Walter *et al.* (1980) have found that exposure of neutrophils to a chemotactic stimulus causes the Fc receptors to localize at the cell's leading edge. Thus, the Fc receptor would be located in precisely the region most likely to first encounter an opsonized microorganism.

4.8. SOLUBILIZATION AND CHARACTERIZATION

Perhaps the ultimate way to study the physical and biochemical properties of the Fc receptor is through solubilization and purification. One of the difficulties facing those who wish to purify Fc receptors is the requirement for an assay to quantitate the isolated fluid-phase receptor. Anderson and Grey (1977, 1978) have devised assays to measure independently IgG2a and IgG2b Fc receptors derived from mouse macrophages. They reported that the IgG2a Fc receptor (FcR I) was not removed by passage of macrophage lysates through a column of aggregated IgG2b, and that the IgG2b Fc receptor (FcR II) was not removed by passage through an IgG2a column. They also found differences in sedimentation values and sensitivities to phospholipase C for the two receptors.

There have been several reports of the partial purification of Fc receptors from mouse macrophages or macrophage cell lines. Although each of the various procedures utilized affinity chromatography on immunoglobulin absorbents, different putative Fc receptor molecules were found. Fc receptor molecules were described as glycosylated polypeptides with molecular weights ranging from 15,000 to 130,000 (Bourgois *et al.*, 1977; Yagawa *et al.*, 1979; Kulczycki *et al.*, 1980). At least three reasons could explain this confusion. First, structurally different Fc receptors may be expressed on different cell types. Second, mouse macrophages and macrophage cell lines appear to express at least three distinct types of Fc receptors. Finally, the third source of confusion may be technical, resulting from either the lack of standardization of cell labeling, or the lack of protection of membrane molecules from proteolysis, or the lack of sufficient prevention of disulfide bond reduction prior to SDS gel analysis. Thus, reports of low-molecular-weight Fc receptors could be due to proteolysis and/or reduction of larger-molecular-weight molecules (Bourgois *et al.*, 1977). It has even been suggested that various molecular weight molecules may represent different molecular forms of the same Fc receptor (Kahn-Perles *et al.*, 1980). To add to the confusion, the Fc receptor from the mouse macrophage-like cell line P388D1 has been characterized as both a lipoprotein (Anderson, 1980) and a glycoprotein (Loube and Dorrington, 1980).

Perhaps a better approach to the problem of receptor isolation has been the tack taken by Mellman and Unkeless (1980). They started with a monoclonal rat anti-mouse Fc receptor antibody that was specific for the trypsin-resistant IgG2b receptor on the mouse macrophage (Unkeless, 1979). The Fab fragment of this antibody (designated 2.4G2 IgG) inhibited rosette formation by IgG1- and IgG2b-sensitized E on mouse macrophages, neutrophils, and spleen cells, as well as on mouse Fc receptor-bearing cell lines of macrophage, B, T, and null lymphocyte origin. Rosette formation by IgG2a-coated E was unaffected. Moreover, binding of [^{125}I]Fab 2.4G2 was unaffected by prior trypsinization of the macrophages. This Fab fragment was used to prepare an affinity reagent to purify Fc receptor from the macrophage cell line J774 to apparent homogeneity. The antigen isolated from J774 cells consisted of two general types of polypeptides with calculated molecular weights of approximately 60,000 and 47,000. The J774 Fc receptor was judged to be a glycoprotein based on the sensitivity of its isoelectric point to neuraminidase digestion, its labeling with galactose oxidase, and its binding to concanavalin A-Sepharose. One particularly interesting finding was that in phosphate-buffered saline, the isolated protein formed large aggregates that retained Fc receptor activity, but with somewhat altered IgG subclass specificity. The isolated Fc receptor agglutinated erythrocytes that were coated with both IgG2b and IgG2a. In addition, iodinated Fc receptor bound to Sephadex beads coated with rabbit IgG, mouse IgG1, IgG2b, and IgG2a, but not to beads coated with mouse IgG3 or rabbit $F(ab')_2$ fragments. The binding of purified receptor to all IgG subclasses was inhibited by 2.4G2 Fab. In contrast, the binding of IgG2a to intact macrophages was inhibited by 2.4G2 Fab by only 15%, whereas rabbit IgG immune aggregate binding was almost completely abolished. Although they used a different approach, the recent data of Schneider *et al.* (1981) fit remarkably well with those of Mellman and Unkeless (1980). P388D1 and J774.2 cells were radiolabeled with ^{125}I, the cells solubilized in NP-40, and the Fc receptor isolated on immunoadsorbents. They reported that the molecular weight of their putative Fc receptor was approximately 50,000 to 65,000. Furthermore, the purified receptor in its isolated state did not discriminate between monomeric IgG2a and IgG2b.

4.9. BIOLOGICAL SIGNIFICANCE

Fc receptors on phagocytic cells play an important role in opsonization and phagocytosis (Newman and Johnston, 1979), ADCC (Walker, 1977), and in the clearance of immune complexes (Lamers *et al.*, 1981). Through these functions, phagocytic leukocytes function to protect the host from infection by pathogenic microorganisms, destroy tumor cells, and clear immune complexes from the circulation.

When bacteria or inert particles (i.e., sheep erythrocytes or latex) coated with IgG are encountered by phagocytic leukocytes, they become bound to the phagocyte membrane through its Fc receptors. Particle binding to the Fc receptor triggers ingestion, and activates phagocytic killing mechanisms such as the generation of superoxide anion, and the release of lysosomal hydrolases (Goldstein *et al.*, 1975; Newman and Johnston, 1979). As mentioned earlier, even when erythrocyte contact is enhanced through binding to CR_1 (C3b receptor), interaction with the Fc receptor is required to trigger ingestion and killing (Scribner and Fahrney, 1976; Newman and Johnston, 1979).

During phagocytosis of an IgG-coated particle, the plasma membrane of the phagocyte is guided by the interaction of its Fc receptors with IgG ligands on the surface of the particle, so that the advancing membrane pseudopod conforms to the shape of the particle (Griffin *et al.*, 1975b). The phagocytic stimulus is confined to the segment of the plasma membrane immediately adjacent to the particle being ingested, and ingestion of one particle does not trigger phagocytosis of other bound particles (Griffin and Silverstein, 1974). Furthermore, repeated triggering of receptors and therefore generation of intracellular phagocytic signals is required to complete the ingestion process (Shaw and Griffin, 1981).

ADCC refers to the *in vitro* ability of nonimmune cells to lyse targets which have been coated with IgG antibody (Walker, 1977). Although the precise mechanism of target cell lysis is not understood, the process is dependent on Fc receptor-bearing effector cell populations.

Fc receptors are mobile within the plane of the phagocyte membrane, and function independently of CR_1 (Griffin *et al.*, 1975a). Macrophages and monocytes that have encountered soluble immune complexes (Griffin, 1980), surface-bound immune complexes (Michl *et al.*, 1979; Ragsdale and Arend, 1980), or IgG-coated particles (Petty *et al.*, 1980b) have shown a subsequent loss of Fc receptor activity. This loss of activity did not appear to be due to Fc receptor migration or interiorization, and was not mediated by cytoskeletal elements. The loss also did not result from damage caused to Fc receptors by lysosomal enzymes or oxygen radicals, but appeared to be modulated by cyclic nucleotide-dependent mechanisms (Ragsdale and Arend, 1980). cAMP has also been shown to be intimately involved in Fc receptor function through its ability to restore Fc receptor-mediated phagocytosis in macrophages (Vogel *et al.*, 1981) and macrophage-like cell lines (Schneck *et al.*, 1981) that possess defects in Fc-mediated phagocytosis. Similarly, lymphokines and BCG have been shown to enhance macrophage ADCC and phagocytosis through their effects on Fc receptors (Koren *et al.*, 1979; Vogel and Rosenstreich, 1979; Ezekowitz *et al.*, 1981; Guyre *et al.*, 1981; Koren *et al.*, 1981). This enhancement may be due to the ability of these molecules to increase intracellular levels of cAMP (Vogel *et al.*, 1981). Finally, Fc receptor-mediated rosette formation and phagocytosis have been shown to require intact microtubules and microfilaments (Passwell *et al.*, 1978; Foris *et al.*, 1981).

It has been suggested that the functions of phagocytosis and ADCC may be performed by different subpopulations of macrophages. Mouse peritoneal macrophages of the IC-21 line were separated into four groups based on their buoyant densities on discontinuous gradients of Percoll (Serio *et al.*, 1979). The results of such experiments indicated that the low-density subpopulations were enriched for cells that mediated ADCC, whereas macrophages from the denser regions of the gradient showed markedly enhanced antibody-dependent phagocytosis activity and only modest ADCC.

5. CONCLUSIONS

Fc and complement receptors provide an excellent system for the study of the relationships between plasma membrane receptors and activation of intracellular processes. Further studies of these receptor systems should provide an understanding of the precise mechanisms involved in ligand binding and receptor regulation. Areas of study that will provide a greater understanding of these receptor systems include determination of the natural ligands and how these ligands are generated and eventually degraded; examination of the pathway of biosynthesis of the receptors, and the mechanisms of receptor insertion and stabilization within the plasma membrane; somatic cell genetic analysis to identify the genetic loci responsible for receptor expression; and identification of the mechanisms by which receptor expression can be enhanced or diminished by changes in intracellular metabolism due to differentiation processes or receptor–ligand interaction.

REFERENCES

Abramson, N., Gelfand, E. W., Jandl, J. H., and Rosen, F. S., 1970, The interaction between human monocytes and red cells: Specificity for subclasses and IgG fragments, *J. Exp. Med.* **132**:1207.

Alexander, M. D., 1980, Specificity of Fc receptors on human monocytes for IgG1 and IgG3, *Int. Arch. Allergy Appl. Immunol.* **62**:99.

An, T., 1980, Fc receptors on human neutrophils: Electron microscopic study of natural surface distribution, *Immunology* **40**:101.

An, T., Hymes, A. J., and O'Neal, C. H., 1981, Natural clusterings of Fc receptors on human neutrophils—not affected by the cytoskeletal reagents, *Immunology* **43**:503.

Anderson, C. L., 1980, The murine macrophage receptor for IgG2b is lipid dependent, *J. Immunol.* **125**:538.

Anderson, C. L., and Abraham, G. N., 1980, Characterization of the Fc receptor for IgG on a human macrophage cell line, U937, *J. Immunol.* **125**:2735.

Anderson, C. L., and Grey, H. M., 1977, Solubilization and partial characterization of cell membrane Fc receptors, *J. Immunol.* **118**:819.

Anderson, C. L., and Grey, H. M., 1978, Physicochemical separation of two distinct Fc receptors on murine macrophage-like cell lines, *J. Immunol.* **121**:648.

Anderson, C. L., and Spiegelberg, H. L., 1981, Macrophage receptors for IgE: Binding of IgE to specific IgE Fc receptors on a human macrophage cell line, U937, *J. Immunol.* **126**:2470.

Arend, W. P., and Mannik, M., 1973, The macrophage receptor for IgG: Number and affinity of binding sites, *J. Immunol.* **110**:1455.

Arnaout, M. A., Melamed, J., Tack, B. F., and Colten, H. R., 1981, Characterization of the human complement (C3b) receptor with a fluid phase C3b dimer, *J. Immunol.* **127**:1348.

Ault, K. A., and Springer, T. A., 1981, Cross-reaction of a rat-anti-mouse phagocyte-specific monoclonal antibody (anti-Mac-1) with human monocytes and natural killer cells, *J. Immunol.* **126**:359.

Beller, D. I., Springer, T. A., and Schreiber, R. D., 1982, Anti-Mac-1 selectively inhibits the mouse and human type three complement receptor, *J. Exp. Med.* **156**:1000.

Berger, M., Gaither, T. A., Hammer, C. H., and Frank, M. M., 1981, Lack of binding of human C3, in its native state, to C3b receptors, *J. Immunol.* **127**:1329.

Bianco, C., Griffin, F. M., Jr., and Silverstein, S. C., 1975, Studies of the macrophage complement receptor: Alteration of receptor function upon macrophage activation, *J. Exp. Med.* **141**:1278.

Bianco, C., Eden, A., and Cohn, Z. A., 1976, The induction of macrophage spreading: Role of coagulation factors and the complement system, *J. Exp. Med.* **144**:1531.

Boltz-Nitulescu, G., and Spiegelberg, H. L., 1981, Receptors specific for IgE on rat alveolar and peritoneal macrophages, *Cell. Immunol.* **59**:106.

Boltz-Nitulescu, G., Bazin, H., and Spiegelberg, H. L., 1981, Specificity of Fc receptors for IgG2a, IgG1/IgG2b, and IgE on rat macrophages, *J. Exp. Med.* **154**:374.

Bourgois, A., Abney, E. R., and Parkhouse, R. M. E., 1977, Structure of mouse Fc receptor, *Eur. J. Immunol.* **7**:691.

Brade, V., Nicholson, A., Bitter-Suermann, D., and Hadding, U., 1974, Formation of the C3-cleaving properdin enzyme on zymosan: Demonstration that factor D is replaceable by proteolytic enzymes, *J. Immunol.* **113**:1735.

Charley, B., and Frenove, B., 1980, Fc and C3 receptors of swine alveolar macrophages, *Res. Vet. Sci.* **28**:380.

Chenoweth, D. E., and Hugli, T. E., 1978, Demonstration of specific C5a receptor on intact human polymorphonuclear leukocytes, *Proc. Natl. Acad. Sci. USA* **75**:3943.

Chenoweth, D. E., and Hugli, T. E., 1980, Human C5a and C5a analogs as probes of the neutrophil C5a receptor, *Mol. Immunol.* **17**:151.

Ciccimarra, F., Rosen, F. S., and Merler, E., 1975, Localization of the IgG effector site for monocyte receptors, *Proc. Natl. Acad. Sci. USA* **72**:2081.

Cooper, N. R., 1969, Immune adherence by the fourth component of complement, *Science* **165**:396.

Czop, J. K., and Austen, K. F., 1980, Functional discrimination by human monocytes between their C3b receptors and their recognition units for particulate activators of the alternative complement pathway, *J. Immunol.* **125**:124.

Czop, J. K., Fearon, D. T., and Austen, K. F., 1978, Membrane sialic acid on target particles modulates their phagocytosis by a trypsin-sensitive mechanism on human monocytes, *Proc. Natl. Acad. Sci. USA* **75**:3831.

Diamond, B., and Scharff, M. D., 1980, IgG1 and IgG2b share the Fc receptor on mouse macrophages, *J. Immunol.* **125**:631.

Diamond, B., and Yelton, D. E., 1981, A new Fc receptor on mouse macrophages binding IgG3, *J. Exp. Med.* **153**:514.

Diamond, B., Bloom, B. R., and Scharff, M. D., 1978, The Fc receptors of primary and cultured phagocytic cells studied with homogeneous antibodies, *J. Immunol.* **121**:1329.

Diamond, B., Birshtein, B. K., and Scharff, M. D., 1979, Site of binding of mouse IgG2b to the Fc receptor on mouse macrophages, *J. Exp. Med.* **150**:721.

Dierich, M. P., and Landen, B., 1978, Demonstration of C5-binding sites on lymphoid cells, *J. Immunol.* **120**:1771.

Dobson, N. J., Lambris, J. D., and Ross, G. D., 1981a, Characteristics of isolated erythrocyte complement receptor type one (CR_1, C4b–C3b receptor) and CR_1-specific antibodies, *J. Immunol.* **126**:693.

Dobson, N. J., Lambris, J. D., Bleau, S. A., and Ross, G. D., 1981b, Role of human neutrophil complement receptors and β1H in the release of superoxide anion, *Fed. Proc.* **40**:1014.

Dorrington, K. J., 1976, Properties of the Fc receptor on macrophages and monocytes, *Immunol. Commun.* **5**:263.

Douglas, S. D., 1978, Alterations in intramembrane particle distribution during interaction of erythrocyte-bound ligand with immunoprotein receptors, *J. Immunol.* **120**:151.

Eddy, A., Newman, S. L., Cosio, F., LeBien, T., and Michael, A. F., 1983, The distribution of CR_3 receptor on human cells and tissue as revealed by a monoclonal antibody, manuscript submitted.

Ehlenberger, A. G., and Nussenzweig, V., 1977, The role of membrane receptors for C3b and C3d in phagocytosis, *J. Exp. Med.* **145**:357.

Einstein, L. P., Schneeberger, E. E., and Colten, H. R., 1976, Synthesis of the second component of complement by long-term primary cultures of human monocytes, *J. Exp. Med.* **143**:114.

Ezekowitz, R. A., Austyn, J., Stahl, P. D., and Gordon, S., 1981, Surface properties of bacillus Calmette-Guerin-activated mouse macrophages: Reduced expression of mannose-specific endocytosis, Fc receptors, and antigen F4/80 accompanies induction of Ia, *J. Exp. Med.* **154**:60.

Fanger, M. W., Shen, L., Push, J., and Bernier, G. M., 1980, Subpopulations of human peripheral granulocytes and monocytes express receptors for IgA, *Proc. Natl. Acad. Sci. USA* **77**:3640.

Fanger, M. W., Push, J., and Bernier, G. M., 1981, The specificity of receptors for IgA on human peripheral polymorphonuclear cells and monocytes, *Cell. Immunol.* **60**:324.

Fearon, D. T., 1979, Regulation of the amplification C3 convertase of human complement by an inhibitory protein isolated from human erythrocyte membrane, *Proc. Natl. Acad. Sci. USA* **76**:5867.

Fearon, D. T., 1980, Identification of the membrane glycoprotein that is the C3b receptor of the human erythrocyte, polymorphonuclear leukocyte, B lymphocyte, and monocyte, *J. Exp. Med.* **152**:20.

Fearon, D. T., Kaneko, I., and Thomson, G. G., 1981, Membrane distribution and absorptive endocytosis by C3b receptors on human polymorphonuclear leukocytes, *J. Exp. Med.* **153:**1615.

Fernandez, H. N., Henson, P. M., Otani, A., and Hugli, T. E., 1978, Chemotactic response to human C3a and C5a anaphylatoxins. I. Evaluation of C3a and C5a leukotaxis *in vitro* under simulated *in vivo* conditions, *J. Immunol.* **120:**109.

Foris, G., Dezso, B., Medgyesi, G., and Bazin, H., 1981, Role of the cytoskeleton in the Fc receptor activity of rat peritoneal macrophages, *Int. Arch. Allergy Appl. Immunol.* **65:**138.

Foster, D. E. B., Dorrington, K. J., and Painter, R. H., 1980, Structure and function of immunoglobulin domains. VIII. An analysis of the structural requirements in human IgG1 for binding to the Fc receptor of human monocytes, *J. Immunol.* **124:**2186.

Ganczankowski, M., and Leslie, R. G. Q., 1979, The binding of rabbit IgG and its enzymatically derived fragments to homologous peritonteal macrophages, *Immunology* **36:**487.

Gerard, C., Chenoweth, D. E., and Hugli, T. E., 1979, Molecular aspects of the serum chemotactic factors, *J. Reticuloendothelial Soc.* **26(Suppl.):**711.

Ghebrehiwet, B., and Müller-Eberhard, H. J., 1979, C3e: An acidic fragment of human C3 with leukocytosis-inducing activity, *J. Immunol.* **123:**616.

Glovsky, M. M., Hugli, T. E., Ishizaka, T., Lichenstein, L. M., and Erickson, B. W., 1979, Anaphylatoxin-induced histamine release with human leukocytes, *J. Clin. Invest.* **64:**804.

Goldstein, I. M., Roos, D., Kaplan, H. B., and Weissman, G., 1975, Complement and immunoglobulins stimulate superoxide production by human leukocytes independently of phagocytosis, *J. Clin. Invest.* **56:**1155.

Gorski, J. P., Hugli, T. E., and Müller-Eberhard, H. J., 1979, C4a: The third anaphylatoxin of the human complement system, *Proc. Natl. Acad. Sci. USA* **76:**5299.

Götze, O., Bianco, C., and Cohn, Z. A., 1979, The induction of macrophage spreading by factor B of the properdin system, *J. Exp. Med.* **149:**327.

Griffin, F. M., Jr., 1980, Effects of soluble immune complexes on Fc receptor- and C3b receptor-mediated phagocytosis by macrophages, *J. Exp. Med.* **152:**905.

Griffin, F. M., Jr., and Mullinax, P. J., 1981, Augmentation of macrophage complement receptor function *in vitro*. III. C3b receptors that promote phagocytosis migrate within the plane of the macrophage plasma membrane, *J. Exp. Med.* **154:**291.

Griffin, F. M., Jr., and Silverstein, S. C., 1974, Segmental response of the macrophage plasma membrane to a phagocytic stimulus, *J. Exp. Med.* **139:**323.

Griffin, F. M., Jr., Bianco, C., and Silverstein, S. C., 1975a, Characterization of the macrophage receptor for complement and demonstration of its functional independence from the receptor for the Fc portion of immunoglobulin G, *J. Exp. Med.* **141:**1269.

Griffin, F. M., Jr., Griffin, J. A., Leider, J. E., and Silverstein, S. C., 1975b, Studies on the mechanism of phagocytosis. I. Requirements for circumferential attachment of particle-bound ligands to specific receptors on the macrophage plasma membrane, *J. Exp. Med.* **142:**1263.

Griffin, J. A., and Griffin, F. M., Jr., 1979, Augmentation of macrophage complement receptor function *in vitro*. I. Characterization of the cellular interactions required for the generation of a T lymphocyte product that enhances macrophage complement receptor function, *J. Exp. Med.* **150:**653.

Guyre, P. M., Crabtree, G. R., Bodwell, J. E., and Munck, A.,1981, MLC-conditioned media stimulate an increase in Fc receptors on human macrophages, *J. Immunol.* **126:**666.

Haeffner-Cavaillon, N., Dorrington, K. J., and Klein, M., 1979b, Studies on the Fcγ receptor of the murine macrophage-like cell line P388D1. II. Binding of human IgG subclass proteins and their proteolytic fragments, *J. Immunol.* **123:**1914.

Haeffner-Cavaillon, N., Dorrington, K. J., and Klein, M., 1979b, Studies on the Fcγ receptor of the murine macrophage-like cell line P388D1. II. Binding of human IgG subclass proteins and their proteolytic fragments, *J. Immunol.* **123:**1914.

Haesert, D. G., 1979, Phagocytic peripheral blood monocytes from rabbits and humans express membrane receptors specific for IgM molecules: Evidence that incubation with neuraminidase exposes cryptic IgM (Fc) receptors, *Clin. Exp. Immunol.* **35:**484.

Hammann, K. P., Raile, A., Schmitt, M., Scheiner, C., Mussle, H. H., Peters, H., and Dierich, M. P.,

1981, Stimulation of murine lymphocytes by human β1H but not by human C3/C3b, *Immunobiology* **158**:126.

Hay, F. C., Torrrigiani, G., and Roitt, I. M., 1972, The binding of human IgG subclasses to human monocytes, *Eur. J. Immunol.* **2**:257.

Hearst, J. E., Warr, G. A., and Jakab, G. J., 1980, Characterization of murine lung and peritoneal macrophages, *J. Reticuloendothelial Soc.* **27**:443.

Henson, P. M., 1969, The adherence of leukocytes and platelets induced by fixed IgG antibody or complement, *Immunology* **16**:107.

Herborn, H. A., Valdimarsson, H., and Wickramasinghe, S. N., 1979, Development of human granulocyte and monocyte Fc receptors, *Scand. J. Haematol.* **22**:364.

Herman, J. J., Rosner, I. K., Davis, A. E., III, Zeigler, R. S., Arnaout, M. A., and Colten, H. R., 1979, Complement dependent histaminase release from human granulocytes, *J. Clin. Invest.* **63**:1195.

Hobbs, M. V., Feldbush, T. L., Needleman, B. W., and Weiler, J. M., 1982, Inhibition of secondary *in vitro* antibody responses by the third component of complement, *J. Immunol.* **128**:1470.

Holland, P., Holland, N. H., and Cohn, Z. A., 1972, The selective inhibition of macrophage phagocytic receptors by anti-membrane antibodies, *J. Exp. Med.* **135**:458.

Huber, H., and Fudenberg, H. H., 1968, Receptor sites of human monocytes for IgG, *Int. Arch. Allergy Appl. Immunol.* **34**:18.

Huber, H., Douglas, S. D., and Fudenberg, H. H., 1969, The IgG receptor: An immunological marker for the characterization of mononuclear cells, *Immunology* **17**:7.

Huber, H., Douglas, S. D., Nusbacher, J., Kochwa, S., and Rosenfield, R. E., 1971, IgG subclass specificity of human monocyte receptor sites, *Nature (London)* **229**:419.

Hugli, T. E., and Erickson, B. W., 1977, Synthetic peptides with the biological activities and specificity of human C3a anaphylatoxin, *Proc. Natl. Acad. Sci. USA* **74**:1826.

Iida, K., Mornaghi, R., and Nussenzweig, V., 1982, Complement receptor (CR_1) deficiency in erythrocytes from patients with systemic lupus erythematosus, *J. Exp. Med.* **155**:1427.

Ishizaka, K., and Ishizaka, T., 1960, Biologic activity of aggregated gamma globulin. II. A study of various methods for aggregation and species differences, *J. Immunol.* **85**:163.

Joseph, M., Capron, A., Butterworth, A. E., Sturrock, R. F., and Houba, V., 1978, Cytotoxicity of human and baboon mononuclear phagocytes against schistosomula *in vitro:* Induction by immune complexes containing IgE and *Schistosoma mansoni* antigens, *Clin. Exp. Immunol.* **33**:48.

Kahn-Perles, B., Sire, J., Boned, A., and Bourgois, A., 1980, Putative conformation of mouse Fc_{γ}-receptor, *J. Immunol.* **125**:1360.

Kay, N. E., and Douglas, S. D., 1981, Detection of shedding of human blood monocyte Fc receptor during *in vitro* culture, *Int. Arch. Allergy Appl. Immunol.* **66**:131.

Kazatchkine, M. D., Fearon, D. T., Appay, M. D., Mandet, C., and Bariety, J., 1982, Immunohistochemical study of the human glomerular C3b receptor in normal kidney and in seventy-five cases of renal diseases. Loss of C3b receptor antigen in focal hyalinosis and in proliferative nephritis of systemic lupus erythematosis, *J. Clin. Invest.* **69**:900.

Kerbel, R. S., 1976, Resistance of activated macrophages to H-2 antibody-mediated cytotoxicity and Fc rosette inhibition, *Nature (London)* **259**:226.

Koide, N., Nose, M., and Muramatsu, T., 1977, Recognition of IgG by Fc receptor and complement: Effects of glycosidase digestion, *Biochem. Biophys. Res. Commun.* **75**:838.

Koren, H. S., Anderson, S. J., and Larrick, J. W., 1979, *In vitro* activation of a human macrophage-like cell line, *Nature (London)* **279**:328.

Koren, H. S., Meltzer, M. S., and Adams, D. O., 1981, The ADCC capacity of macrophages from C3H/HeJ and A/J mice can be augmented by BCG, *J. Immunol.* **126**:1013.

Kulczycki, A., Jr., Krause, U., Killion, C. C., and Atkinson, J. P., 1980, Purification of the Fcγ receptor from rabbit alveolar macrophages that retains ligand-binding activity, *J. Immunol.* **124**:2772.

Lachmann, P. J., 1981, Studies with monoclonal antibodies to complement components, *Immunol. Today* **2**:144.

Lambris, J. D., and Ross, G. D., 1982, Characterization of the lymphocyte membrane receptor for factor H (β1H-globulin) with an antibody to anti-factor H idiotype, *J. Exp. Med.* **155**:1400.

Lambris, J. D., Dobson, N. J., and Ross, G. D., 1980, Release of endogenous C3b inactivator from lymphocytes in response to triggering membrane receptors for β1H globulin, *J. Exp. Med.* **152:**1625.

Lamers, M. C., DeGroot, E. R., and Roos, D., 1981, Phagocytosis and degradation of DNA–anti-DNA complexes by human phagocytes. I. Assay conditions, quantitative aspects and differences between human blood monocytes and neutrophils, *Eur. J. Immunol.* **11:**757.

Lane, B. C., Kan-Mitchell, J., Mitchell, M. S., and Cooper, S. M., 1980, Structural evidence for distinct IgG subclass-specific Fc receptors on mouse peritoneal macrophages, *J. Exp. Med.* **152:**1147.

Lay, W. H., and Nussenzweig, V., 1968, Receptors for complement on leukocytes, *J. Exp. Med.* **128:**991.

Lay, W. H., and Nussenzweig, V., 1969, Ca^{++}-dependent binding of antigen–19S antibody complexes to macrophages, *J. Immunol.* **102:**1172.

Leslie, R. G. Q., and Cohen, S., 1976, Comparison of the cytophilic activities of guinea pig IgG1 and IgG2 antibodies, *Eur. J. Immunol.* **6:**848.

Loos, M., Muller, W., Boltz-Nitulescu, G., and Forster, D., 1980, Evidence that Clq, a subcomponent of the first component of complement, is an Fc receptor of peritoneal and alveolar macrophages, *Immunobiology* **157:**54.

Loube, S. R., and Dorrington, K. J., 1980, Isolation of biosynthetically-labeled Fc-binding proteins from detergent lysates and spent culture fluid of a macrophage-like cell line (P388D1), *J. Immunol.* **125:**970.

Lucas, D. L., Bowles, C. A., and Robinson, D. M., 1980, Characterization of canine monocytes *in vitro:* Increased receptor activity for Fc, C3, heterologous erythrocytes, *Transplantation* **29:**133.

Medof, M. E., Iida, K., Mold, C., and Nussenzweig, V., 1982, Unique role of the complement receptor CR_1 in the degradation of C3b associated with immune complexes, *J. Exp. Med.* **156:**1739.

Mellman, I. S., and Unkeless, J. C., 1980, Purification of a functional mouse Fc receptor through the use of a monoclonal antibody, *J. Exp. Med.* **152:**1048.

Messner, R. P., and Jelinek, J., 1970, Receptors for human γG globulin on human neutrophils, *J. Clin. Invest.* **49:**2165.

Michl, J., Pieczonka, M. M., Unkeless, J. C., and Silverstein, S. C., 1979, Effects of immobilized immune complexes on Fc- and complement-receptor function in resident and thioglycollate-elicited mouse peritoneal macrophages, *J. Exp. Med.* **150:**607.

Muller, W., Anausje-Abel, H., and Loos, M., 1978, Biosynthesis of the first component of complement by human and guinea pig peritoneal macrophages: Evidence for independent production of C1 subunits, *J. Immunol.* **121:**1578.

Munthe-Kaas, A. C., 1976, Phagocytosis in rat Kupffer cells *in vitro, Exp. Cell Res.* **99:**319.

Nelson, R. A., Jr., 1953, The immune adherence phenomenon: An immunologically specific reaction between microorganisms and erythrocytes leading to enhanced phagocytosis, *Science* **118:**733.

Newman, S. L., and Johnston, R. B., Jr., 1979, Role of binding through C3b and IgG in polymorphonuclear neutrophil function: Studies with trypsin-generated C3b, *J. Immunol.* **123:**1839.

Newman, S. L., Musson, R. A., and Henson, P. M., 1980, Development of functional complement receptors during *in vitro* maturation of human monocytes into macrophages, *J. Immunol.* **125:**2236.

Newman, S. L., Dobson, N. J., Lambris, J. D., Ross, G. D., and Henson, P. M., 1981, Specificity and function of human macrophage complement receptors for different fragments of C3, *Fed. Proc.* **40:**1017.

Newman, S. L., Devery-Pocius, J., Ross, G. D., and Henson, P. M., 1983, Phagocytosis by human monocyte-derived macrophages. Independent function of CR_1 and CR_3, manuscript in preparation.

Okafor, G. O., Turner, M. W., and Hay, F. C., 1974, Localization of monocyte binding site of human immunoglobulin G, *Nature (London)* **248:**228.

Ovary, Z., Saluk, P. H., Quijada, L., and Lamm, M. E., 1976, Biological activities of rabbit immunoglobulin G in relation to the domains of the Fc region, *J. Immunol.* **116:**1265.

Passwell, J. H., Schneeberger, E., and Merler, E., 1978, Cellular requirements for the formation of EA rosettes by human monocytes, *Immunology* **35:**863.

Perez, H. D., Goldstein, I. M., Webster, R. O., and Henson, P. M., 1981, Enhancement of the chemotactic activity of human C5a des arg by an anionic polypeptide ("cochemotaxin") in normal serum and plasma, *J. Immunol.* **126**:800.

Perlmann, H., Perlmann, P., Schreiber, R. D., and Müller-Eberhard, H. J., 1981, Interaction of target cell-bound C3bi and C3d with human lymphocyte receptors: Enhancement of antibody-mediated cellular cytotoxicity, *J. Exp. Med.* **153**:1592.

Petty, H. R., Smith, L. M., Fearon, D. T., and McConnell, H. M., 1980a, Lateral distribution and diffusion of the C3b receptor of complement, HLA antigens, and lipid probes in peripheral blood leukocytes, *Proc. Natl. Acad. Sci. USA* **77**:6587.

Petty, H. R., Hafeman, D. G., and McConnell, H. M., 1980b, Specific antibody-dependent phagocytosis of lipid vesicles by RAW264 macrophages results in the loss of cell surface Fc but not C3b receptor activity, *J. Immunol.* **125**:2391.

Rabellino, E. M., and Metcalf, D., 1975, Receptors for C3 and IgG on macrophage, neutrophil, and eosinophil colony cells grown *in vitro*, *J. Immunol.* **115**:688.

Rabellino, E. M., Ross, G. D., Trang, H. T. K., Williams, N., and Metcalf, D., 1978, Membrane receptors on mouse leukocytes. II. Sequential expression of membrane receptors and phagocytic capacity during leukocyte differentiation, *J. Exp. Med.* **147**:434.

Rabinovitch, M., 1967, The role of antibodies in the ingestion of aldehyde-treated erythrocytes attached to macrophages, *J. Immunol.* **99**:232.

Ragsdale, C. G., and Arend, W. P., 1980, Loss of Fc receptor activity after culture of human monocytes on surface-bound immune complexes: Mediation by cyclic nucleotides, *J. Exp. Med.* **151**:32.

Ralph, P., Nakoinz, I., Diamond, B., and Yelton, D., 1980, All classes of murine IgG antibody mediate macrophage phagocytosis and lysis of erythrocytes, *J. Immunol.* **125**:1885.

Reynolds, H. Y., Atkinson, J. P., Newball, H. H., and Frank, M. M., 1975, Receptors for immunoglobulin and complement on human alveolar macrophages, *J. Immunol.* **114**:1813.

Rhodes, J., 1975, Macrophage heterogeneity in receptor activity: The activation of macrophage Fc receptor function *in vivo* and *in vitro*, *J. Immunol.* **114**:976.

Rosenfeld, S. I., Kelly, M. E., and Leddy, J. P., 1976a, Hereditary deficiency of the fifth component of complement in man. I. Clinical, immunochemical, and family studies, *J. Clin. Invest.* **57**:1626.

Rosenfeld, S. I., Baum, J., Steigbigel, R. T., and Leddy, J. P., 1976b, Hereditary deficiency of the fifth component of complement in man. II. Biological properties of C5-deficient human serum, *J. Clin. Invest.* **57**:1635.

Ross, G. D., and Polley, M. J., 1975, Specificity of human lymphocyte complement receptors, *J. Exp. Med.* **141**:1163.

Ross, G. D., and Lambris, J. D., 1982, Identification of a C3bi-specific membrane complement receptor that is expressed on lymphocytes, monocytes, neutrophils, and erythrocytes, *J. Exp. Med.* **155**:96.

Ross, G. D., and Lachman, P. J., 1983, Membrane complement receptor type three (CR_3) is a lectin analogous to bovine conglutinin that functions as the zymosan receptor of neutrophils and monocytes as well as an iC3b receptor, submitted for publication.

Ross, G. D., Polley, M. J., Rabellino, E. M., and Grey, H. M., 1973, Two different complement receptors on human lymphocytes: One specific for C3b and one specific for C3b inactivator-cleaved C3b, *J. Exp. Med.* **138**:798.

Ross, G. D., Jarowski, C. I., Rabellino, E. M., and Winchester, R. J., 1978, The sequential appearance of Ia-like antigens and two different complement receptors during the maturation of human neutrophils, *J. Exp. Med.* **147**:730.

Ross, G. D., Lambris, J. D., Cain, J. A., and Newman, S. L., 1982, Generation of three different fragments of bound C3 with purified factor I or serum. I. Requirements for factor H versus CR_1 cofactor activity, *J. Immunol.* **129**:2051.

Ross, G. D., Newman, S. L., Lambris, J. D., Devery-Pocius, J., Cain, J. A., and Lachmann, P. J., 1983a, Generation of three different fragments of bound C3 with purified factor I or serum. II. Location of binding sites in the C3 fragments for factors B and H, complement receptors, and bovine conglutinin, *J. Exp. Med.* **158**:334.

Ross, G. D., Thompson, R. A., Walport, M. J., Ward, R. H. R., Lida, J., Newman, S. L., Harrison, R. A., and Lachmann, P. J., 1983b, Identification of a genetic deficiency of leukocyte membrane complement receptor type three (CR_3, an iC3b receptor) and its association with increased susceptibility to bacterial infections, submitted for publication.

Schlesinger, M., and Chaouat, M., 1975, The association of H-2 antigens and EAC receptors on the surface of peritoneal cells, *Eur. J. Immunol.* **5**:27.

Schneck, J., Rosen, O. M., Diamond, B., and Bloom, B. R., 1981, Modulation of Fc-receptor expression and Fc-mediated phagocytosis in variants of a macrophage-like cell line, *J. Immunol.* **126**:745.

Schneider, R. J., Atkinson, J. P., Krause, V., and Kulczycki, A., Jr., 1981, Characterization of ligand-binding activity of isolated murine Fcγ receptor, *J. Immunol.* **126**:735.

Schopf, R. E., Hammann, K. P., Scheiner, O., Lemmel, E. M., and Dierich, M. P., 1982, Human β1H globulin and C3b stimulate the respiratory burst in human monocytes, *Mol. Immunol.* **19**:1401.

Schreiber, R. D., Pangburn, M. K., Bjornson, A. B., Brothers, M. A., and Müller-Eberhard, H. J., 1982, The role of C3 fragments in endocytosis and extracellular cytotoxic reactions by polymorphonuclear leukocytes, *Clin. Immunol. Immunopathol.* **23**:335.

Scribner, D. J., and Fahrney, D., 1976, Neutrophil receptors for IgG and complement: Their roles in the attachment and ingestion phases of phagocytosis, *J. Immunol.* **116**:892.

Segal, D. M., and Hurwitz, E., 1977, Binding of affinity cross-linked oligomers of IgG to cells bearing Fc receptors, *J. Immunol.* **118**:1338.

Serio, C., Gandour, D. M., and Walker, W. S., 1979, Macrophage functional heterogeneity: Evidence for different antibody-dependent effector cell activities and expression of Fc-receptors among macrophage subpopulations, *J. Reticuloendothelial Soc.* **25**:197.

Shaw, D. R., and Griffin, F. M., Jr., 1981, Phagocytosis requires repeated triggering of macrophage phagocytic receptors during particle ingestion, *Nature (London)* **289**:409.

Shin, H. S., Smith, M. R., and Wood, W. B., Jr., 1969, Heat labile opsonins to pneumococcus. II. Involvement of C3 and C5, *J. Exp. Med.* **130**:1229.

Snyderman, R., Durack, D. T., McCarty, G. A., Ward, F. E., and Meadows, L., 1979, Deficiency of the fifth component of complement in humans: Clinical, genetic and immunologic studies in a large kindred, *Am. J. Med.* **67**:638.

Spiegelberg, H. L., 1974, Biological activities of immunoglobulins of different classes and subclasses, in: *Advances in Immunology* (F. J. Dixon and H. G. Kunkel, eds.), p. 259, Academic Press, New York.

Spiegelberg, H. L., and Melewicz, F. M., 1980, Fc receptors specific for IgE on subpopulations of human lymphocytes and monocytes, *Clin. Immunol. Immunopathol.* **15**:424.

Stecher, V. J., Morse, J. H., and Thorbecke, G. J., 1967, Sites of production of primate serum proteins associated with the complement system, *Proc. Soc. Exp. Biol. Med.* **124**:433.

Strunk, R. C. and Kunke, K., 1982, Human peripheral blood monocyte-derived macrophages (Mϕ) produce hemolytically active C3, *Fed. Proc.* **41**:732.

Sugiyama, N., Tamoto, K., and Koyama, J., 1981, Evidence for two distinct Fc receptors on guinea pig peritoneal macrophages, *Mol. Immunol.* **18**:999.

Sulica, A., Medesan, C., Laky, M., Onica, D., Sjoquist, J., and Ghetie, V., 1979a, Effect of protein A of *Staphylococcus aureus* on the binding of monomeric and polymeric IgG to Fc receptor-bearing cells, *Immunology* **38**:173.

Sulica, A., Gherman, M., Medesan, C., Sjoquist, J., and Ghetie, V., 1979b, IgG binding sites on macrophage cell membrane. I. Identification of two distinct Fc receptors on mouse peritoneal macrophages, *Eur. J. Immunol.* **9**:979.

Sulica, A., Gherman, M., Medesan, C., Ghetie, V., and Sjoquist, J., 1979c, IgG binding sites on macrophage cell membrane. II. Mobility of Fc receptors induced by the interaction with their corresponding IgG ligands, *Eur. J. Immunol.* **9**:985.

Sundsmo, J. S., 1983, Lymphocyte complement: A possible role for C5 in lymphocyte activation, *J. Immunol.* **131**:886.

Sundsmo, J., and Götze, O., 1979, A possible role for C5 in the induction of monocyte spreading by factor B, *Fed. Proc.* **38**:1467.

Sundsmo, J. S., and Götze, O., 1981, Human monocyte spreading induced by factor Bb of the alternative pathway of complement activation: A possible role for C5 in monocyte spreading, *J. Exp. Med.* **154:**763.

Sundsmo, J. S., and Wood, L. M., 1981, Activated factor B (Bb) of the alternative pathway of complement activation cleaves and activates plasminogen, *J. Immunol.* **127:**877.

Tack, B. F., Segal, D. M., and Schechter, A. N., 1978, Interaction of the third component of human complement (C3) with erythrocytes and leukocytes, *J. Immunol.* **120:**1800.

Tenner, A. J., and Cooper, N. R., 1980, Analysis of receptor-mediated Clq binding to human peripheral blood mononuclear cells, *J. Immunol.* **125:**1658.

Uher, F., Dobronyi, I., and Gergel, J., 1981, IgM-Fc receptor-mediated phagocytosis of rat macrophages, *Immunology* **42:**419.

Unkeless, J. C., 1977, The presence of two Fc receptors on mouse macrophages: Evidence from a variant cell line and differential trypsin sensitivity, *J. Exp. Med.* **142:**931.

Unkeless, J. C., 1979, Characterization of a monoclonal antibody directed against mouse macrophage and lymphocyte Fc receptors, *J. Exp. Med.* **150:**580.

Unkeless, J. C., 1980, Mouse macrophage Fc receptors, *J. Reticuloendothelial Soc.* **28:**11s.

Unkeless, J. C., and Eisen, H. N., 1975, Binding of monomeric immunoglobulins to Fc receptors of mouse macrophages, *J. Exp. Med.* **142:**1520.

Vogel, S. N., and Rosenstreich, D. L., 1979, Defective Fc receptor-mediated phagocytosis in C3H/HeJ macrophages. I. Correction by lymphokine-induced stimulation, *J. Immunol.* **123:**2842.

Vogel, S. N., Weedon, L. L., Oppenheim, J. J., and Rosenstreich, D. L., 1981, Defective Fc-mediated phagocytosis in C3H/HeJ macrophages. II. Correction by cAMP agonists, *J. Immunol.* **126:**441.

Walker, W. S., 1977, Mediation of macrophage cytolytic and phagocytic activities by antibodies of different classes and class specific Fc receptors, *J. Immunol.* **119:**367.

Walter, R. J., Berlin, R. D., and Oliver, J. M., 1980, Asymmetric Fc receptor distribution on human PMN oriented in a chemotactic gradient, *Nature (London)* **286:**724.

Ward, P. A., Cochrane, C. G., and Müller-Eberhard, H. J., 1966, Further studies on the chemotactic factor of complement and its formation *in vivo*, *Immunology* **11:**141.

Weigle, W. O., Morgan, E. L., Goodman, M. G., Chenoweth, D. E., and Hugli, T. E., 1982, Modulation of the immune response by anaphylatoxin in the microenvironment of the interacting cells, *Fed. Proc.* **41:**3099.

Wetsel, R., and Kolb, W. P., 1982, Complement independent activation of the fifth component (C5) of human complement: Limited trypsin digestion resulting in the expression of biological activity, *J. Immunol.* **128:**2209.

Whaley, K., 1980, Biosynthesis of the complement components and the regulatory proteins of the alternative complement pathway by human peripheral monocytes, *J. Exp. Med.* **151:**501.

Wilson, J. G., Wong, W. W., Schur, P. H., and Fearon, D. T., 1982, Mode of inheritance of decreased C3b receptors on erythrocytes of patients with systemic lupus erythematosus, *N. Engl. J. Med.* **307:**981.

Yagawa, K., Onoue, K., and Aida, Y., 1979, Structural studies of Fc receptors. I. Binding properties, solubilization, and partial characterization of Fc receptors of macrophages, *J. Immunol.* **122:**366.

Yasmeen, D., Ellerson, J. R., Dorrington, K. J., and Painter, R. H., 1973, Evidence for the domain hypothesis: Location of the site of cytophilic activity toward guinea pig macrophages in the C_H3 homology region of human immunoglobulin G, *J. Immunol.* **110:**1706.

Yodoi, J., Masuda, T., Miyama, M. Maeda, M., and Ichikawa, Y., 1978, Interaction of lymphocytes and macrophage cell line cells (M1 cells). I. Functional maturation and appearance of Fc receptors in M1 cells, *Cell. Immunol.* **39:**5.

Zuckerman, S. H., and Douglas, S. D., 1978, Optimal conditions for Fc receptor ligand interaction, *Int. Arch. Allergy App. Immunol.* **57:**269.

Zuckerman, S. H., and Douglas, S. D., 1979, Characterization and functional significance of plasma membrane Fc receptors, *CRC Crit. Rev. Microbiol.* **7:**1.

12

Antigen-Nonspecific Factors Elaborated by Macrophages Which Stimulate Lymphocytes

Interleukin-1

DAVID D. WOOD

1. INTRODUCTION

The essential role of macrophages in supporting lymphocyte responses in culture has been well established since the initial demonstration that neither antibody production nor T-cell proliferation takes place in the absence of macrophages (Mosier, 1967; Oppenheim *et al.*, 1968). At least three functions of the macrophage have been described which contribute to the vigor of the immune response. The most easily demonstrated of these is a feeder layer effect which can be replaced almost entirely by the addition of 2-mercaptoethanol to the culture (Chen and Hirsch, 1972). It has been suggested that the mercaptoethanol replaces the macrophage by modifying some high-molecular-weight component present in fetal calf serum (Opitz *et al.*, 1977) or by keeping glutathione reduced (Hoffeld and Oppenheim, 1980).

If the lymphocytes are depleted still further of macrophages, they become unresponsive even in the presence of mercaptoethanol. These cultures can be reconstituted by syngeneic, allogeneic, or even xenogeneic macrophages or their supernatants. The active factors in these supernatants have generally been found to be antigen nonspecific and genetically nonrestricted. While their role as immunostimulants *in vitro* depends upon their ability to stimulate both T and B

DAVID D. WOOD • Department of Immunology, Ayerst Research Laboratories, Princeton, New Jersey, 08540.

lymphocytes, their importance to the whole organism depends upon their ability to stimulate many nonlymphoid cell types as well. This review will deal with these factors, the monokines.

Finally, very thorough depletion of the macrophages yields lymphoid cultures which will respond only if they are reconstituted with macrophages or dendritic cells which share determinants of the major histocompatibility complex with the lymphocytes. It is believed that this last effect reflects an absolute dependence for antigen presentation on the macrophage surface or via antigen-specific, genetically restricted factors released from macrophages. These genetically restricted events are reviewed elsewhere in this volume.

1.1. LYMPHOCYTE-ACTIVATING FACTOR

Lymphocyte-activating factor (LAF) was first defined by Gery and his coworkers (Gery and Waksman, 1972; Gery *et al.*, 1972) as a T-cell mitogenic factor produced by the adherent cells obtained from the mouse spleen or human blood. These crude supernatants could be shown to be directly mitogenic to murine thymocytes and splenocytes and to potentiate the proliferative response of murine thymocytes, nonadherent murine splenocytes, and human blood lymphocytes to lectins. Most authors now assay LAF by its ability to enhance the incorporation of [^{3}H]thymidine by murine thymocytes which are cultured for 2 to 3 days in media containing the factor in the presence of both a lectin and mercaptoethanol.

It was shown that LAF could be derived from the macrophages of all the species investigated. The published examples include murine alveolar and peritoneal macrophages (Gery and Handschumacher, 1974; Blyden and Handschumacher, 1977), rat peritoneal macrophages (Ramic *et al.*, 1979b; Kierszenbaum and Waksman, 1977), rabbit alveolar and bone marrow macrophages (Ulrich, 1977; Efremov *et al.*, 1978; Simon and Willoughby, 1981), guinea pig peritoneal, splenic, and alveolar macrophages (Ramic *et al.*, 1979a; Stosic-Grujicic and Simic, 1979; Blyden and Handschumacher, 1977), dog alveolar and blood macrophages (Blyden and Handschumacher, 1977), and monkey splenic, blood, and alveolar macrophages (Blyden and Handschumacher, 1977). Finally, it has been found that LAF could be obtained from a number of murine macrophage cell lines (Lachman *et al.*, 1977a; Meltzer and Oppenheim, 1977; Mizel *et al.*, 1978a,b) and human myelomonocytic leukemias (Lachman *et al.*, 1978).

1.2. B-CELL-ACTIVATING FACTOR

Shortly after Gery's observation was published, Schrader (1973) reported that macrophage supernatants could also stimulate the development of antibody-secreting B cells in splenocyte cultures from athymic (nude) mice in the presence of the thymus-dependent antigen, fowl gamma globulin. In the absence of these supernatants, few antibody-secreting cells were observed. Since the macrophages used for these experiments were obtained from the peritoneal exudates of nude mice, it seemed probable that this T-cell-replacing activity was the product of a macrophage rather than a T cell.

Subsequently, it was demonstrated that a similar monokine could be derived from human blood monocytes (Wood and Gaul, 1974). This factor, later termed B-cell-activating factor (BAF), was defined by its ability to stimulate the plaque response to heterologous erythrocytes in 4-day cultures of T-cell-deficient murine splenocytes (either nude or normal splenocytes which were T cell depleted with anti-Thy-1 serum and complement) (Wood and Cameron, 1975). Because of the simplicity of the assay and the dramatic increase in response caused by the addition of monokines, the latter assay has become the most widely used to evaluate the role of monokines on the B-cell response. In this review, the term BAF will be used to indicate the ability of a monokine to induce the anti-erythrocyte response in T-cell-deficient cultures.

A detailed discussion of LAF and BAF will follow after a review of their biochemistry.

2. BIOCHEMICAL CHARACTERIZATION OF LAF AND BAF

2.1. MOLECULAR WEIGHT

The most commonly reported molecular species of LAF elutes from gel filtration columns at a position which is characteristic for globular proteins with molecular weights between 12,000 and 18,000 (12–18K). This species has been reported to be present in the culture supernatants of murine peritoneal adherent cells (Gery and Handschumacher, 1974; Calderon *et al.*, 1975), murine macrophage cell lines (Mizel *et al.*, 1978b,c; Mizel, 1979c), rabbit alveolar macrophages (Ulrich, 1977; Simon and Willoughby, 1981), and human blood monocytes (Gery and Handschumacher, 1974; Lachman *et al.*, 1977b; Blyden and Handschumacher, 1977; Koopman *et al.*, 1978; Togawa *et al.*, 1979). Independent methods have provided similar estimates of the molecular weight. Economou and Shin (1978), having measured the sedimentation and diffusion constants, estimated the molecular weight of the LAF from murine peritoneal macrophages to be 17K. Subsequently, Mizel (1979c), using disc gel electrophoresis in SDS and 2-mercaptoethanol, reported a weight of 12K for LAF from the murine macrophage cell line P388D1.

In addition to the 12–18K LAF, several larger species have also been observed. The smallest of these, eluting from gel filtration at 20–28K, overlaps so much with the lower MW species that its existence will be overlooked in all but high-resolution columns. It has been described in the supernatants of murine peritoneal macrophages and continuous cell lines (Economou and Shin, 1978; Mizel, 1979b; Mishell *et al.*, 1979) and, although not explicitly discussed, it has been clearly seen in the supernatants of rabbit alveolar macrophages (Simon and Willoughby, 1981) and human monocytes (Oppenheim *et al.*, 1980c). Both human and rabbit supernatants show a second peak of LAF in the region of

30–40K (Wood, 1979b; Simon and Willoughby, 1981) while a 39K species has been reported in the lysates of the murine cell line P388D1 (Mizel and Rosenstreich, 1979). Finally, one or two peaks of LAF activity have been observed above 50K in murine (Gery and Handschumacher, 1974; Lachman *et al.*, 1977a; Lachman and Metzgar, 1980a; Mizel and Rosenstreich, 1979), rabbit (Simon and Willoughby, 1981), guinea pig (Iribe *et al.*, 1982), and human macrophage supernatants (Gery and Handschumacher, 1974; Wood *et al.*, 1976; Blyden and Handschumacher, 1977; Lachman *et al.*, 1977b; Koopman *et al.*, 1978; Wood, 1979a; Togawa *et al.*, 1979).

Upon gel filtration, the BAF activity derived from human monocytes has been shown to elute with an apparent MW of 15–23K and coincident with 15K LAF (Wood *et al.*, 1976; Koopman *et al.*, 1978; Wood, 1979a,b). Indeed, the 30K LAF also exhibits BAF activity but is usually not present in sufficient quantity to be detected in the crude supernatants (unpublished results). Although similar data have never been published for murine BAF, it has also been claimed to exhibit an apparent MW of 15K (Calderon *et al.*, 1975; Hoffmann *et al.*, 1979; Hoffmann, 1980).

2.2. ISOELECTRIC POINT

When the fractionation is based upon ionic characteristics, LAF is again found to be heterogeneous. Upon isoelectric focusing of the 10–20K material from human monocytes, the major peak of both BAF and LAF activity coelute at an isoelectric point of 6.5–7.0 (Lachman *et al.*, 1977b; Wood, 1979a,b). Several minor peaks of activity are observed at lower pHs, typically at pI 4.5–5.2 and 5.5–6.0 (Lachman *et al.*, 1977b, 1980; Wood, 1979b). Isoelectric focusing of the LAF species eluting at approximately 35K yields similar profiles with a single peak at pH 6.5–7.5 and a broad, split peak at pH 4.5–5.5 (Ihrie and Wood, unpublished observations). An example of this molecular heterogeneity is shown in Fig. 1.

Similar heterogeneity has been observed among the monokines prepared from rabbit alveolar macrophages. Isoelectric focusing of the 10–20K fractions recovered from gel filtration resolved a major peak of LAF activity at pI 7.3–7.4 and several peaks of activity in the region of pI 4.5–4.8 (Murphy *et al.*, 1980; Simon and Willoughby, 1981). MW calculation using the Svedberg equation revealed that the pI 4.6–4.7 species were larger than the pI 7.4 species (14.4K vs. 11.6K).

In the mouse, no LAF activity has been found with a neutral isoelectric point. Economou and Shin (1978) have reported that the LAF eluting from gel filtration at 17K has a pI of 5.3 while the 22K fraction has a pI of 4.8. Similarly, Mizel (1979c) reported that P388D1 cell line-derived 12K LAF possessed pI values in the range of 5.0–5.6. Using P388D1 and three other murine macrophage lines, Lachman and his colleagues (Lachman *et al.*, 1977a; Lachman and Metzgar, 1980a) reported that high-MW LAF has a pI of 4.6–5.0 while low-MW LAF exhibits a broad peak of activity from pI 4.0 to 6.0. Chromatography of murine

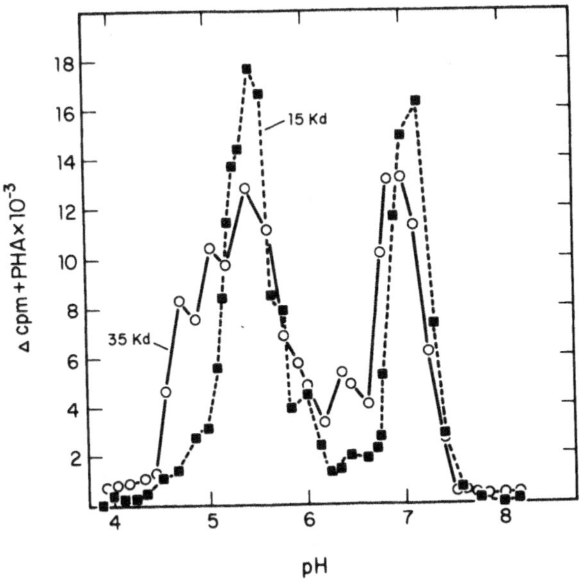

FIGURE 1. Molecular heterogeneity of human LAF. Endotoxin-stimulated mononuclear cell supernatants from a patient with chronic myelomonocytic leukemia were fractionated by gel filtration over Sephadex G-75. The LAF active products eluting with apparent MW of 10–17K (■) and 28–40K (○) were pooled and further analyzed by isoelectric focusing. All fractions were assayed at a dilution of 1 : 2000.

low-MW LAF on DEAE yielded one peak which failed to bind in 10 mM Tris and two or three peaks which were resolved in the salt gradient (Mizel *et al.*, 1978b; Mizel, 1979c). If the cultures were freed of contaminating lymphocytes, the breakthrough peak was missing, making it unclear whether this peak is a lymphokine or monokine. The heterogeneity of the 15K LAF is also reflected in the observation of multiple peaks (termed α, β, and γ) on Tris-glycinate disc PAGE (Mizel, 1979b; Mizel and Mizel, 1981).

Recently, Mizel and Mizel (1981) reported the isolation of the low-MW P388D1 LAF free of detectable contaminants. The factor was purified by sequential ammonium sulfate precipitation, hydrophobic chromatography on phenyl Sepharose, gel filtration on Ultrogel AcA54, and isoelectric focusing. The final product showed two major and two minor bands on two-dimensional gel electrophoresis using the highly sensitive silver stain. The bands presumably correspond to the α, β, and γ peaks of activity resolved by electrophoresis in Tris-glycinate disc gels. The estimated specific activity was 10^6 U/mg, meaning that approximately 50% maximal proliferation can be induced with 1 ng LAF/10^6 thymocytes. A partial amino acid analysis of this acidic LAF showed a relatively high proportion of acid residues with no proline and only one methionine residue (Mizel and Mizel, 1981).

2.3. INTERLEUKIN-1

It was concluded in 1979 that the same 15K monokine probably possessed both LAF and BAF activities, since the activities had been shown to coelute by gel filtration and isoelectric focusing (Koopman *et al.*, 1978; Wood, 1979b). Therefore, in order to simplify the nomenclature, it was suggested that the term interleukin-1 (IL-1) be introduced to designate the 12–18K molecule which exhibits a pI of 4.5–5.5 in the mouse and 6.5–7.5 in man (Aarden *et al.*, 1979). Throughout the remainder of this review, I will use the term IL-1 to refer to these molecular species and will use the other acronyms to designate the assay under discussion. It should be borne in mind, however, that these designations are a matter of convenience and do not rest upon rigorous scientific proof. In particular, it is quite possible that the protein designated as IL-1 in man differs significantly from the one designated IL-1 in the mouse. This topic will be discussed in detail later in this review.

Although the work of Koopman *et al.* (1977) was orginally considered to be evidence for the identity of LAF and BAF, that conclusion is suspect. Using supernatants of human mixed leukocyte reactions, Koopman *et al.* (1977) showed that the thymocyte-mitogenic (LAF) and PFC-stimulatory (BAF) activities fractionated together by gel filtration, DEAE ion-exchange, CM-cellulose chromatography, and electrophoresis on polyacrylamide. Although this work did convincingly demonstrate that a factor exists which shares LAF and BAF activity, it is likely that Koopman and co-workers were studying the T-cell product known as T-cell growth factor or interleukin-2 (IL-2) and not IL-1. It is well known that T cells do release IL-2 during the mixed lymphocyte reaction (Chen and DiSabato, 1976; Harwell *et al.*, 1976), and Farrar (1974, 1975) had shown earlier that T cells were required to obtain BAF activity in human MLC supernatants. Further, human IL-1 and IL-2 are not readily distinguished biochemically. Human IL-2, as measured by its ability to maintain the growth of cloned T cells, exhibits an apparent MW of 15K and a pI of 6.0–6.5 just as does human IL-1 (Gillis *et al.*, 1980; Watson *et al.*, 1980). Therefore, in this review, in order to avoid confusing the understanding of IL-1 with results which may be due to the presence of IL-2, I have ignored those data derived from work on supernatants prepared from mixed macrophage–lymphocyte cultures stimulated with T-cell activators.

2.4. CHEMICAL PROPERTIES

There is little evidence to suggest that the 15K monokine contains carbohydrates. On cesium chloride density gradients, the factor exhibits the buoyant density of a typical protein whether it is derived from the mouse (Economou and Shin, 1978), rabbit (Simon and Willoughby, 1981), or man (Wood, 1979a). Second, although Lachman and Metzgar (1980b) reported that human LAF is sensitive to treatment with the classical sugar oxidant, sodium periodate, most authors have found that neither mouse (Calderon *et al.*, 1975; Mizel, 1979b) nor human LAF (Blyden and Handschumacher, 1977) is affected by treatment with sodium periodate. Neither the mouse (Mizel, 1979c) nor human (Wood, unpublished observations) factor binds to Con A-derivatized Sepharose. Finally, mouse LAF (Calderon *et al.*, 1975) is insensitive to neuraminidase.

One of the most useful chemical properties for the identification of IL-1 is its sensitivity to mild treatment with phenylglyoxal. Reacting with the guanidinium group of arginine, phenylglyoxal is not considered to be a broad-spectrum enzyme inhibitor, and yet it strongly inhibits the activity of both human and mouse IL-1 (Mizel, 1980; Mizel *et al.*, 1981).

3. IMMUNOSTIMULATORY ACTIVITY OF THE MONOKINES

3.1. T-CELL MITOGENIC ACTIVITY

It is well known that macrophages are required in order to obtain significant mitogenic responses by T cells to mitogens or antigens *in vitro*. In cultures of macrophage-depleted murine lymph node or splenic lymphocytes, the mitogenic response to lectins (Gery *et al.*, 1972) and to antigens (Rosenstreich and Wilton, 1975; Rosenwasser and Rosenthal, 1978a) is markedly increased by the addition of monokines, but not by 2-mercaptoethanol. Indeed, as long as the macrophage depletion is not too thorough, the reconstituting monokines are active even when they are derived from allogeneic (Rosenwasser and Rosenthal, 1978b) or xenogeneic (Gery *et al.*, 1972; Rosenwasser *et al.*, 1979) macrophages.

3.1.1. Antigen-Dependent Proliferation

The first evidence that IL-1 could restore the proliferative response of macrophage-depleted murine lymphocytes to antigen was published by Rosenwasser *et al.* (1979). They showed that a 15K human monokine could restore the response of primed murine lymph node lymphocytes to the priming antigen almost as effectively as did the supernatants of syngeneic peritoneal macrophages. It was subsequently shown that highly purified IL-1 from the P388D1 cell line had the same activity (Mizel and Ben-Zvi, 1980). In both cases, the mitogenic effect was antigen dependent but not antigen specific (Rossenwasser and Rosenthal, 1978b; Mizel and Ben-Zvi, 1980). In other words, IL-1 stimulates the response of antigen-primed lymphocytes only to the priming antigen.

Although IL-1 could restore the antigen-dependent proliferative response of conventionally macrophage-depleted cultures, it could not restore the response if the cultures were depleted by both passage over nylon wool columns and subsequent treatment with antimacrophage serum and complement (Mizel and Ben-Zvi, 1980). In the latter case, as few as 100 irradiated, syngeneic peritoneal cells were sufficient to restore the response of 4×10^5 lymph node lymphocytes to IL-1. Presumably, the few macrophages which remain after the conventional depletion technique are sufficient to present antigen to the lymphocytes so that the response is limited only by the lack of the macrophage-derived antigen-nonspecific factors (IL-1). When more thorough macrophage depletion is achieved, the T cells are not "activated" because of the lack of antigen presentation and, therefore, remain unresponsive to the amplifying effects of IL-1. In this context, it is interesting to note that the monokines are reportedly incapable of restoring the response to genetically restricted antigens (poly-L-glutamyl-L-lysyl-L-tyrosine) even in conventionally macrophage-depleted cultures (Rosenwasser and Rosenthal, 1978b).

Recently, this interpretation was challenged by the observation that IL-1 could restore the proliferative response of cultures depleted of Ia-bearing cells (Durum and Gershon, 1982). The authors concluded that IL-1 was sufficient to initiate antigen-dependent proliferation even in the absence of Ia-dependent antigen presentation. The more likely explanation is that during the 4-day culture a sufficient number of Ia^- macrophages differentiated into Ia^+ cells to provide the necessary antigen presentation.

3.1.2. Thymocyte Proliferation

The idea that T cells must be "activated" by some previous signal before they respond to IL-1 is consistent with the information available from thymocyte cultures. When murine thymocytes are first placed in culture, they show a high rate of thymidine incorporation; if they are exposed to macrophage supernatants or purified IL-1 immediately a marked enhancement of proliferation is seen on day 3 (Gery *et al.*, 1972; Mizel *et al.*, 1978b; Beller and Unanue, 1979). In contrast, if the macrophage supernatants are added at 24 hr, a time when the spontaneous proliferation of the thymocytes is quite small, very little enhancement is observed (Beller and Unanue, 1979; Oppenheim *et al.*, 1980a). These unresponsive thymocytes can be "activated" again by briefly pulsing them with either Con A or wheat germ agglutinin, treatments which do not themselves promote thymocyte proliferation (Beller and Unanue, 1979). Reversing the order of application of the lectin and monokine was ineffective (Beller and Unanue, 1979). These results again suggest that the monokine itself does not deliver a sufficient signal to initiate proliferation; presumably, an "activation" signal must precede the monokine and bring the thymocyte into a responsive state. In this sense, LAF is really an amplification signal, not an activator.

Consistent with these conclusions, monokines (but not necessarily IL-1) have been shown to synergize the lectins to enhance the proliferative response of most of the T-cell populations tested. In addition to murine thymocytes, these include murine splenic T cells (Gery *et al.*, 1972), human thymocytes (Maizel *et al.*, 1981a), guinea pig thymocytes (Ramic *et al.*, 1979a), and rat lymph node and thymic T cells (Ramic *et al.*, 1979b; Kierszenbaum and Waksman, 1977; Katz *et al.*, 1980). The response is due to a true increase in mitosis and can be detected either by measuring the incorporation of radiolabeled thymidine or by counting the number of cells in metaphase after a colcemide block of division (Diamantstein and Ulmer, 1976). The monokines also have been shown to promote the growth of PHA-stimulated human and murine T-cell colonies in soft agar (Claesson *et al.*, 1977; Sredni *et al.*, 1978). The lectin appears to promote blastogenesis with the characteristic increase in cell size and alterations in nuclear size and polysome formation of the T cells but does not trigger DNA synthesis (Maizel *et al.*, 1981b). The addition of IL-1 stimulates these G phase cells and drives them into the S phase (Maizel *et al.*, 1981b).

In contrast to the other T-cell types discussed above, there is controversy over the ability of monokines to enhance the proliferation of human peripheral blood T cells to lectins. Oppenheim *et al.* (1980a,b) reported that the ability of PHA to stimulate both proliferation and lymphokine release by monocyte-depleted human T cells can be restored with the 50–150K monokines but not by the 15K IL-1. Subsequently, Maizel *et al.* (1981a) reported that low-MW IL-1 enhanced the proliferative response of similarly monocyte-depleted human T cells to both PHA and Con A. Finally, Lipsky *et al.* (1983) attempted to block PHA and Con A responses of unfractionated peripheral blood leukocytes with anti-Il-1 without success. The explanation for these differences is unclear, but since the 15K IL-1 does affect other human T-cell functions such as the formation of E rosettes (Ben-Zvi *et al.*, 1981), the human T cell does appear to recognize IL-1. One possible explanation is that IL-1 has both stimulatory and inhibitory effects depending upon the exact mixture of cell types used in the test. For example, Dinarello *et al.* (1983) have reported that IL-1 stimulates PGE secretion by monocytes which would inhibit the T-cell proliferation. The results reported may be a balance of the stimulatory effects of IL-1 upon the T cells and the inhibitory effect of monocyte-derived PG; a similar controversy exists in the fibroblast and mesangial cell literature (see Section 4).

If IL-1 only serves as a second signal to initiate the DNA synthesis by lectin- or antigen-"activated" T cells, then the assay of IL-1 based upon its direct mitogenic effect is inappropriate and potentially misleading. For example, it is generally recognized that the direct mitogenic effect of IL-1 is much more pronounced with the thymocytes from some mouse strains than in others (Farr *et al.*, 1977; Mizel, 1979b; Wood, 1979b). This may be due to strain-dependent differences in the "activation" state of the thymocytes at the time of sacrifice. Similar differences in the spontaneous activation state may account for the failure of some authors to observe a direct mitogenic effect of monokines on splenocytes and lymph node cells (Rosenstreich and Wilton, 1975; Kierszenbaum and Waksman, 1977; Mizel and Ben-Zvi, 1980) while others have reported moderate stimulation (Gery *et al.*, 1972; Kammer and Unanue, 1980). Finally, the observation that high-MW human LAF is more active as a direct mitogen for both murine thymocytes (Wood, 1979b) and human T cells (Oppenheim *et al.*, 1980a,b) than is the 15K IL-1 might suggest that the high-MW fractions are contaminated with a material which can enhance the activation state of the T cells and thereby synergize with a small amount of IL-1. Indeed, we have recently found that upon isoelectric focusing or chromatography over solid-phase anti-IL-1, the direct mitogenic activity of the high-MW LAF can be resolved from the majority of the PHA comitogenic activity confirming the hypothesis of a contaminant (Ihrie and Wood).

The requirement for the preactivation of the T cells is also compatible with the observations that IL-1 predominantly stimulates the division of mature thymocytes. Presumably, the mature thymocytes are more likely to have been activated *in situ* than the immature cells. The dense, peanut agglutinin $(PNA)^+$, Lyt-2^+ immature cells which predominate in the cortex of the thymus fail to respond to IL-1 (Oppenheim *et al.*, 1980b; Piantelli *et al.*, 1981; Luger *et al.*, 1982). In contrast, the low-density, cortisone-resistant, PNA^-, Lyt-2^- mature thymocytes respond strongly to both IL-1 and the high-MW monokines (Gery *et al.*,

1972; Blyden and Handschumacher, 1977; Oppenheim *et al., 1980b; Otterness et al.*, 1980; Luger *et al.*, 1982).

3.1.3. Effects of Monokines Other Than IL-1

Although the 15K IL-1 may be the only monokine necessary to explain the effects of macrophage supernatants on murine T-cell proliferation, other cultures have been described which require other monokines. For example, the proliferative response of macrophage-depleted guinea pig lymphocytes to PHA could be partially restored if they were cultured in a two-chambered "Marbrook" vessel separated from peritoneal macrophages by a cell-impermeable Nucleopore membrane (Rosenstreich *et al.*, 1976).

Surprisingly, neither the IL-1-producing cell line P388D1 nor purified P388D1 derived IL-1 substituted for the peritoneal macrophages (Rosenstreich and Mizel, 1978). When the macrophage supernatants were fractionated by ultrafiltration, all of the activity was retained by a membrane with a nominal 50K exclusion cutoff (Rosenstreich and Mizel, 1978). Subsequently, Iribe *et al.*, (1981) have demonstrated that the proliferation of macrophage-depleted guinea pig T cells to PHA was maximally stimulated by homologous monokines eluting from Sephadex with an apparent MW of 53–85K. The same high-MW monokine has also been demonstrated to stimulate the release of lymphokines (MIF) from immune guinea pig lymph node lymphocytes in the presence of antigen (Yamamoto *et al.*, 1978; Yamamoto and Onoue, 1979). If the lymph nodes were doubly depleted of macrophages by passage over a Tetron fiber column followed by passage over nylon, the lymphocytes became unresponsive to the factor. The readdition of 0.01% syngeneic macrophages restored the response in the presence of the factor, but the macrophages were inactive alone (Yamamoto and Onoue, 1979). As in the case of IL-1, the factor was active across allogeneic barriers and was antigen dependent but not antigen specific in its effect.

T-cell proliferation is also induced using proteases. In serum-free cultures of rat lymph node cells, it can be shown that proteolytic enzymes enhance the mitogenic effect of PHA (Katz *et al.*, 1980). Indeed, inhibitors of carboxypeptidase B inhibit the mitogenic activity of crude rat macrophage supernatants, and the mitogenic activity of these supernatants correlates with the carboxypeptidase activity (Katz *et al.*, 1980). Similarly, the ability of human monocyte supernatants to stimulate the release of lymphokines can be blocked by inhibitors of carboxypeptidase B (Bendtzen, 1981) although these same inhibitors failed to inhibit the pyrogenic activity of IL-1 (Dinarello *et al.*, 1982). The interpretation of these results remains unclear.

3.2. THE INDUCTION OF LYMPHOKINE RELEASE

It is now clear that another of the activities of monokines is to induce the release of IL-2. Lectin- or alloantigen-stimulated murine T cells produce a soluble factor which, like IL-1, stimulates the proliferative response of thymocytes (Di-

Sabato *et al.*, 1975; Chen and DiSabato, 1976). Unlike IL-1, however, this factor also has the property of maintaining the viability and growth of cytotoxic T-cell clones in long-term culture (Watson *et al.*, 1980; Smith *et al.*, 1979). Because of this characteristic, the factor was originally named T-cell growth factor (TCGF) and subsequently has been renamed interleukin-2 (Aarden *et al.*, 1979).

The ability of splenic T cells to produce IL-2 in the presence of Con A is dependent upon the presence of either macrophages or macrophage supernatants (J. Farrar *et al.*, 1980; Smith *et al.*, 1980b). At least one of the active monokines is IL-1 since preparations of purified IL-1 of both human and murine origin have been shown to stimulate IL-2 release (Smith *et al.*, 1980a,b; Shaw *et al.*, 1980; Larsson *et al.*, 1980; Gillis and Mizel, 1981). In an even more definitive test of the identity of IL-1 and the IL-2 inducer, P388D1 supernatants were fractionated by gel filtration and multiple fractions were assayed across the peak of activity (J. Farrar *et al.*, 1980). It was found that the LAF activity and IL-2-inducing activity coeluted with an apparent MW of 24K. Only a shoulder of activity was found at the more typical 15K position. Larsson *et al.* (1980) also reported that the IL-2 inducer eluted at 22K. This is somewhat disturbing since IL-1 has typically been reported at 12–18K; however, the discrepancy may result from the fact that in all of the above studies the IL-2 inducer was obtained from serum-free cultures. The identity of IL-1 with the IL-2 inducer is also supported by the observation that they share similar isoelectric points (Smith *et al.*, 1980b) and are both destroyed by phenylglyoxal (Gillis and Mizel, 1981). It is noteworthy that the amount of IL-1 required for half-maximal IL-2 production is about 5% of the amount needed for half-maximal thymocyte proliferation in the presence of PHA (Gillis and Mizel, 1981).

Just as in the case for the mitogenic activity of IL-1, the ability of IL-1 to stimulate the production of IL-2 depends upon the presence of a second signal. Con A (Larsson *et al.*, 1980; Smith *et al.*, 1980a), PHA (Gillis and Mizel, 1981), and autologous HLA-DR antigens (Palacios and Moller, 1981) have been shown to serve as adequate second signals. It can be expected that alloantigens and antigens to which the T cells have been primed will also be shown to serve as adequate second signals.

While it is clear that two signals are normally required to initiate IL-2 release, two different pathways can be imagined. The IL-1 and the second signal could affect the same cell or could affect different cells that then must interact to initiate IL-2 production. This question was addressed using a clone of an IL-2 producing lymphoma (LBRM-33 1A5) which failed to produce IL-2 in response to mitogen alone (Gillis and Mizel, 1981). Incubation of this cell line with IL-1 for as little as 4 hr at 37°C caused it to produce IL-2 upon subsequent stimulation with PHA. Because 1A5 is a cloned cell line, it can be assumed that IL-1 and PHA can stimulate IL-2 release by their coordinate effects upon a single cell.

The T cell which releases IL-2 in response to IL-1 appears to be the classical helper T cell. In the thymus, only the mature PNA^- thymocytes, which respond to the mitogenic effects of IL-1, produce significant amounts of IL-2 under the influence of IL-1. The PNA^+ thymocytes are unresponsive in both assays (Piantelli *et al.*, 1981). In the murine lymph node, the IL-2 producing cell has been shown to be Lyt-$1^+2^-5^+6^-7^+$ (Shaw *et al.*, 1980) while in man it is OKT 4^+8^- (Palacios and Moller, 1981).

Since IL-2 is active in the LAF assay, it has been suggested that IL-1 has no direct mitogenic activity, but rather expresses its LAF activity by causing the release of IL-2 (Smith *et al.*, 1980b). Indeed, preliminary reports have shown that the addition of monoclonal anti-IL-2 to thymocyte cultures does block the LAF activity of IL-1 suggesting that IL-2 may mediate the LAF effect (Conlon *et al.*, 1982; Oppenheim and Gery, 1982). Unfortunately, because neither report provided evidence to exclude a nonspecific effect of antibody on T cell proliferation, the role of IL-2 in the LAF effect still remains conjectural.

Finally, it should be recognized that the ability of IL-1 to induce the secretion of IL-2 by Lyt 1^+2^- T cells is only one example of a general induction of helper factors. Indeed, IL-1 can also be shown to secrete other distinct T cell factors such as those which induce the differentiation of cytotoxic cells and induce antibody secretion (Rao *et al.*, 1983) as well as LIF (Bendtzen, 1981).

3.3. T-CELL SURFACE MODIFICATIONS

3.3.1. Increase of Membrane Viscosity

The ability of IL-1 to serve as a second signal to drive T cells into S phase and to induce IL-2 release clearly demonstrates that IL-1 induces the differentiation of T cells. Therefore, it is not surprising that IL-1 can also be shown to modify the characteristics of the T cell membrane. Within 2 hr of incubation of splenic T cells with LPS-stimulated supernatants of the P388D-1 murine macrophage cell line, there is an increase in the frequency of antigen binding cells and in the membrane viscosity (Puri *et al.*, 1980).

It is likely that IL-1 is responsible for both these effects. Upon gel filtration, the active factors coelute with those which exhibit LAF activity as measured by the thymocyte mitogenic assay in the presence of PHA (Puri *et al.*, 1980). Peaks of activity were found with the apparent molecular weights of 16 and 50K. Chromatography of the 16K fractions on DEAE resulted in the elution of a factor which increased both antigen binding and membrane viscosity at the position where LAF activity has been reported by others (Puri *et al.*, 1980). Finally, it is the LAF responsive Lyt-1^+2^- cells, not the IL-2 responsive Lyt-1^+2^+ cells, which exhibit both the increased antigen binding and the increased membrane viscosity (Lonai and Steinman, 1977; Puri *et al.*, 1980).

The mechanistic relation between the three phenomena is interesting. An examination of the genetic restriction of the antigen binding showed that the supernatant could enhance the binding of only those antigens for which the T cell was a genetic responder whereas the peritoneal macrophages used to generate the monokines could be of either the responder or nonresponder genotype (Puri and Lonai, 1980). Therefore, the increased membrane viscosity does not create new antigen binding specificities. On the other hand, the addition of cholesterol to the T cells in the absence of monokines increased both the membrane viscosity and the antigen binding (Puri *et al.*, 1980) suggesting that the increased viscosity may cause an increase in the antigen-binding activities which are genetically programmed into the cell.

3.3.2. Enhanced Expression of Membrane Antigens

Monokines have been demonstrated to increase the expression of at least three T cell membrane antigens: Ia, Lyt-1, and H-2. An increase in Ia can be detected after 2–20 hr of incubation with monokines (Lonai and Steinman, 1977). For these experiments, the monokines were prepared by culturing resident murine peritoneal cells for 48 hr in the absence of any intentional stimulation. No attempt was made to biochemically characterize the factor involved. Although these conditions have not been found by other authors to yield significant amounts of IL-1, Puri *et al.* (1980) were able to show LAF activity in these supernatants. Further, like the LPS stimulated P388D-1 supernatants, these supernatants increased both the frequency of antigen binding and the membrane viscosity. Using quantitative absorption as the assay, the increase in Ia could be demonstrated in both thymocytes and splenic T cells, but not on B cells (Puri *et al.*, 1980). As was the case for the antigen binding, the effect was not dependent upon the Ia of the supernatant donor but was controlled by the Ia genotype of the T cell.

Oppenheim *et al.* (1980b) reported an increased expression of Lyt-1 antigen on thymic lymphocytes after 18 hr of incubation with supernatants derived from LPS-stimulated human mononuclear leukocytes. The active fractions eluted in the void volume of a Sephadex G-150 column (MW > 150K) whereas fractions eluting with an apparent MW of 15K were not significantly active.

Although the incubation of thymocytes with macrophage supernatants failed to induce any changes in H-2 or Thy-1 in 1 day (Lonai and Steinman, 1977; Beller and Unanue, 1977), a fivefold increase in H-2 could be demonstrated after 48 hr by quantitative absorption (Beller and Unanue, 1977). If the thymocytes were fractionated into immature and mature cell populations by density equilibrium centrifugation on BSA gradients, it could be shown that the increase in H-2 occurred in the immature population. It should be recalled that this population has been shown to be relatively unresponsive to the mitogenic activity of IL-1 (Oppenheim *et al.*, 1980c).

The supernatants used by Beller and Unanue were derived from 24-hr cultures of murine peritoneal cells from mice injected 7 days earlier with *Listeria monocytogenes*. Although these supernatants contained the typical peak of thymocyte mitogenic activity eluting at 15K, the fractions eluting at 15K failed to alter the H-2 expression. Instead, the factor which affects the expression of H-2 (termed T-cell-differentiating factor, TDF) eluted together with a minor peak of thymocyte mitogenic activity in the region of 35–40K. No further attempt was made to resolve the mitogenic activity from TDF; however, the TDF activity clearly does not depend upon a monokine-mediated stimulation of thymocyte proliferation since the increased expression of H-2 occurs equally well in the presence or absence of mitomycin C (Beller and Unanue, 1977).

The identity of the TDF is unclear. It could be interferon, a T-cell product, an aggregate of the 15K IL-1, or yet another factor. The possibility that TDF may be a T-cell product such as IL-2 and not a macrophage products stems from the fact that peritoneal cells from *Listeria*-primed mice were used to derive the factor. Although the macrophages were washed free of most of the lymphocytes before culture, the heightened LAF activity of these cultures has been shown to result from the interaction of a small number of T cells with the macrophages (Unanue *et al.*, 1976), and therefore the supernatants might well contain small amounts of T-cell products. Since murine IL-2 is a thymocyte mitogen and is reported to elute from Sephadex with an apparent MW of 35K (Watson *et al.*, 1980; Shaw *et al.*, 1980), it has several of the properties reported for TDF. On the other hand, although IL-2-rich supernatants have been shown to induce a very similar increase in H-2 expression by thymocytes, the H-2-inducing activity can be distinguished from IL-2 by its molecular weight and pH stability (DiSabato *et al.*, 1979).

A second possibility is that TDF is macrophage-derived interferon. It is generally agreed that fibroblast interferon (IFN-β) will induce a similar increase of H-2 on thymocytes (Lonai and Steinman, 1977; Beller and Unanue, 1977). Beller and Unanue (1977) have, however, argued that TDF is not interferon because the interferon activity, but not the TDF activity, of the supernatant was lost by heating at 56°C for 60 min. Whatever the final conclusion is of this question, it is clear that IL-1 does not alter the expression of H-2 on T cells.

3.3.3. Functional Maturation

The changes in the T-cell membrane are paralleled by changes in the functional maturation of the T cells. Immature thymocytes normally respond poorly in an MLC. In contrast, following 1 or 2 days of incubation in macrophage supernatants, the thymocytes could be washed free of monokines and still respond strongly in an MLC (Oppenheim *et al.*, 1976; Beller and Unanue, 1977). Both the stimulator and responder activity of the thymocytes were enhanced by the preincubation (Oppenheim *et al.*, 1976). The active factor has not been biochemically characterized.

3.3.4. Membrane TL Antigen

Lastly, Beller and Unanue (1977) demonstrated a decrease in the sensitivity of the immature thymocytes to lysis with anti-TL serum and complement after 3 days of culture with the macrophage supernatants. They suggested that this change might be due to a redistribution of TL on the membrane, rather than to a loss of TL, since no change is detected using a quantitative absorption assay. Again, the factor(s) responsible for this effect was uncharacterized.

In summary, it is likely that monokines exist which can induce a series of changes in thymocytes *in vitro*. Within 2 hr, increases in membrane viscosity and antigen binding are observed which are probably caused by IL-1. Within a day the amount of Ia and Lyt-1 on the T-cell surface increases, eventually leading to the increase in both the stimulator and responder activity of the thymocytes in an MLC. Whether the other maturational effects discussed above are the result of monokines remains to be proven. The implications of these observations to T-cell maturation in the thymus will be discussed in detail later.

The ability of monokines to modify expression of membrane antigens of T cells other than murine thymocytes is just beginning to be investigated. In the first report using human peripheral blood T cells, Ben-Zvi *et al.* (1981) showed that incubation of the T cells with human or murine IL-1 could markedly enhance the frequency of T cells forming "stable" rosettes with sheep erythrocytes. Although a detectable increase in the rosette frequency was observed within 6 hr, the frequency continued to rise through the entire 70 hr of culture examined. The concentration of IL-1 required for half-maximal E-rosette activity was approximately equal to that required to induce a half-maximal thymocyte mitogenic response in mice.

3.4. INDUCTION OF CYTOTOXIC LYMPHOCYTES

The requirement for macrophages in the induction of cytotoxic T lymphocytes to both alloantigens and syngeneic tumors has been well documented (Wagner *et al.*, 1972; Taniyama and Holden, 1979), and once again the requirement for macrophages can be circumvented by the addition of monokines but not by mercaptoethanol (Bach *et al.*, 1970; Gorczynski, 1977; Igarashi *et al.*, 1977; W. Farrar *et al.*, 1980). IL-1 is probably one of the monokines which augments the induction of cytotoxic T cells to alloantigens. This was first demonstrated by Gorczynski (1977) who showed that the larger macrophages recovered from the normal murine peritoneal cavity secreted a 10–15K factor which could reconstitute the cytotoxic response of macrophage-depleted murine splenic T cells to allogeneic B cells. The monokine acted across allogeneic barriers. Subsequently, it was shown that even more active supernatants could be prepared by stimulating peritoneal macrophages or the P388D1 cell line with phorbol myristate acetate (W. Farrar *et al.*, 1980). The active factor in these supernatants eluted together with LAF activity upon gel filtration, DEAE-cellulose chromatography, or polyacrylamide electrophoresis (W. Farrar *et al.*, 1980). As expected, the IL-1 was found to stimulate the cytotoxic response only when the alloantigen was present and only to the alloantigen presented (W. Farrar, *et al.*, 1980). The amount of IL-1 necessary to obtain half-maximal cytotoxic response was similar to that needed to obtain half-maximal mitogenic effect with PHA-stimulated thymocytes (W. Farrar, *et al.*, 1980).

At the moment it is unclear how IL-1 stimulates the cytotoxic response. It has been shown that the addition of IL-2 to macrophage-depleted cultures will restore the cytotoxic response (Farrar *et al.*, 1981) which suggests that IL-1 may stimulate the response by stimulating the release of IL-2. On the other hand, macrophage-derived products and IL-2 can be shown to synergize in this assay (Lutz *et al.*, 1981). While the apparent synergy could have resulted from the use of suboptimal amounts of IL-2, the observation raises the possibility that IL-1 has a direct effect on the cytotoxic response in addition to its effect upon IL-2 production.

Two observations appear to be incompatible with the hypothesis that the cytotoxic T-cell inducer is IL-1. First, Finke *et al.* (1981) have shown that IL-1 fails to stimulate the cytotoxic response of nylon wool-nonadherent T cells cultured with heated allogeneic thymocytes. In this case the required monokine exhibits an apparent MW of 38K. Second, Price and Gorczynski (1979) have claimed that the cytotoxic inducer is associated with β_2-microglobulin (β_2m). They showed that human urinary β_2 could restore the cytotoxic response of macrophage-depleted murine splenocytes as well as did the 15K monokine. Further, they showed that the activity of the 15K murine monokine could be inhibited by preincubation with goat anti-human β_2m and could be bound to and eluted from columns of Sepharose-bound anti-β_2m. I have performed similar tests using human IL-1. In my hands, human β_2m fails to exhibit either BAF or LAF activity, nor does anti-human β_2m inhibit the BAF or LAF activity of purified human IL-1 (unpublished experiments). It remains to be determined whether these widely differing results reflect experimental errors or fundamental differences in the triggering requirements of cytotoxic cell precursors exposed to different targets.

In addition to the above monokines, two peaks of cytotoxic T-cell inducer activity have been reported at 30–45 and 70–90K in murine peritoneal macrophage supernatants (Gorczynski, 1977; Gorczynski and Price, 1979) which are active only with histocompatible T cells. The 70–90K factor displays a restriction for the *K/D* end of the major histocompatibility complex while the 30–45K factor is restricted to the *I* region (Gorczynski and Price, 1979).

Monokines have also been reported to stimulate the secondary cytotoxic response to alloantigens and to syngeneic tumor antigens (Igarashi *et al.*, 1979; Klimpel, 1980) and the polyclonal cytotoxic response in the presence of 2-mercaptoethanol (Igarashi *et al.*, 1977; Okada *et al.*, 1978). The biochemistry of these monokines has not been described.

3.5. STIMULATION OF NK CELLS

NK cells represent an antigen-nonspecific class of cytotoxic lymphocytes. *In vitro* assays have shown that both IL-2 and interferon can stimulate the cytotoxic activity of partially purified human NK cells whereas IL-1 alone is inactive (Dempsey *et al.*, 1982). On the other hand, IL-1 is capable of augmenting the NK activation when it is used together with IL-2 or interferon or both (Dempsey *et al.*, 1982). The mechanism of this effect is unknown but may reflect IL-1-induced changes in the sensitivity of the NK cells to the stimulatory lymphokines.

3.6. ENHANCEMENT OF GLUCOCORTICOID RESISTANCE

Under conditions of stress (fasting, exposure to cold, inflammation, etc.), glucocorticosteroid hormones are released from the adrenals and exert strong effects on the viability and metabolism of a number of cell types. The macrophage appears to be capable of antagonizing at least a few of the steroid-induced phenomena through the release of the monokines termed glucocorticosteroid response-modifying factor (GRMF) and glucocorticoid-antagonizing factor (GAF).

3.6.1. GRMF

Of particular interest to the immunologist is the strong immunosuppressive effect which results from the administration of glucocorticosteroids both *in vivo* and *in vitro*. This effect is the result of the ability of steroids to depress the functional capacity of both T cells and macrophages (Cohen and Claman, 1971; Balow and Rosenthal, 1973; Lee *et al.*, 1975). These effects include the dramatic loss of cortical thymocytes as well as the suppression of both cellular and humoral immune responses. In this context, it was of interest to find that monokines could partially reverse the effect of steroids upon the proliferative response of human lymphocytes to pokeweed mitogen (Blomgren, 1974) and upon the *in vitro* antibody response of murine splenocytes (Mishell *et al.*, 1979). The effect on the humoral response has been investigated in detail and the monokine responsible has been termed GRMF.

Biochemically, GRMF has not been resolved from LAF and BAF. Fractionation of the supernatants derived from activated murine peritoneal macrophages by gel filtration resolves two peaks of GRMF activity at 13–16 and 23–28K which coincide with the peaks of LAF activity (Mishell *et al.*, 1979; Mizel, 1979a). Similar results were obtained when supernatants of activated human monocytes were analyzed (Fig. 2). For these experiments, GRMF assays were run by Grabstein and Mishell while the BAF and LAF assays were performed in my laboratory. The lowest MW peak of GRMF activity eluted together with the 15K LAF and BAF activity. If the fractions were assayed on C3H/HeJ splenocytes, two higher MW peaks were observed. The one eluting at a position corresponding to 60K coincided with fractions which stimulate the proliferation of thymocytes in the absence of lectins but which have rather little BAF activity. The other peak of GRMF activity eluted between 34 and 40K coincident with fractions which enhance the plaque response of C57BL/10CR splenocytes, but not of nude splenocytes. Relatively little further biochemical characterization has been reported which might distinguish GRMF from IL-1.

The standard GRMF assay involves the coculture of T and B cells with GRMF and the glucocorticoid. Therefore, GRMF could give the appearance of reversing the steroid effect either by protecting the helper T cells or by directly stimulating the B cells, i.e., by a BAF effect. Indeed, there is no evidence which demonstrates that T-cell-replacing (BAF) activity does not contribute to the final response; however, using a two-step procedure, Mishell *et al.* (1980b) have shown that GRMF does protect the helper T cells from inhibition by the steroid. For these experiments, splenocytes primed with SRBC *in vivo* 12 days earlier were cultured with dexamethasone and GRMF for 2 days and the residual T-helper activity measured. Preculture of the T cells in dexamethasone (10^{-6}M) reduced the helper activity by more than 95%. The inclusion of GRMF along

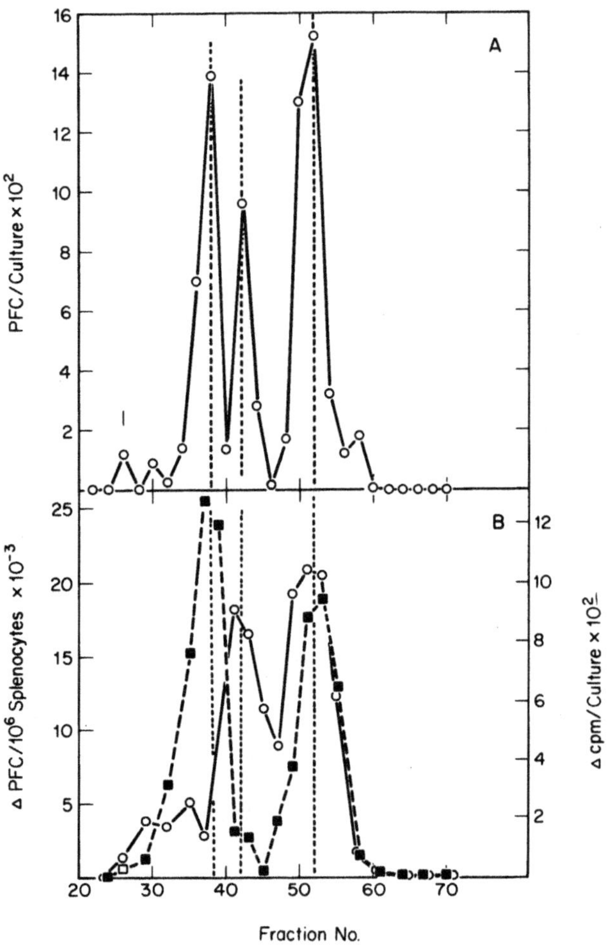

FIGURE 2. Cochromatography of GRMF, LAF, and BAF. Five hundred milliliters of LPS-stimulated monocyte supernatant were concentrated and chromatographed on Sephadex G-75 in RPMI-1640. Fractions (6.9 ml) were collected and assayed under different conditons. (A) 5 × 10^6 C3H/HeJ splenocytes were cultured with 10^{-6} M dexamethasone and sheep erythrocytes in the presence of a 1 : 5 dilution of the column fractions. After 5 days the cultures were assayed for direct PFC. (Assays performed by Grabstein and Mishell, University of California, Berkeley.) (B) Other fractions were assayed at a 1 : 10 dilution for their ability to enhance the direct plaque response of C57BL/10CR splenocytes to horse erythrocytes (○) or at a 1 : 40 dilution for their ability to enhance the proliferative response of C3H/HeJ thymocytes cultured in the absence of lectins (■). Further analysis of this set of fractions was previously described (Wood, 1979b).

with dexamethasone in the preculture prevented the loss of 25 to 50% of the helper activity and resulted in a 20-fold increase in the plaque response above that of dexamethasone alone (Mishell *et al.*, 1980a,b). These results indicate that GRMF protects against steroid suppression by a mechanism other than merely serving as a T-cell-replacing factor. Similar experiments have shown that GRMF can protect the helper activity of PNA^- thymocytes from steroid suppression (Mishell *et al.*, 1979a).

Despite the dramatic protection which GRMF provides to steroid-treated helper T cells, it does not protect all T cells. For example, the proliferative response of murine T cells to PHA, Con A, or alloantigens is dexamethasone sensitive and is not protected by GRMF (Mishell *et al.*, 1979, 1980a). The same is true for S49.1, a steroid-sensitive murine T-cell line whose growth inhibition by dexamethasone is not reversed by GRMF (Mishell *et al.*, 1980b). Finally, GRMF fails to protect suppressor T cells from dexamethasone (Bradley and Mishell, 1981).

In light of the observation that IL-1 can induce the release of helper factors, it is possible that the steroid protection afforded by GRMF is an indirect effect dependent on the presence of IL-2. Nevertheless, direct tests of IL-2 in the two-step GRMF assay have shown it to be inactive (Mishell *et al.*, 1980a), indicating that the steroid-protecting activity of IL-1 is not mediated by IL-2. In contrast, IL-2 can be shown to reverse the inhibition of mitogen-induced proliferation caused by glucocorticoids (Crabtree *et al.*, 1980) where IL-1 is ineffective (Mishell *et al.*, 1980a).

Finally, Mishell *et al.* (1982) have shown that IL-1 also prevents the inhibition of granulocyte/monocyte colony formation by dexamethasone. Again, the steroid-protecting effect of IL-1 is not shared by IL-2.

3.6.2. GAF

The second monokine which can modulate the body's response to steroids is GAF. The isolation and characterization of GAF has been monitored by its ability to block the induction of the enzyme phosphoenolpyruvate carboxykinase by hydrocortisone in rat hepatoma cell cultures (Goodrum and Berry, 1979) or in the liver *in vitro* (Moore *et al.*, 1978). This factor is reviewed in detail in Chapter 1 in Volume 7B of this series by Moore and Berry. Unlike GRMF, GAF elutes from Sephadex in one or two peaks in the region corresponding to 100–200K (Moore *et al.*, 1978; Goodrum and Berry, 1979). The existence of GAF is consistent with the suggestion that the macrophage may play a role in the modulation of the response to glucocorticosteroids *in vivo.*

3.7. ENHANCEMENT OF THE ANTIBODY RESPONSE

3.7.1. Particulate Antigens

In addition to the many responses which monokines elicit from T cells, the monokines also appear to induce the differentiation of B cells. The most dramatic of these effects is the induction of IgM antierythrocyte secreting cells (direct PFC) in cultures of T-cell-depleted or nude murine splenocytes. Typically, monokines will elicit a 10- to 100-fold increase in the number of PFC detected (Wood and Cameron, 1975, 1976; Hoffman *et al.*, 1979). The monokine responsible for the effect (BAF) has been demonstrated in the supernatants and lysates of human monocytes (Wood and Cameron, 1975, 1976), murine peritoneal macrophages (Calderon *et al.*, 1975; Hoffmann *et al.*, 1979; Hoffmann and Watson, 1979), rat peritoneal macrophages (Wood, unpublished observations), and rhesus monkey monocytes (Wood, unpublished observations). As discussed earlier, human BAF cofractionates with the 15K LAF upon both gel filtration and isoelectric focusing. Therefore, it has been assumed that BAF is identical with the 15K LAF or IL-1.

The stimulation of the antibody response of T-cell-deficient cultures by IL-1 has been demonstrated not only with heterologous erythrocytes, but also to haptenated heterologous and haptenated isologous erythrocytes (Cameron and Wood, 1978; Hoffmann *et al.*, 1979). In the absence of any added antigen, monokines induce a polyclonal response which is approximately 1/10th that of the antigen-dependent response (Wood and Cameron, 1975; Hoffmann *et al.*, 1979). IL-1 stimulates little or no B-cell proliferation (Wood and Cameron, 1975, 1978; Hoffmann *et al.*, 1979).

This is not to suggest that the macrophage does not make a monokine which enhances the division of B cells. On the contrary, Kurland *et al.* (1977) have shown that a monokine exists which substantially increases the frequency and size of murine B-cell clones grown in soft agar. This monokine has not been characterized.

As was the case for the stimulation of the proliferative response of T cells to antigens, the enhancement of the antibody response by IL-1 depends on the presence of a few macrophages. Partial depletion of the macrophages by adherence to plastic (Wood, 1979b) or by passage over Sephadex G-10 in balanced salt solutions (Hoffmann *et al.*, 1976; Hoffmann and Watson, 1979; Hoffmann, 1980) failed to significantly reduce the response of T-cell-deficient splenocytes to IL-1. If, however, the splenocytes are more thoroughly depleted of macrophages by passage over Sephadex G-10 in minimal essential medium, the responsiveness of the splenocytes to BAF is abolished (Wood, 1979b). The response of the macrophage-depleted splenocytes can be reconstituted fully by either irradiated G-10-adherent cells (Wood, 1979c) or irradiated adherent peritoneal macrophages (Wood, unpublished results). Although 2-mercaptoethanol has been shown to replace macrophages in the primary antibody response of normal splenocytes (Chen and Hirsch, 1972), 2-mercaptoethanol does not replace the requirement for BAF in T-cell-depleted cultures or the requirement for macrophages in the BAF assay. Indeed, all the experiments described in this section were performed using media supplemented with mercaptoethanol. Instead, it is likely that the macrophage requirement in the presence of BAF represents the requirement for the appropriate presentation of antigen.

The number of B cells which can serve as precursors for a clone of antibody-secreting cells can be determined by a limiting dilution analysis. Using this technique it was shown that the frequency of precursors was greater in the presence of both IL-1 and T cells (or T-cell products) than in the presence of either one alone (Wood, 1977; Hoffmann, 1980). Similarly, the total number of plaque-forming cells developed in the culture is substantially greater when both T cells and IL-1 are present than when either one is added alone (Wood, 1977,

1979c; Hoffmann *et al.*, 1979; Hoffmann and Watson, 1979). These facts imply that two populations of B cells must exist with different requirements for induction. It appears that these two populations may be distinguished by the presence of a complement receptor. Those B cells which express the complement receptor (CR^+) can differentiate into antibody-secreting cells if stimulated by helper T cells in the absence of monokines (Hoffmann *et al.*, 1976). In contrast, the CR^- B cells are only stimulated by helper T cells if IL-1-rich preparations are added as well (Hoffmann *et al.*, 1976, 1977). Since these same IL-1-rich preparations can be shown to induce the differentiation of bone marrow cells from Ia^- to Ia^+ and from CR^- to CR^+ (Hoffmann *et al.*, 1977, 1979), it was assumed that IL-1 caused the differentiation of CR^- splenocytes to the CR^+ state which allowed them to respond to T-cell help.

In addition to its direct effect upon B cells, IL-1 may induce the release of helper factors from the few residual T cells present in the populations of splenocytes treated with anti-Thy-1 and complement or from the immature T cells of the nude. When both exogenous IL-1 and T-cell-derived helper factors are added to cultures of T-cell-depleted splenocytes a synergy of 6- to 10-fold can be observed (Hoffmann and Watson, 1979). A large synergy can also be seen if the splenocytes are exposed to IL-1 for 2 days, washed, and recultured with T-cell factors for the last 2 days before harvesting (Hoffmann, 1980). Thus, the production of even small amounts of endogenous helper factor might significantly augment the response to IL-1.

Taken together, these results suggest that IL-1 can elicit two important responses in splenocyte cultures. First, it can induce the differentiation of CR^- B cells into a mature state (CR^+) which allows them to respond directly to T-cell-derived factors. Second, IL-1 stimulates Lyt-1^+2^- T cells to release helper factors. It remains uncertain whether the response of T-cell-deficient cultures to IL-1 alone depends upon the release of minute amounts of T-cell-derived factors or upon the ability of IL-1 itself to differentiate a small number of B cells all the way into antibody secretors. The fact that the addition of monokines for only the first day or two gives a smaller plaque response than addition for the last 2 days (Wood and Cameron, 1975; Hoffmann, 1980; Hoffmann and Watson, 1979) suggests that IL-1 alone exerts its principal effect upon the terminal differentiation. This would support the latter model; however, it may well be that both mechanisms are at play.

Recently, Shiozawa *et al.* (1980) have described cultures in which as few as 2000 rosette purified virgin B cells can yield an average of 500 PFC against chicken erythrocytes. In this culture, both the T cells and macrophages can be replaced by soluble factors. Although the active monokine has not yet been identified, the preliminary experiments suggest that it is not IL-1 (Diener, personal communication).

3.7.2. Soluble Antigens

Although Schrader (1973) reported that unfractionated murine monokines could dramatically stimulate the primary antibody response of nude splenocytes to fowl gamma globulin, my laboratory has been unable to achieve more than a twofold stimulation in the response of T-cell-depleted splenocytes to dinitrophenylated keyhole limpet hemocyanin (DNP-KLH) with purified human IL-1 (Cameron and Wood, unpublished observations). It is possible that Schrader's results reflect an exceptionally intense polyclonal effect induced by monokines or the activity of a monokine other than IL-1. In contrast, it can be shown that crude monokines can augment the secondary plaque response to haptenated KLH in the presence of primed T cells but not in T-cell-depleted cultures (Calderon *et al.*, 1975).

In the presence of pokeweed mitogen (PWM), monokines stimulate both the polyclonal and antierythrocyte antibody response of human peripheral blood lymphocytes in culture (Dimitriu and Fauci, 1978; (Rosenberg and Lipsky, 1980, 1981). Human B cells, when partially depleted of monocytes and T cells, fail to respond to PWM with either proliferation or immunoglobulin secretion. The addition of monokines restored the immunoglobulin secretion but not the proliferative response (Rosenberg and Lipsky, 1980, 1981). In the absence of PWM, the monokines were ineffective. If the B cells were further purified, the activity of the monocyte supernatants became dependent upon the addition of a few T cells (Rosenberg and Lipsky, 1980) and macrophages (Rosenberg and Lipsky, 1981). As in the case for LAF and BAF, the active monokine in this system was released during the first 24 hr of monocyte culture with little, if any, activity released upon subsequent culture. After 24 hr, the "aged" macrophages were unable to reconstitute the immunoglobulin response of the PWM-stimulated B cells; however, the "aged" macrophages together with the monocyte supernatants reconstituted the response very well even in cultures of highly macrophage-depleted B cells. Presumably, this phenomenon reflects the need for both IL-1 and antigen presentation. Tests with partially purified human IL-1 (15K, pI 6.6) showed that it was sufficient to replace the monocyte supernatant (Rosenberg and Lipsky, 1981). Similarly, addition of rabbit anti-IL-1 to the cultures inhibited the PWM-induced B-cell proliferation and immunoglobulin secretion, but not the T-cell proliferation (Lipsky *et al.*, 1983). This inhibition could be reversed by the addition of exogenous IL-1. In summary, the ability of human B cells to respond to PWM with immunoglobulin secretion appears to depend on the presence of IL-1 as well as the presence of both T cells and macrophages. The cells may be required for helper factor production and antigen presentation, respectively.

3.8. INDUCTION OF T-HELPER CELLS

Monokines have also been shown to enhance the differentiation of macrophage-depleted lymph node or mature thymic T cells into becoming helper cells. One of these factors (GRF) is a genetically restricted factor which is reviewed by Katz, Sunshine, and Feldmann (Chapter 8). The second is known as nonspecific macrophage factor (NMF). NMF induces helper T cells in the presence of particulate, but not soluble, antigens (Erb and Feldmann, 1975a,b) and stimulates Lyt-$1^{+}2^{-}$ T cells as does IL-1 (Erb *et al.*, 1977). Unlike most of the IL-1 activities, however, the activity of NMF in this assay can be replaced by the addition of 2-mercaptoethanol to the culture (Erb and Feldmann, 1975a). Therefore, the mechanism of action of NMF in the induction of help (the NMF assay) differs from the action of IL-1 in the induction of PFC in T-cell-depleted cultures (the BAF assay). Nevertheless, the monokine which possesses NMF activity may be identical to IL-1.

3.9. SUMMARY

Based upon the biochemical and immunological studies just reviewed, it would appear that the 15K IL-1 is the principal immunoregulatory monokine. A schematic illustration of its principal immunoregulatory effects are shown in Fig. 3. IL-1 is capable of stimulating the T-cell proliferation to both antigens and lectins as long as sufficient macrophages remain in the culture to adequately present the antigen. This proliferative effect seems to be mediated by IL-2, a product of the IL-1-responsive Lyt-$1^{+}2^{-}$ lymphocytes. IL-1 also appears to modify the viscosity of the T-cell membrane, the display of its surface antigens, and its steroid sensitivity. While the ability of IL-1 to stimulate the release of helper factors may well contribute to its ability to enhance the proliferation and differentiation of B cells, the induction of cytotoxic T cells, and the stimulation of NK cells, it remains likely that IL-1 also exerts some of its effects directly on the B cells and NK cells at least.

In addition to IL-1, a number of other immunoregulatory monokines have been reported whose biochemical properties and biological effects are less well characterized. Among these are the 50–150K LAF which has been reported to alter membrane viscosity and improve steroid resistance (Table I). Unfortunately, until this material has been better characterized, it remains quite likely that it is a mixture of aggregated LAF with other mitogenic or stimulatory materials

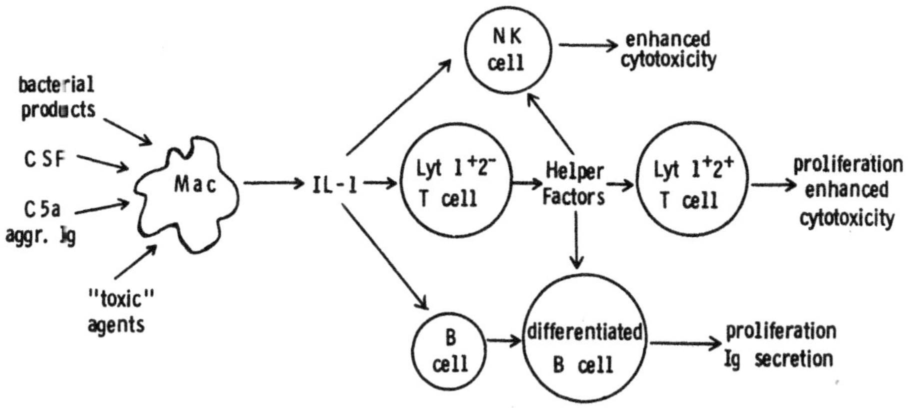

FIGURE 3. Pathway of the immunostimulatory effects of IL-1.

TABLE 1. THE ACTIVITIES OF HIGH- AND LOW-MOLECULAR-WEIGHT MONOKINES

Activity	Molecular weight 15K	50–150K
Enhancement of thymocyte proliferation to PHA (LAF)	+	+
Increased membrane viscosity	+	+
Enhanced steroid resistance (GRMF)	+	+
IL-2 induction	+	?
Cytotoxic T-cell induction	+	?
B-cell differentiation	+	?
Proliferative response of guinea pig T cells to PHA	–	+
Induction of Lyt-1 on murine thymocytes	–	+

such as GAF. Thus, the reported ability of these fractions to serve as a direct mitogen for T cells or to stimulate guinea pig T cells may be properties unrelated to the LAF activity present in the same fractions. In addition, macrophage supernatants also seem to contain proteases, a 35K factor which affects T-cell maturation and cytotoxic T-cell induction, and a factor that affects B-cell colony formation. The relation of these factors to each other and to IL-1 remains to be determined.

4. NONIMMUNOLOGICAL ACTIVITIES OF IL-1

In addition to its effects on the immune system, IL-1 appears to exert important effects on a large number of nonlymphoid cells. Obviously, any real understanding of the physiological role of IL-1 requires an appreciation of these nonimmunological activities and consequently these have been reviewed briefly below. More extensive reviews of several of these activities can be found in Volume 7B of this series by Mitchell and Kampschmidt (Chapter 7) and by Bernheim (Chapter 14). The effects include a coordinated series of physiological responses which constitute the body's response to infection (fever, synthesis of acute-phase proteins, muscle breakdown, neutrophilia, neutrophil activation, and serum ion changes) as well as the stimulation of several mesenchymal cell types.

4.1. THE INDUCTION OF FEVER

The study of the pyrogenicity of monokines actually predated the observations of Gery by two decades. In 1948, Beeson reported that a fever-producing substance could be obtained from the glycogen-induced peritoneal exudate cells of a rabbit. This factor, known as leukocytic or endogenous pyrogen (EP), could be distinguished from bacterial endotoxin by at least three parameters. The injection of EP into rabbits induced a monophasic fever with a latency of only 20 min in contrast to the biphasic fever and 1-hr latency typical of endotoxin-induced fevers. Second, EP was heat sensitive while endotoxin was not. Lastly, repeated injections of endotoxin into rabbits rendered them unresponsive to the pyrogenic effects of endotoxin whereas such "endotoxin-tolerant" rabbits responded normally to EP. It was subsequently shown that the only EP-producing cell in these exudates was the macrophage (Hanson *et al.*, 1980). As was the case for LAF, it could be shown that the macrophages derived from many other tissues and many other species also produced EP (see review by Bernheim in Chapter 14, Volume 7B of this series and by Bernheim *et al.*, 1979).

Recently, it has been recognized that the same molecules probably possess both LAF and pyrogenic activity. Upon gel filtration, rabbit EP exhibits an apparent MW of 13–16K (Cebula *et al.*, 1979) as does rabbit LAF (Simon and Willoughby, 1981). Upon isoelectric focusing, the 13–16K EP separates into a neutral (pI 7.3) and an acidic (pI 5.1) fraction. When the acid fractions were refocused on more shallow gradient, two to four peaks of activity could be resolved (Cebula *et al.*, 1979; Murphy *et al.*, 1981a). Peaks of LAF activity coincided with each of the peaks of EP activity with a resolution of approximately 0.02 pH unit (Murphy *et al.*, 1980). Further, both the EP and LAF activity of the pI 7.3 monokine bound to thiol-Sepharose and could be eluted with mercaptoethanol (Murphy *et al.*, 1980). Finally, both the EP and LAF activity of the pI 7.3 monkine could be blocked with a goat anti-rabbit EP (Murphy *et al.*, 1980). It is estimated that the amount of rabbit EP required to induce a 1°C fever (1 pyrogen unit) is 250 times the amount needed to produce a half-maximal LAF response (1 LAF unit) (Murphy *et al.*, 1980).

Similar data have also been obtained with human pyrogen where 1 pyrogen unit would appear to equal 10–100 LAF units (Rosenwasser and Dinarello, 1981). Depending upon the experimental protocol, human monocytes release variable amounts of a 15K, pI 6.8–7.1 pyrogen and a 38–40K, pI 5.1–5.2 pyrogen (Dinarello *et al.*, 1974; Dinarello and Wolff, 1977). The acidic EP reportedly elicits a more delayed but more sustained fever than does the neutral pyrogen (Dinarello *et al.*, 1974). Preparations of each of these pyrogens were found to have LAF activity and to stimulate antigen-dependent T-cell proliferation (Rosenwasser *et al.*, 1979; Rosenwasser and Dinarello, 1981). Further, a rabbit anti-human monokine serum which binds both the neutral and acidic pyrogen (Dinarello *et al.*, 1977) blocked the LAF activity of the neutral factor (results with acidic LAF were not reported, Rosenwasser and Dinarello, 1981).

Despite the substantial biochemical evidence favoring the identity of IL-1 and EP, they may be subtlely distinct. Damais *et al.* (1982) have shown that macrophages when stimulated with a butyl ester of MDP release a thymocyte comitogen but no pyrogen. The final proof of this apparent separation of the two activities must await careful evaluation of the properties of comitogen purified from these supernatants.

EP has been shown to induce fever through its action on the temperature-sensitive neurons in the preoptic anterior hypothalamus (Cooper *et al.*, 1967; Cabanac *et al.*, 1968), midbrain (Nakayama and Hori, 1973), and medulla oblongata (Sakata *et al.*, 1981). Unit studies in the hypothalamus have shown that the warm receptors are the most numerous (Nakayama *et al.*, 1963). These receptors increase their spontaneous discharge rate with a Q10 of 5–15. The less numerous cold receptors increase their discharge rate with decreasing temperature (Nakayama *et al.*, 1963; Hardy *et al.*, 1964; Eisenman and Jackson, 1967). Exposure of the temperature-sensitive neurons to EP is believed to increase the "set-point" of this neural thermostat. In other words, EP decreases the discharge rate of the warm receptors and increase the rate of the cold receptors (Sakata *et al.*, 1981). In order to return the discharge rate of the neurons to "normal," the body temperature must be raised. That the body temperature is indeed regulated during fever has been shown by exercise studies. When febrile patients exercise, their body temperature rises above the febrile level. When the exercise ceases, the temperature falls back to the preexisting febrile level, not to normal (MacPherson, 1959; Cooper *et al.*, 1964).

4.2. STIMULATION OF ACUTE-PHASE PROTEIN SYNTHESIS

The injection of monokines into mice and rats has been shown to cause a flux of amino acids into the liver and an increase in the synthesis of several serum proteins (Wannemacher *et al.*, 1972, 1975; Sipe *et al.*, 1979; Kampschmidt, 1981). The monokine responsible for this effect has been named leukocytic endogenous mediator (LEM) and has been extensively reviewed by Mitchell and Kampschmidt in this series. The affected proteins are known as the acute-phase proteins. Those acute-phase proteins which are normally present in substantial concentrations such as haptoglobin and fibrinogen are increased in concentration by only two- or threefold following the injection of monokines (Kampschmidt and Upchurch, 1974; Thompson *et al.*, 1976; Bornstein and Walsh, 1978). Other serum proteins which normally occur at low concentrations such as α_2-macrofetoprotein, C-reactive protein, serum amyloid P-component, and serum amyloid A (SAA) protein increase several hundredfold after the injection of LEM (Eddington *et al.*, 1972; Merriman *et al.*, 1975; Thompson *et al.*, 1976; Le *et al.*, 1982; Sztein *et al.*, 1981).

Although there is some evidence that neutrophils and splenocytes can synthesize SAA (Rosenthal and Sullivan, 1978; Cohen *et al.*, 1965), the liver appears to be the major source of the acute-phase proteins (Sipe *et al.*, 1978; Benson and Kleiner, 1980). Further, although there is some indirect evidence that the increase in acute-phase proteins is modified by the endocrine system and the central nervous system (Thompson *et al.*, 1975; Turchik and Bornstein, 1980), the observations that LEM can augment the synthesis of acute-phase proteins by cultured hepatocytes (Kampschmidt and Upchurch, 1974; Rupp and Fuller, 1979; Selinger *et al.*, 1980) has led most investigators to conclude that LEM affects the hepatocytes directly. Finally, the observations that LEM increases the uptake of amino acids and the synthesis of ribosomal RNA by the liver (Wannemacher *et al.*, 1975) are consistent with the idea that it is the liver which synthesizes the acute-phase proteins in response to LEM.

The evidence that LEM is identical with IL-1 and with EP is fairly extensive. LEM can be obtained from the same macrophage populations following the same stimuli which induce the release of IL-1 and EP (Kampschmidt, 1982; Sztein *et al.*, 1981). It should be noted, however, that the literature of LEM is somewhat confusing because it refers to LEM as a product of neutrophils. Like the similar claim made for EP, this statement has never been verified with studies using pure neutrophils and has been assumed to be false in this review based on the demonstration that neutrophils do not make EP (Hanson *et al.*, 1980).

Biochemically, LEM has proven to be inseparable from the LAF and pyrogenic activities. The fibrinogen-inducing activity of a rabbit leukocyte extract exhibited the same relation to pyrogenicity in the crude extract as it did after purification by gel filtration, ion-exchange chromatography, and isoelectric focusing at pI 7.7–7.9 (Merriman *et al.*, 1977). In addition, both the acidic and neutral rabbit pyrogens have been found to induce SAA (Sztein *et al.*, 1981). Similarly, the SAA-inducing activity derived from murine macrophage supernatants was found to roughly correspond with LAF activity through gel filtration, ion-exchange chromatography, and phenyl-Sepharose chromatography (Sztein *et al.*, 1981). Partially purified human LAF also showed SAA-inducing activity (Sztein *et al.*, 1981; McAdam and Dinarello, 1981). Finally, the pI 7.3 rabbit LEM is blocked by goat anti-rabbit pyrogen just as is the pI 7.3 LAF and pyrogenic activity (Sztein *et al.*, 1981).

4.3. STIMULATION OF MUSCLE BREAKDOWN

Another common sequela of infection is a negative nitrogen balance due to the loss of muscle protein. This effect can be viewed as part of the coordinated response which allows the liver to increase its uptake of amino acids and its output of the acute-phase proteins. Baracos *et al.* (1983) have recently shown that IL-1 *in vitro* stimulates the breakdown of protein from muscle. This treatment of muscle with IL-1 results in a three- to fivefold increase in the production of PGE_2 which in turn stimulates the muscle catabolism. Raising the incubation temperature to 39°C increases the rate of PGE_2 synthesis and of protein breakdown. Inhibitors of cyclooxygenase block the effect.

4.4. EFFECTS ON THE NEUTROPHIL

4.4.1. Neutrophilia

The injection of monokines into mice, rats, and rabbits caused a rapid release of neutrophils from the bone marrow into the blood (Merriman *et al.*, 1975; Kampschmidt and Upchurch, 1980a; Kampschmidt *et al.*, 1980). In rats the number of blood neutrophils may increase up to eightfold within 1 hr. The active rabbit monokine shows a similar sensitivity to sulfhydryl reagents as does the neutral rabbit pyrogen (Kampschmidt *et al.*, 1973b) and copurifies with EP by gel filtration, ion-exchange chromatography, and isoelectric focusing (Merriman *et al.*, 1977).

4.4.2. Neutrophil Activation

In addition to the induction of neutrophilia, monokines have several other effects on the neutrophil. The incubation of human neutrophils with human EP causes an increased release of specific granules, an increase in glucose metabolism through the hexose monophosphate shunt, and an increase in the generation of superoxide as measured by an increase in the reduction of either ferricytochrome C or nitroblue tetrazolium (Klempner *et al.*, 1978, 1979). For these experiments the monokine was isolated by elution from an anti-EP immunoabsorbent column, gel filtration, and DEAE ion-exchange using pyrogenicity as the assay. In all the assays, 10 rabbit pyrogen doses per milliliter gave near-maximal stimulation.

The percentage of human neutrophils which reduced nitroblue tetrazolium increased roughly linearly with increasing amounts of factor. Only 4% of the untreated cells reduced the dye whereas after incubation for 30 min with 4 rabbit pyrogen doses per milliliter, 83% were positive. Similarly, the amount of ferricytochrome C reduced also increased linearly to a maximal sixfold stimulation in the presence of 10 rabbit pyrogen doses per milliliter. These neutrophils also showed an increased rate of glucose metabolism through the hexose monophosphate shunt. Despite the frequent association of the hexose monophosphate shunt with increased phagocytosis, Klempner *et al.* (1979) did not observe an increase in the rate at which IL-1-treated neutrophils phagocytize bacteria.

4.4.3. Neutrophil Migration

Monokines have also been shown to enhance the migration of neutrophils. The activity described by Stevenson (1976) causes a 40–80% increase in the area of the corona formed by human neutrophils migrating out of a capillary tube, whereas Merrill *et al.* (1980) have described a factor with true chemotactic activity. Stevenson and Gray (1976) reported that the migration stimulator had a molecular weight of 10–15K; however, their data showed it eluting together with the amino acids on Sephadex G-100. The chemotactic factor was reported to have an apparent MW near 10K and a pI of 5.0 (Merrill *et al.*, 1980). Saunder *et al.* (1983) have further characterized the chemotactic factor and have found it to be inseparable from either LAF or pyrogenic activity by gel filtration or isoelectric focusing. Further, a crude antiserum containing anti-leukocytic pyrogen was able to block the chemotactic activity. Therefore, again at least one of the chemotactic monokines is IL-1.

4.5. ALTERATION OF SERUM CATION CONCENTRATIONS

The injection of LEM into mice, rats, and rabbits also causes a pronounced decrease in the concentration of plasma iron and zinc and an increase in plasma copper (Kampschmidt and Upchurch, 1969a; Pekarek *et al.*, 1972a; Merriman *et al.*, 1975; Kampschmidt *et al.*, 1980). This activity copurifies with EP through gel filtration, ion-exchange chromatography, and isoelectric focusing (Merriman *et al.*, 1977). Further, the pI 7 ion regulatory factor from rabbits can be inactivated with reagents that react with free sulfhydryl groups and reactivated with dithiothreitol just like the pI 7 EP (Kampschmidt *et al.*, 1973b).

It is generally assumed that the changes in ion concentration are secondary to other effects of LEM. The iron appears to be lost from the plasma to the liver and spleen (Pekarek *et al.*, 1972b; Kampschmidt, 1979). This ion redistribution is presumably mediated both by the effect of LEM on the liver and by the release of lactoferrin from the neutrophils. The elevation in serum copper is believed to reflect the enhanced synthesis and secretion of ceruloplasmin by the liver (Pekarek *et al.*, 1972a).

4.6. EFFECTS ON MESENCHYMAL CELLS

Macrophages and related cell types have recently been recognized to enhance the release of proteases from a number of mesenchymal cell types. Vaes (1980) recently reviewed the cellular aspects of these interactions, concluding that many of the interactions are mediated by monokines. For some of these cell types (the vascular smooth muscle and vascular endothelium, for example) the principal monokine responsible may not be IL-1 (Martin *et al.*, 1981). In contrast, it is clear that IL-1 can influence the activity of the synoviocyte. In still other cases, such as chondrocyte, fibroblast, bone, and corneal cells, the role of IL-1 is still controversial.

4.6.1. Synoviocyte Stimulation

In the active synovitis which characterizes rheumatoid arthritis, vigorous collagen destruction and bone resorption occurs under the advancing pannus. The cells which comprise the rheumatoid synovium can be dispersed using proteolytic enzymes. The adherent cells derived from the resulting cell suspension secrete large quantities of both prostaglandins and collagenase. The collagenase activity in early cultures can be sufficient to degrade 70 μg of collagen/min per 10^6 cells per day. The prostaglandin synthesis, which is 85% PGE_2, can be as high as 1.2 μg/10^6 cells per day (Dayer *et al.*, 1980a). These cell products are of interest because collagenase can degrade the undenatured collagen present in the joint structures while the prostaglandins may have several effects including promoting bone resorption and increasing local vascular dilation and permeability.

The adherent synovial cells when first isolated are a mixed population (Dayer *et al.*, 1976). The predominant population is a large (approximately 30-μm diameter), slow-growing stellate cell type which reacts positively by immunofluorescence with anticollagenase antibody (Woolley *et al.*, 1978). The cells are readily distinguished from both macrophages and fibroblasts. A minor population of cells resembling monocytes/macrophages contaminate the synovial preparations (Dayer *et al.*, 1980a). Upon repeated treatment with trypsin and passage, the macrophage population disappears, and a decline is noted in the amount of collagenase and prostaglandin released (Dayer *et al.*, 1976). If the stellate cells are exposed to supernatants of human monocytes, the amounts of prostaglandin and collagenase released increase to levels near those of fresh explants.

It is likely that IL-1 is one of the monocyte products which account for the synoviocyte stimulation. Upon chromatography of the supernatants on Ultragel AcA 54, the activities which enhance the secretion of collagenase, prostaglandin, plasminogen activator, and glycosaminoglycans elute together at a position corresponding to a globular protein of 12–14K (Dayer *et al.*, 1977a,b, 1979; McGuire-Goldring *et al.*, submitted; Wood *et al.*, 1983a). When tested in the thymocyte proliferation assay, these column fractions had LAF activity (Mizel *et al.*, 1981; McGuire-Goldring *et al.*, submitted; Wood *et al.*, 1983a). Both the LAF and the synoviocyte-stimulating activity could be recovered after denaturation with 8 M urea but both were destroyed by papain digestion in 8 M urea and by phenylglyoxal (Mizel *et al.*, 1981). The synoviocyte-stimulating factor also elutes from DEAE in low salt as does IL-1 (Dayer *et al.*, 1980a). Finally, if IL-1 from P388D1 was subjected to PAGE (Mizel *et al.*, 1981) or human IL-1 resolved by isoelectric focusing (McGuire-Goldring *et al.*, submitted; Wood *et al.*, 1983a), the synoviocyte-stimulating activity again cofractionates with the LAF activity. The only difference noted was that the basic component of P388D1 IL-1 was relatively more active as a synoviocyte stimulator than was the acidic component. Recently, Dayer *et al.* (1981) have further purified the synoviocyte-stimulating factor by DEAE, phenyl-Sepharose, and high-performance liquid chromatography.

The molecular heterogeneity of the monokines can be observed with this assay as with the other assays described earlier. Figure 4 shows the results obtained when Dayer assayed the synoviocyte-stimulating activities of fractionated monocyte supernatants prepared in my laboratory. The presence of a peak of activity coincident with the BAF activity is evident; nevertheless, the majority of the activity observed eluted from Sephadex with an apparent MW above 15K. The explanation for the differences between these preparations and those of Dayer is unknown, but the observation suggests that caution should be exercised before assuming that the 15K IL-1 is the only monokine which affects the human synoviocytes.

Unlike many of the other effects of IL-1, the stimulation of the stellate cells requires only brief exposure and exerts a prolonged effect. A fourfold enhancement of collagenase secretion can be observed following only 5 min of exposure

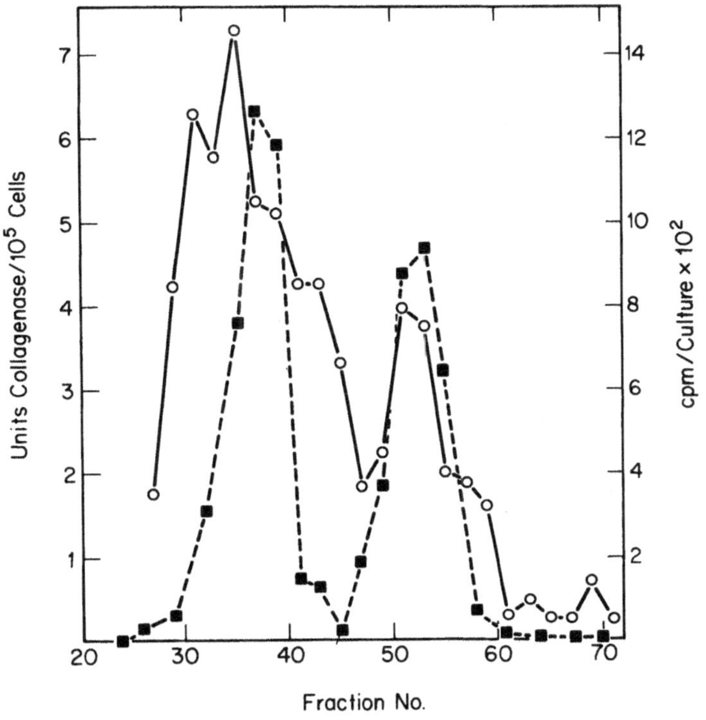

FIGURE 4. Fractionation of synoviocyte-stimulating and direct thymocyte mitogenic activity by gel filtration. LPS-stimulated human monocyte supernatants were concentrated and fractionated on Sephadex G-75. The fractions were assayed either for their ability to enhance the release of collagenase by human synoviocytes by Dayer (○) or for their mitogenic activity on the thymocytes of C3H/HeJ mice (Wood, 1979b) (■).

of the adherent synovial cells to IL-1, and the effect can persist for up to 15 days (Dayer *et al.*, 1980a).

4.6.2. Chondrocyte Stimulation

In experiments analogous to those with human synoviocytes, it can be shown that monokines can stimulate the secretion of prostaglandin, collagenase, and plasminogen activator by rabbit and human articular chondrocytes *in vitro* (Deshmukh-Phadke *et al.*, 1978; Ridge *et al.*, 1980; Jasin and Dingle, 1981; McGuire-Goldring *et al.*, submitted). Paradoxically, the macrophage supernatants also cause an increase in the rate of incorporation of proline and sulfate presumably into collagen and proteoglycan (Deshmukh-Phadke *et al.*, 1980). Therefore, the net effect of the stimulation may be increased turnover of cartilage rather than increased catabolism. On the other hand, since the monokines also inhibit the proliferation of chondrocytes *in vitro* even in the absence of prostaglandins, they could ultimately lead to cartilage destruction (Gowens, unpublished observations).

The monokine responsible for increasing the secretion of proteases by chondrocytes has been demonstrated in LPS-stimulated supernatants from rabbit peritoneal macrophages, rabbit blood monocytes, and human monocytes (Ridge *et al.*, 1980; Phadke *et al.*, 1981; McGuire-Goldring *et al.*, submitted; Gowens *et al.*, 1985a). As expected, the crude macrophage supernatants could be shown to contain IL-1 by both the direct thymocyte mitogenic assay and the PHA synergistic assay (Phadke *et al.*, 1981). Further, upon gel filtration, the chondrocyte stimulator eluted in the range of 13–15K (Deshmukh-Phadke *et al.*, 1980). Despite these similarities with IL-1, however, Phadke *et al.* (1981) reported that purified IL-1 was inactive as a chondrocyte stimulator. Unfortunately, Phadke and colleagues reported their data relative to the dilution of IL-1 tested rather than in LAF units; therefore, it remained possible that IL-1 stimulated chondrocytes but was merely tested at excessively high dilutions.

We have reinvestigated this question using human monokines on human chondrocytes. In our hands, the monokine which stimulated both prostaglandin and neutral protease (plasminogen activator, collagenase, and proteoglycanase) release from chondrocytes cofractionated with LAF activity by both gel filtration and isoelectric focusing. Further, all three activities were inhibited by treatment with phenylglyoxal (McGuire-Goldring *et al.*, submitted; Gowens *et al.*, 1985a). Therefore, it seems likely that IL-1 is the principal monokine affecting chondrocyte metabolism.

4.6.3. Fibroblast Stimulation

Macrophage supernatants have also been shown to stimulate the rate of division (Martin *et al.*, 1981) and collagenase production (Huybrechts-Godin *et al.*, 1979) by fibroblasts; however, the identity of the active factor is controversial. Martin *et al.* (1981) were able to show that one factor which enhances fibroblast proliferation was separable from IL-1, eluting in the void volume of Sephadex G100 (≥ 100K). Further, Wharton *et al.* (1982) were able to separate the proliferation stimulant derived from the P388D1 macrophage line from IL-1 by chromatography on DEAE-Sephadex. Finally, one monokine which stimulates collagenase release from fibroblasts is lost upon dialysis (Huybrechts-Godin *et al.*, 1979) and, therefore, is probably too small to be IL-1. On the other hand, Jalkanen (1981) has described a rat monokine with a pI of 4.6–5.3 which enhances the secretion of glycosaminoglycans from fibroblasts. Although this is an appropriate pI for mouse IL-1, no IL-1 assay was reported. Other authors have shown that purified IL-1 does have the capacity to stimulate fibroblast proliferation (Schmidt *et al.*, 1982; Melcion *et al.*, 1982) and collagenase production (Postlethwaite *et al.*, 1983; Melcion *et al.*, 1982). A possible explanation for these divergent results comes from the work of Korn *et al.* (1980). They demonstrated that a 12–20K product of adherent non-T human mononuclear cells inhibits fibroblast proliferation in part by inducing the secretion of PGE. It is possible that this activity might mask the fibroblast mitogenic activity of IL-1. In conclusion, although IL-1 apparently exhibits some fibroblast-stimulating activity, it is not necessarily the only active monokine. Obviously, further research will be necessary before the effects of monokines on fibroblasts are resolved.

4.6.4. Bone Metabolism

IL-1 also exerts a number of effects on bone. In bone fragment culture, IL-1 can be shown to enhance the rate of calcium release (Gowens *et al.*, 1985b). When added to cultures of purified osteoblasts, however, IL-1 stimulates the secretion of prostaglandins and glycosaminoglycans but not neutral proteases (Gowens *et al.*, 1985a). In all these cases, the evidence for the identity of the bone-stimulating activity with IL-1 rests upon cofractionation by gel filtration and isoelectric focusing as well as inhibition by phenylglyoxal.

4.6.5. Corneal Effects

It has been demonstrated that LPS-stimulated supernatants of unfractionated human leukocytes stimulate protein and DNA synthesis in corneal keratocytes (Ben-Ezra and Gery, 1979) as well as collagenase production by normal and alkali-burned corneas (Newsome and Gross, 1979). Because LPS is the stimulant, it is possible that these may be additional activities of IL-1; however, neither the cell of origin nor the molecular weight of these factors has been determined.

4.6.6. Mesangial Cells

The mesangial cell is a mesenchyme-derived multipotential vascular pericyte. Exposure of mesangial cell cultures to macrophage supernatants or to IL-1-enriched fractions has been reported to stimulate proliferation in some cases (Melcion *et al.*, 1982) and to inhibit it in others through a partially PG-mediated mechanism (Ooi *et al.*, 1983). The difference in the results is reminiscent of the controversy regarding the ability of IL-1 to affect the proliferation of fibroblasts and human T cells and remains as yet unexplained. IL-1 also stimulated the synthesis of total protein and of collagen in these cultures (Melcion *et al.*, 1982).

4.7. SUMMARY

Based upon the observations reviewed above, it seems clear that IL-1 or a molecule biochemically very similar to IL-1 can affect a large number of cell types other than lymphocytes. These include at least the temperature-sensitive neurons, the hepatocyte, muscle, polymorphonuclear leukocytes, and a variety of mesenchymal cells. In each case the measured response to IL-1 is different reflecting the role the particular cell plays in the physiology of the host. The differences in the activity of IL-1 upon its various target cells can even be seen within the various mesenchymal cells discussed (see Table 2). For example,

TABLE 2. EFFECTS OF IL-1 ON MESENCHYMAL CELLS

Response to IL-1	Target cell			
	Synoviocyte	Chondrocyte	Fibroblast	Osteoblast
Proliferation	↑	↓	↑	↑
PGE_2	↑	↑	?	↑
Neutral protease	↑	↑	?	0
Collagen	↑	↓	↑	↑
Glycosaminoglycan	↑	↑	↑	↑

although IL-1 stimulates the release of neutral proteases from synoviocytes and chondrocytes, it has no effect on the release of proteases from osteoblasts. Similarly, although it reportedly stimulates collagen production from several cell types, it appears to suppress collagen synthesis by chondrocytes (Gowens, unpublished observation).

5. MECHANISM OF IL-1 EFFECTS

The mechanism by which IL-1 exerts its effects upon its target cells is as yet poorly defined. Gillis and Mizel (1981) reported that IL-1 can be absorbed by a glutaraldehyde-fixed T-cell line suggesting that a cell surface receptor may exist. The biochemical events which follow the interaction of IL-1 with the cell have yet to be studied extensively. Some, such as fever and the enhancement of muscle catabolism, are blocked by inhibitors of cyclooxygenase suggesting mediation through prostaglandins (Baracos *et al.*, 1983); however, other effects of IL-1, such as the changes in acute-phase proteins and serum ions, mesenchymal cell responses, and the LAF response, are insensitive to these inhibitors (Wood and Staruch, unpublished observations; Tocco *et al.*, 1983; Gowens *et al.*, 1985b; Meats *et al.*, 1980; Dinarello *et al.*, 1983). Finally, Dinarello *et al.* (1983) have claimed that the LAF effect is sensitive to lipoxygenase inhibitors suggesting that the products of the lipoxygenase pathway may mediate the T-cell proliferation. Obviously, the biochemistry of the action of IL-1 remains a rich field for study.

At a cellular level, the immunoregulatory effects of IL-1 are now beginning to form a coherent picture. IL-1 appears to increase the viscosity of the membrane of Lyt-1^+2^- T cells. It seems likely that this single effect could explain the enhanced binding of lectins and antigens to the membrane, expression of Ia, and steroid resistance. Possibly, a similar event could explain the enhanced expression of Ia and the complement receptor on B cells. The increased binding of antigen on the T cell may promote the release of T-cell-derived helper factors. Finally, it is probably the induced helper factors, in conjunction with antigen and IL-1-induced maturation of the IL-2 responder cell, account for the induction of cytotoxic T cells and antibody-secreting B cells by IL-1. Because of the requirement for adequate antigen presentation, it is not surprising that a few macrophages are necessary to allow many of the IL-1 responses to occur, i.e., antigen-dependent T-cell proliferation, antierythrocyte PFC induction, and PWM-induced antibody secretion by human B cells.

6. ORIGIN OF THE BIOCHEMICAL HETEROGENEITY

As described throughout this review, there appears to be considerable biochemical heterogeneity among the monokines. In addition to the 10–25K factors, biological activities have also been reported with at least two higher molecular weights. Further, the analysis of the 10–25K factors by isoelectric focusing resolves active factors with both acidic and neutral isoelectric points. The amount of each of these molecular species recovered from a particular supernatant seems to depend upon the producing cell type, the induction procedure used, and the animal from which the cells are derived.

While the origin of this biochemical heterogeneity is unknown, several possible explanations must be considered. First, it is possible that the various LAF species are different proteins which share certain biological activities. Alternatively, they may all be derivatives of a single common precursor being generated by incomplete protein processing and artifacts of isolation. For example, Mizel and Rosenstreich (1979) reported that the lysate of stimulated P388D1 cells yielded LAF activity at 220, 50–70, 39, 26, and 13K whereas supernatants of these cultures contain only the 13K species. These results suggest that the higher-MW species have been incompletely processed from larger precursors.

Several observations also exist which suggest artifactual modification. For example, Economou and Shin (1978) have reported that the LAF obtained from the supernatants of murine peritoneal macrophages which were cultured for 24 hr in the presence of lipopolysaccharide (LPS) but the absence of serum was much more heterogeneous than that derived from a 90-min incubation of preactivated macrophages in the presence of a protease inhibitor. This result suggests that some of the heterogeneity may be an artifact of proteolysis. Second, Togawa *et al.* (1979) have demonstrated that aggregation can also contribute to the heterogeneity. They found that when the low-MW LAF was reconstituted with 2% serum, concentrated 10-fold by ultrafiltration, and rechromatographed on Bio-Gel P-100, a significant portion of the LAF activity eluted with an MW of 50–70K. A similar shift in the elution profile was not observed if the low-MW LAF was concentrated in the absence of serum. Further, they observed that a portion of the high-MW LAF obtained from human monocytes was dissociated upon rechromatography into the low-MW form (Togawa *et al.*, 1979; Oppenheim *et al.*, 1980a). These results have been confirmed in my laboratory with human monocyte supernatants; however, in their work with guinea pig LAF, Iribe *et al.* (1982) were unable to dissociate the 50–90K LAF even on SDS-PAGE.

Nevertheless, even if the high-MW species are aggregates, they may still be biologically significant. Indeed, in the earlier sections of this review a number of differences in the biological activities of the 15K and the very large LAF were cited (see Table 1). A further indication that the high-MW factors may represent biologically significant aggregates comes from the work of Gorczynski and Price (1979). They demonstrated that the supernatants of unstimulated murine peritoneal cells yielded three immunostimulatory factors eluting at 15, 30–45, and 70–90K. These factors stimulated both the induction of cytotoxic lymphocytes and the plaque response to TNP-KLH in cultures of macrophage-depleted splenocytes supplemented with 2-mercaptoethanol. As has been shown by others, they found that the 15K factor showed no genetic restrictions in its immunostimulatory activity. On the other hand, the higher-MW factors were highly restricted. The 30–45K factor was found to stimulate only lymphocytes homologous in the *IA* or *IB* region of the major histocompatibility complex with the macrophages from which the monokine was derived, and it could be absorbed with anti-Ia antibody. In contrast, the 70–90K factor stimulated only lymphocytes homologous at *H-2K* or *H-2D*. Since incubation of the 70–90K factor with 2-mercaptoethanol led to the appearance of some 15K activity, Gorczynski and Price (1979) suggested that the larger factors might be aggregates of the 15K factor with Ia or H-2D or K antigens. If this observation is relevant to the heterogeneity of the human monokines, it must be assumed that spontaneous dissociation accounts for the activity observed in cultures of xenogeneic cells.

It is important to emphasize that not all the observed heterogeneity is readily explained away. In our hands, the 30K LAF is a very stable species which fails to dissociate even in 6 M urea (unpublished results). Further, there are as yet no documented explanations for the heterogeneity of the isoelectric points although they could obviously be generated by either proteolysis or posttranslational modification.

The best evidence that the acidic and neutral LAFs are structurally distinct proteins has been obtained in studies of rabbit pyrogen. Both the acidic and neutral endogenous pyrogens are inactivated by phenylglyoxal suggesting that they may have similar active sites (Murphy *et al.*, 1981a). On the other hand, the pI 7.3 pyrogen is blocked by a goat antiserum and contains a free sulfhydryl group which is essential to its biological activity. Neither of these properties is shared by the acidic pyrogens (Murphy *et al.*, 1981a). Since no evidence for glycosylation could be found to explain the biochemical or antigenic differences (Murphy *et al.*, 1981b), it is likely that the differences between these molecules reflect true structural differences.

In conclusion, it seems likely that many of the IL-1 species reported are simply derived from modifications of a common precursor, but it is likely that the macrophage may in addition produce other distinct proteins with immunoregulatory activity.

7. INDUCTION AND RELEASE OF IL-1

7.1. SECRETING CELLS

Until recently the only cells which had clearly been shown to produce IL-1 were those in the monocyte-macrophage lineage. These included not only the monocytes and macrophages of the peritoneum, alveolae (Atkins *et al.*, 1967; Simon and Willoughby, 1981), and spleen (Atkins *et al.*, 1967; Wyler *et al.*, 1979) but also Kupffer cells (Dinarello *et al.*, 1968; Kampschmidt *et al.*, 1973a; Haeseler *et al.*, 1977) and bone marrow (Gery and Waksman, 1972; Efremov *et al.*, 1978). In addition, both murine and human macrophage cell lines have been reported to secrete IL-1 (Bodel, 1978; Lachman *et al.*, 1977a; Mizel *et al.*, 1978a; Palacios *et. al.*, 1982; Amento *et al.*, 1982a). Fibroblasts, L1210 cells, lymphoblasts, HeLa cells, baby hamster kidney, 3T3, and Vero cells are all reportedly incapable of IL-1 secretion (Root *et al.*, 1970; Bodel and Miller, 1977; Blyden and Handschumacher, 1977; Calderon *et al.*, 1975). The literature on endogenous pyrogen and LEM heavily references the production of IL-1 by neutrophils based upon an early experiment of Beeson (1948) showing that the PMN-rich peritoneal exudates of the rabbit produce pyrogen. However, whenever the neutrophils are isolated from macrophages, they have been found to release no IL-1 (Wood and Gaul, 1974; Hanson *et al.*, 1980), and indeed, the IL-1 released by unfractionated human leukocytes or rabbit peritoneal exudates can be entirely accounted for by the amount released by the contaminating monocytes (Hanson *et al.*, 1980). By the same token, monocyte contamination also explains the claim that eosinophils release IL-1 (Mickenberg *et al.*, 1972).

There is also some evidence that macrophage subsets differ in their ability to secrete IL-1. When the normal peritoneal macrophages of the mouse are stimulated by LPS, only the larger cells secrete substantial amounts of IL-1 (Gorczynski, 1977; Lee *et al.*, 1981). These cells are predominately peroxidase negative suggesting that they were mature macrophages (Lee *et al.*, 1981). The smaller macrophages, including those which are Ia^+ and peroxidase positive, secrete substantially less IL-1 (Gorczynski, 1977; Lee *et al.*, 1981).

Recently, IL-1 production also has been reported in cell types whose relation to the macrophage is unlikely. The best characterized of these is ETAF, an IL-1-like factor secreted by murine keratinocytes and keratinocyte cell lines (Luger *et al.*, 1981; Saunder *et al.*, 1982). This factor exhibits LAF activity, enhances IL-2 release from lectin-stimulated T cells, stimulates PMN chemotaxis, stimulates fibroblast proliferation, and promotes the secretion of acute-phase proteins (Luger *et al.*, 1981, 1982; Saunder *et al.*, 1983; Sztein *et al.*, 1982). Further, ETAF is biochemically similar to IL-1 by gel filtration, isoelectric focusing, DEAE ion-exchange, or phenyl-Sepharose chromatography (Luger *et al.*, 1981, 1982; Sztein *et al.*, 1982). Similar observations have been made for supernatants of rat mesangial cells (Lovett *et al.*, 1983) and of LPS-stimulated murine glial cells and the C6 glioma cell line (Fontana *et al.*, 1982b). In these cases, the factor has been shown to exhibit LAF activity, enhance IL-2 release, and have an MW of 13.5–18K upon gel filtration.

Finally, there are several cases in which the relation of the IL-1-producing cell to the macrophage is unknown. These include rabbit corneal epithelial cells and corneal cell lines (Grabner *et al.*, 1982), human synovial cells (Wood *et al.*, submitted), and dendritic cells (Rollinghoff *et al.*, 1982).

7.2. CELL BIOLOGY

The production of IL-1 is a highly regulated response. Normal macrophages do not contain stores of biologically active IL-1 (Bodel, 1970; Wood and Cameron, 1976; Blyden and Handschumacher, 1977; Unanue and Kiely, 1977; Dayer *et al.*, 1977a). Instead, when activated, the macrophage appears to synthesize IL-1 *in vivo* as evidenced by the success of attempts to biosynthetically radiolabel IL-1 (Moore *et al.*, 1973; Cebula *et al.*, 1979) and to inhibit its production with puromycin or cycloheximide (Bodel, 1970; Nordlund *et al.*, 1970; Diamantstein and Ulmer, 1976; Unanue and Kiely, 1977). Subsequently, IL-1 appears to be processed (Mizel and Rosenstreich, 1979) in the microsomes (Unanue and Kiely, 1977). Since some agents (such as LPS and latex in murine peritoneal macrophages) can induce the appearance of intracellular IL-1 without stimulating much release of the factor (Gery *et al.*, 1981a), the synthesis and release of IL-1 appear to be independently regulated events. Once triggered, IL-1 release typically continues for 24 hr (Bodel, 1974; Wood and Cameron, 1975, 1976; Finelt and Hoffmann, 1979; Dayer *et al.*, 1980b). Finally, because inhibitors of RNA and protein synthesis can augment the secretion of IL-1 if added after the macrophages are activated (Unanue and Kiely, 1977; Mizel and Mizel, 1981), it has been suggested that IL-1 release is terminated by an active process. However, it remains unclear whether these phenomena reflect an enhancement of the conversion of an inactive precursor to active IL-1 or a reduction in the rate of degradation of intracellular IL-1.

7.3. STIMULANTS OF IL-1 RELEASE

7.3.1. Stimulation by Bacterial Products

A large number of agents have been described which stimulate the release of IL-1. These agents have recently been reviewed by Dinarello (1979), Bernheim *et al.* (1979), Oppenheim *et al.* (1979a), and Gery (1982). The most physiologically relevant of these are: bacterial cell wall components, T-cell products, and the products of inflammation. Among the bacterial products, the endotoxic LPS is certainly the most potent. Most preparations of human monocytes respond to as little as 1 ng/ml of LPS with maximal IL-1 release (Wood and Cameron, 1978). In contrast, murine peritoneal macrophages release relatively little IL-1 when stimulated with LPS (Unanue *et al.*, 1976; Meltzer and Oppenheim, 1977; Tenu *et al.*, 1980; Oppenheim *et al.*, 1980a), although LPS does markedly increase the amount of intracellular IL-1 (Gery *et al.*, 1981a,b). These LPS-stimulated macrophages will subsequently release the intracellular IL-1 if they are exposed to toxic agents such as carrageenan, silica, glucocerebroside, or colchicine (Stamenkovic *et al.*, 1979; Gery *et al.*, 1981a; Bodel, 1975; Oppenheim *et al.*, 1979a). In fact, it has been persuasively argued that the trigger for IL-1 release depends upon the ability of the stimulant to injure the cell thereby prolonging the G_1 phase (Gery *et al.*, 1981a; Luger *et al.*, 1982). Murine macrophages will also release IL-1 in the presence of LPS if they have been preactivated with BCG or *C. parvum* (Meltzer and Oppenheim, 1977), organisms which increase the sensitivity of the macrophage to LPS by 500- to 1000-fold (Weinberg *et al.*, 1978).

Once macrophages have become sensitive to subnanogram quantities of

LPS, it is difficult to determine their sensitivity to anything else. Most biological reagents are contaminated with more than enough LPS to stimulate these macrophages. Indeed, many lots of sera (Wood and Cameron, 1978) and several of the common media (for example, RPMI-1640 from GIBCO but not Microbiological Associates; Wood, unpublished observations) contain enough LPS to maximally stimulate human monocytes.

In addition to LPS, the ubiquitous muramyl dipeptide (MDP) portion of bacterial peptidoglycan has been shown to induce IL-1 release (Oppenheim *et al.*, 1980a; Wood and Staruch, 1980; Tenu *et al.*, 1980; Mishell *et al.*, 1981). In cultures of LPS-sensitive macrophages, as little as 100 ng/ml of LPS-free MDP stimulates nearly maximal IL-1 release (Wood and Staruch, 1980; Tenu *et al.*, 1980). Finally, the components, porin, protein H, and protein I from *P. aeruginosa* as well as heat-killed staphylococci have also been shown to induce IL-1 release (Chao *et al.*, 1977; Mishell *et al.*, 1981). The biological relevance of these observations should not be overlooked. LPS is a common component of the cell wall of all gram-negative bacteria; MDP is even more ubiquitous being present in the peptidoglycan of most bacteria (Kotani *et al.*, 1975). The sensitivity of human monocytes to these two agents suggests that the release of IL-1 may be one of the first responses of the leukocytes to the invasion of bacteria *in vivo*.

7.3.2. Stimulation by Lymphokines

In addition to exogenous stimulants, IL-1 release can also be stimulated by activated T cells (Atkins *et al.*, 1972; Farr *et al.*, 1977; Mizel *et al.*, 1978a; Dayer *et al.*, 1979; Atkins *et al.*, 1980) and by the lymphokines secreted by T cells (Meltzer and Oppenheim, 1977; Rosenstreich and Mizel, 1978; Atkins *et al.*, 1978; Atkins and Francis, 1978; Ramic *et al.*, 1979a; Stosic-Grujicic and Simic, 1979; Bernheim *et al.*, 1980; Dinarello, 1981). At least one of the lymphokines which stimulates the release of IL-1 is the colony-stimulating factor (CSF) for macrophages and granulocytes. Whether the CSF is derived from L-cell conditioned medium or from the supernatants of splenocytes stimulated with Con A, 1000–3000 U of CSF activity is necessary to induce IL-1 (Moore *et al.*, 1980). When chromatographed on Sephadex G-200, two peaks of CSF activity were observed in Con A-stimulated splenocyte supernatants at apparent MW of 25 and 35K, both of which had IL-1-inducing activity (Moore *et al.*, 1980). Similarly, when supernatants from the L929 cell line were chromatographed on Sephadex G-150, both CSF and IL-1-inducing activity eluted in the void volume of the column (Oppenheim *et al.*, 1980a). Other lympohokines are apparently also active as IL-1 inducers since gel filtration of both the Con A-stimulated splenocyte supernatants and the L929 supernatants resolved fractions which actively stimulated IL-1 release but showed no CSF activity (Moore *et al.*, 1980; Oppenheim *et al.*, 1980a). Surprisingly, it has been shown that the injection of 10–20K monokine preparations into mice causes a dramatic increase in the activity of CSF in the serum (Kampschmidt *et al.*, 1980) suggesting the presence of a positive feedback loop.

For reasons which are not clear, other authors have reported that activated

T cells could enhance IL-1 release only when the T cells and macrophages were in contact (Unanue *et al.*, 1976; Farr *et al.*, 1977; Mizel *et al.*, 1978a). Farr *et al.* (1977) also reported a genetic restriction for the T–macrophage interaction. In view of the lack of genetic restriction of the CSF, it seems likely that the genetic restrictions observed by Farr and co-workers were imposed by the need for histocompatible macrophages to present the antigen to the T cells which then became activated releasing CSF.

Despite these results, the caveat should be kept in mind that the lymphokines themselves may not actually be triggering the secretion of IL-1. Lympholines are known to enhance the responsiveness of macrophages to both MDP and LPS (Mishell *et al.*, 1981), and it may be that they appear to induce IL-1 release merely because they make the macrophages sensitive to the LPS which contaminates the cultures.

7.3.3. Stimulation by the Products of Inflammation

Finally, two products commonly found in sites of inflammation, C5a and aggregated immunoglobulin, may stimulate IL-1 release. The conclusion that the anaphylatoxic fragment of the fifth component of complement (C5a) stimulates IL-1 release is based on the observation that C5a stimulates the appearance of both BAF and LAF activity in macrophage supernatants (Goodman *et al.*, 1982); however, until this factor has been biochemically characterized, its identity with IL-1 will remain questionable.

Secondly, aggregated human IgG has been shown to cause a striking increase in the synoviocyte-stimulating activity of monocyte supernatants (Dayer *et al.*, 1980b). Nonaggregated IgG or its Fab fragment failed to stimulate the monocytes; however, Fc fragments markedly stimulated release with a 50% effective dose of 10 mg/ml. Although endotoxin is a ubiquitous stimulator, it is unlikely that the phenomenon was due to endotoxin contamination since the monomeric IgG and Fab fragments prepared from the same digest as the Fc fragments did not stimulate and since polymyxin B, which inhibits the stimulation by endotoxin, failed to inhibit the stimulation by Fc fragments. Since the synovial fluids of the rheumatoid joints are often rich in aggregated IgG, they could stimulate the monocytes and macrophages to release the synoviocyte stimulator which could in turn promote collagen degradation and bone resorption.

If indeed Fc fragments can stimulate the release of IL-1 from macrophages, the phenomenon may well be important in a number of diseases in which the RES is exposed to large amounts of immune complexes. Unfortunately, this possibility cannot yet be accepted as proven because there is as yet no evidence that the activity in the Fc-induced supernatants is in fact IL-1. One possible alternative explanation is that the synoviocytes are actually responding to subfragments of the Fc. In this regard, macrophages can be shown to digest the Fc fragments of human IgG into a 14K subfragment (Morgan and Weigle, 1980;

Thoman *et al.*, 1980) which is highly immunostimulatory. Since the latter subfragments can be purified by affinity chromatography over anti-Fc columns (Morgan and Weigle, 1980) and can be generated by the digestion of Fc fragments with pepsin or papain (Morgan *et al.*, 1982), it is clear that the activity of the Fc subfragments is not due to contamination by LEM.

7.3.4. Artifacts of Supernatant Assays

The single most significant failing in the study of IL-1 has been the lack of an available and reliable immunoassay for IL-1. In its absence, investigators have been forced to rely upon the bioactivity of IL-1. This constraint has made the study of the biology of IL-1 secretion considerably more complex than it should have been. Two examples serve to illustrate the point. In 1978, Bodel observed that the human myelomonocytic cell line U937 secreted leukocytic pyrogen, but the observation went essentially unused by LAF biologists until Amento *et al.* (1982b) showed that the LAF activity was inhibited by another high-MW product of U937.

The second type of artifact is typified by the effect of phorbol myristic acetate (PMA). Since it was first reported by Mizel *et al.* (1978c) to stimulate P388D1, PMA has become one of the stimulants of choice. Unfortunately, it has only recently been recognized that PMA synergizes with IL-1 in the LAF assay and cannot be readily removed by either dialysis or charcoal absorption (Krakauer *et al.*, 1982). Therefore, it is actually quite difficult to know whether PMA is really a bona fide stimulant of IL-1 release. In conclusion, until more definitive assays are available, studies of the induction of IL-1 secretion should be made with caution.

8. THE ROLE OF MONOKINES *IN VIVO*

It is clear from the preceding review that a number of different monokines exist which display activities upon lymphoid and nonlymphoid cells. Although most of these factors may eventually prove to be important, only IL-1 has been studied thoroughly enough to permit serious speculation about its role in physiology and disease. IL-1 stands out because of its remarkably broad spectrum of activity. It appears to cause the differentiation of both T and B cells, to induce the release of IL-2, to amplify the division rate of activated T cells, and to modulate the sensitivity of T cells to steroids. In addition, it appears to cause fever, the release of acute-phase proteins, and the stimulation of neutrophils and mesenchymal tissue. While the weight of evidence certainly supports the belief that all the above activities are the property of a single molecule, it must be remembered that there could be a family of biochemically similar molecules, released in concert, which collectively exert the above effects. In either case, the ultimate physiological response will be the same.

8.1. RELEASE OF IL-1 *IN VIVO*

The existence of EP in the serum of LPS-treated animals was first demonstrated in rabbits by the transfer of the febrile response to LPS-tolerant recipients (Beeson, 1948). More recently the serum of rodents injected with LPS or bacteria has been shown to contain a factor which induces SAA, decreases the plasma iron concentration, and causes a neutrophilia (Kampschmidt *et al.*, 1973a; Sipe *et al.*, 1979). In contrast, the immunostimulatory activities of IL-1 have been more difficult to demonstrate in sera. Tanabe *et al.* (1977) reported a BAF-like activity in the sera of LPS-treated mice although others have failed to repeat the observation (Hoffmann *et al.*, 1978). On the other hand, if mice are preinfected with BCG prior to the challenge with LPS, the serum can be shown to contain high titers of BAF, B-cell-differentiating activity, and factors which cause an increase in H-2 and a decrease in TL in immature thymocytes (Hoffmann *et al.*, 1978; Abbott *et al.*, 1981).

Mannel *et al.* (1980) have analyzed the molecular characteristics of the BCG-LPS-induced factor. Under the typical conditions of gel filtration in low-ionic-strength buffers, the BAF activity of these sera eluted predominantly at 125–150K and 60K with a minor peak at 13K. If, on the other hand, the serum was precipitated with ammonium sulfate and chromatographed in 1.6 M salt, virtually all of the activity eluted at an apparent MW of 13K. In this case, the plaque-inducing (BAF) and PHA-synergizing (LAF) activity coeluted.

In man, attempts to demonstrate the presence of EP in the serum of febrile patients using the febrile response of rabbits have been unsuccessful (Dinarello and Wolff, 1979; Dinarello *et al.*, 1981). In contrast, Wannemacher *et al.* (1972) were able to show that the transfer of serum from patients during the first day of typhoid fever caused a decrease in serum iron and zinc and an elevation in cycloleucine uptake into liver of rats. Sera taken before infection or after heating the sera (90°C 30 min) were inactive.

The short half-life of IL-1 in blood probably contributes to the difficulty which has been encountered in demonstrating the presence of IL-1 *in vivo*. Exogenous LEM is cleared from the blood of rats with a $t½$ of 6–10 min (Kampschmidt and Upchurch, 1980b). The liver is believed to be the principal site of clearance with little LEM activity detectable in the urine (Lorber *et al.*, 1971).

8.2. DEFENSE AGAINST INFECTION

The observation that animals do respond to bacterial infection or LPS with the release of IL-1 into the serum suggests that IL-1 may play a role in the defense of the host against infection. Indeed, the facts that are known about IL-1 suggest that this may be its primary function (Fig. 5).

Monocytes release IL-1 upon exposure to minute quantities of bacterial products [1 ng/ml of endotoxin (Wood and Cameron, 1978) or 100 ng/ml of MDP (Wood and Staruch, 1980)]. The IL-1 then induces fever, neutrophilia, and the synthesis of acute-phase proteins as well as amplifying the immune response.

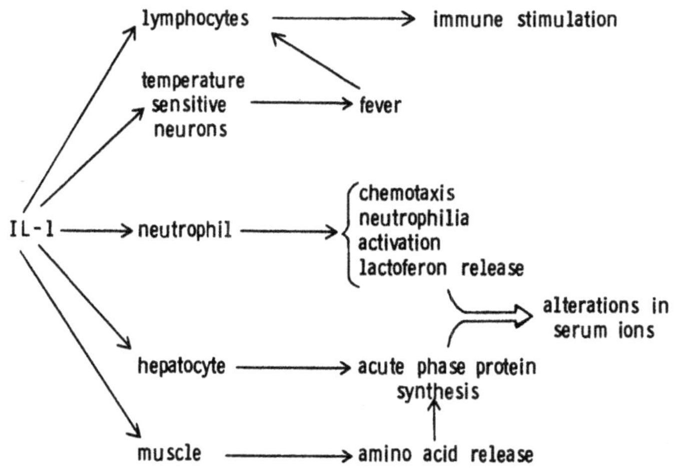

FIGURE 5. Effects of IL-1 on the processes of natural resistance.

The importance of the febrile response in the defense against infection is suggested by its evolutionary conservation. It can be shown that reptiles produce a pyrogen which is active in rabbits (Bernheim and Kluger, 1976) and respond to infection by basking in a warmer environment. Because the fever can be controlled externally in animals which regulate their temperature behaviorally, they can be used to evaluate the protective value of fever. If iguana were infected with *Aeromonas hydrophila* and maintained in a 42°C environment, all survived; however, if they were held in a 35°C environment, most died (Kluger *et al.*, 1975). Similar results have been obtained with infected fish (Covert and Reynolds, 1977).

Although the above observations point to the protective effect of fever, it is still unknown how fever benefits the host. Recently two groups have demonstrated that fever may be immunostimulatory since the responses to both LAF and IL-2 increase significantly with an elevation in temperature (Hanson *et al.*, 1983; Duff and Durum, 1983). The Q_{10} for the LAF response is estimated to be between 50 and 300 and that for IL-2 close to 9. The effect of elevated temperatures appears to be largely upon the initiation of the immune response since Duff and Durum (1983) showed that effect was largely complete after the first day of culture after which the cultures could be returned to 37°C. Elevation of the temperature on the last day of culture had little effect. It has not yet been determined whether elevated temperature modifies the other activities of IL-1.

Alterations in the serum ion concentrations also have antibacterial effects although the mechanism is not well understood. Infected febrile lizards become hypoferremic and survive; however, when they were injected with exogenous sources of iron, their mortality rate increased significantly (Grieger and Kluger, 1978). Presumably, the increased sequestration of iron by the liver and the acute-phase proteins (transferrin and lactoferrin) serve to deprive the bacteria of the iron needed for maximal growth (Weinberg, 1978). Interestingly, when lactoferrin becomes iron saturated, it inhibits the release of CSF (Broxmeyer *et al.*, 1978); and, since CSF stimulates IL-1 release, this activity might be expected to reduce the production of IL-1 in a feedback loop. Probably, the lowered concentration of serum zinc promotes the migration, phagocytosis, and oxygen radical production by neutrophils (Chvapil, 1976; Chvapil *et al.*, 1977). Therefore, the effect of lowering the zinc concentration may be to amplify the antibacterial effect of the neutrophilia and increased oxygen radical production induced by IL-1.

Finally, since bacterial infection also causes the release of steroids, the selective effect of IL-1 in protecting helper T cells but not suppressor T cells from steroids (Bradley and Mishell, 1981) would be expected to further enhance the immune response.

The observations that keratinocytes secrete IL-1 which in turn promotes fibroblast proliferation become more meaningful in the context of infection. Certainly, the principal portal of entry for bacteria into the host is through wounds, and therefore an IL-1-mediated mechanism to enhance wound healing is consistent with its other functions. Indeed, Luger *et al.* (1981, 1982) have reported that confluent keratinocyte cultures secrete relatively little IL-1 but increase the secretion if the cell layer is disrupted, a manipulation analogous to wounding.

The objective of future research will be to determine which of the many IL-1 effects are really relevant to antibacterial resistance. Kampschmidt and Pulliam (1975) have reported that the injection of LEM protects rats from an otherwise fatal dose of *Salmonella typhimurium*. In this case the protection is apparently not associated with fever, since rats do not show a febrile response to LEM (Kampschmidt and Upchurch, 1969b). Nor is it likely to be due principally to the transient hyperferremia or acute-phase protein changes since significant protection can be obtained with injections of LEM given 48 hr before the infection (Kampschmidt and Pulliam, 1975). The actual mechanism of this effect remains to be elucidated.

8.3. MALARIA

The release of IL-1 is no doubt beneficial when it occurs in response to the small bacterial challenges normally encountered by the host; however, when the response is excessive the effects may be debilitating. This may be the case in malaria.

Like *C. parvum* and BCG, *Plasmodium* infections sensitize mice to endotoxin and a challenge with endotoxin results in the release of tumor-necrotizing factor, interferon, and IL-1 into the serum (Clark *et al.*, 1981). It is possible that many of the symptoms of malaria are due to the periodic release of endotoxin into the circulation of the infected patient. Indeed, Tubbs (1980) reported finding endotoxin in the plasma of all 16 patients studied with acute infections with *P. falciparum* and in only 2 of 18 controls. If this is the case, it is reasonable to assume that the release of IL-1 may account for the fever, the increased serum amyloid levels, and the T-cell-dependent splenomegaly observed in malaria

(Roberts and Weidanz, 1978). While both the splenomegaly and secondary amyloidosis are fairly rare consequences of malaria, they do occur together with a high frequency in one population group in Papua, New Guinea (Pryor, 1967; McAdam *et al.*, 1979). It is interesting to speculate that these individuals may produce excessive amounts of IL-1.

8.4. ADJUVANTICITY

Many of the agents which have been shown to enhance the antibody response to soluble antigens are known to affect macrophages and induce an expansion of T cells. The adjuvants fitting this description include LPS (Biozzi *et al.*, 1955; Skopinska, 1972), double-stranded RNA (Braun and Nakano, 1967; Cone and Johnson, 1972), the polyene antibiotics (Lin *et al.*, 1977; Shirley and Little, 1979), the vitamin A analogs (Block *et al.*, 1978; Taub *et al.*, 1970), and MDP (Wahl *et al.*, 1979; Tanaka *et al.*, 1979; Wood and Staruch, 1980; Lowy *et al.*, 1977; Sugimoto *et al.*, 1978). Since IL-1 is a product of stimulated macrophages and since IL-1 can be expected to enhance the proliferation of antigen-activated T cells, it is attractive to hypothesize that the adjuvanticity of many materials depends upon their ability to induce the secretion of IL-1.

The "side effects" of adjuvant treatment are consistent with the hypothesis that the adjuvants cause the release of IL-1 *in vivo*. In addition to LPS, which is well known to be an IL-1 inducer, the polyenes have been shown to induce neutrophilia and an increase in SAA (Lin *et al.*, 1977; Staruch and Wood, unpublished observations). MDP induces fever (Kotani *et al.*, 1976) and enhances SAA titers (Staruch and Wood, 1983). Double-stranded RNA induces fever (Lindsay *et al.*, 1969) and acute-phase protein synthesis (McAdam and Ryan, 1978). Further, *in vitro* the ability of MDP analogs to induce monokine release correlates with their adjuvanticity *in vivo* (Iribe *et al.*, 1981).

Finally, some adjuvants have been reported to inhibit the immune response if injected 1 or 2 days prior to the antigen. This phenomenon can also be explained with the above hypothesis. IL-1 is detectable in the serum of rabbits from 2 to 6 hr after the injection of LPS (Atkins and Wood, 1955); the time period during which adjuvanticity is observed. In contrast, the early acute-phase proteins reach their maximal blood concentration at 10–40 hr (Rupp and Fuller, 1979; Sipe *et al.*, 1979). Since several of the acute-phase reactants [lactoferrin (Duncan and McArthur, 1981), α-globulin (Glaser and Nelken, 1972), and SSA (Benson and Aldo-Benson, 1979)] are reportedly immunosuppressive, they may contribute to the observed adjuvant-induced suppression.

Consistent with the hypothesis, it has recently been shown that IL-1 does exhibit adjuvant effects *in vivo* (Staruch and Wood, 1983). The amount of IL-1 which is necessary to produce a significant stimulation of the antibody response corresponds to the amount needed to significantly increase the titer of the acute-phase proteins. It is interesting that the immune response is maximally stimulated when the IL-1 is injected 2 hr after the priming antigen. This corresponds to the time delay seen *in vitro* between the stimulation of macrophages and the first appearance of IL-1.

On the other hand, some evidence exists which appears to refute the hypothetical involvement of IL-1 as the principal mediator of adjuvant action. Casein, for example, is known to strongly stimulate SAA production suggesting that it stimulates IL-1 release *in vivo* (Benson *et al.*, 1977) but is not known to be an adjuvant. The reverse is also reported. Several analogs of MDP and LPS are known which are potent adjuvants but are only weakly pyrogenic (Kotani *et al.*, 1976; Schenck *et al.*, 1969; Chedid *et al.*, 1975; Damais *et al.*, 1982).

8.5. THYMIC FUNCTION

The monokines produced by the macrophages of the thymic reticulum may play a role in the T-cell maturation process. Beller and Unanue (1978) have shown that immature thymocytes when cultured together with thymic macrophages exhibit the same maturational changes which were observed when thymocytes were cultured with the supernatants of peritoneal macrophages (Beller and Unanue, 1977), i.e., an increase in H-2 antigen, a loss of TL antigen, and an increased responsiveness in a mixed lymphocyte reaction. Therefore, it is likely that thymic macrophages can release the monokines which promote differentiation.

Indeed, the location of thymic macrophages in the corticomedullary junction of the thymus (Raviola, 1975) is consistent with such a role in differentiating cortical thymocytes into medullary cells. The patterns of steroid resistance also fit this hypothesis. In cultures lacking macrophages, the PNA^- mature medullary thymocytes are no more resistant to steroids than are the immature cortical thymocytes (Triglia and Rothenberg, 1981), but the former cells become steroid resistant in the presence of GRMF (Mishell *et al.*, 1979). It is, therefore, likely that the steroid resistance of the medullary thymocytes *in situ* is the result of IL-1 (GRMF) release by the thymic macrophages of the corticomedullary junction.

8.6. AUTOIMMUNE AND CONNECTIVE TISSUE DISEASE

The role of IL-1 in the autoimmune and connective tissue diseases has just begun to receive attention, but already its role in arthritis and peridontitis appears to be important. Suggestions also exist that IL-1 may be relevant to Crohn's disease and systemic lupus erythematosus.

Recently, the exudates present in the inflamed joints of patients with rheumatoid arthritis have been reported to contain IL-1 (Fontana *et al.*, 1982a; Ise *et al.*, 1982; Wood *et al.*, 1983b). It is interesting that in our study the fluids were prefractionated by affinity chromatography over a column of rabbit anti-human leukocytic pyrogen. This column allow us to separate the LAF activity from IL-2 and from nonspecific inhibitors. Using this technique we found that IL-1 could be detected not only in rheumatoid joint fluids but in those of other inflamed joints as well including psoriatic arthritis and osteoarthritic joints. These results correspond well with the earlier observation of Bodel and Hollingsworth (1968) that leukocytic pyrogen could be isolated from both rheumatoid and osteoarthritic joint fluids. The failure of other investigators to detect IL-1 in osteoarthritic effusions (Fontana *et al.*, 1982a; Ise *et al.*, 1982) may have been due to the presence of contaminating inhibitors.

Since IL-1 was found even in the absence of a mononuclear infiltrate, it seems likely that the synovium itself might serve as the source of the factor. Indeed, normal synovium as well as rheumatoid or osteoarthritic synovium secretes a factor which is indistinguishable from IL-1 by gel filtration, isoelectric focusing, antigenicity, or biological activity (Dingle *et al.*, 1979; Meats *et al.*, 1980; Saklatvala and Dingle, 1980; McGuire *et al.*, 1980; Wood *et al.*, submitted).

In view of the activities of IL-1 previously described, it seems quite reasonable to hypothesize that the presence of IL-1 in the joint space could lead to enhanced cartilage breakdown due to the release of neutral proteases from both the synovium and the chondrocyte and to enhanced bone resorption either stimulated by IL-1 itself or indirectly through the release of PGE_2 by the synoviocyte and chondrocyte. If this construct is true, IL-1 could be an important mediator of arthritis.

The possible presence of IL-1 in the inflammed joint is also supported by the observation that IL-1 enhances the frequency of stable erythrocyte-rosetting T cells (Ben-Zvi *et al.*, 1981) which are found at an abnormally high percentage in the synovial fluid of patients with rheumatoid arthritis, ankylosing spondylitis, psoriatic arthritis, and postinfective arthritis (Galili *et al.*, 1981). In addition to its T-cell stimulatory effects, IL-1 might contribute to the characteristically high titers of anti-IgM (rheumatoid factor) seen in patients with rheumatoid arthritis. This is especially true since in chronic inflammation, when elevated steroid levels persist, the ability of IL-1 to protect helper T cells but not suppressors from steroids may contribute to the establishment of autoimmunity.

Peridontitis is a second common disease in which IL-1 may serve as a mediator. Charon *et al.* (1982) have shown that IL-1 can be detected in human gingival fluid and its activity is roughly twice as high from inflamed sites as from the noninflamed areas. In view of the multiple effects of IL-1 on connective tissue, it is not unlikely that IL-1 might contribute to the ultimate loosing of the teeth which characterizes chronic gingival disease.

In Crohn's disease, patients with acute exacerbation have lower plasma zinc concentrations than do normals (Solomons *et al.*, 1978). Furthermore, the transfer of serum from patients with Crohn's disease, but not normal individuals, caused a decrease in the serum zinc concentration in rats (Solomons *et al.*, 1978). While these observations suggest that IL-1 may be present in the serum of patients with Crohn's disease, it is unknown whether the IL-1 plays a significant role in the disease or merely reflects the leakage of bacterial products from the inflammed ileum.

In the above disease states, the pathology correlated with the overproduction of IL-1; in systemic lupus erythematosus (SLE), the converse is true. Following the incubation with PMA, SLE monocytes yielded less than 25% of the normal IL-1 activity (Linker-Israeli *et al.*, 1983). This defect was not correlated with prior steroid therapy.

9. CONCLUSIONS

This review has stressed the molecular heterogeneity of the biologically active proteins secreted by the monocyte-macrophage. Nonetheless, it remains possible that all the varied phenomena described here are the results of only a few proteins or possibly even a single protein which exists in several chemically modified states. Indeed, only a few years ago, many of the relationships which are now accepted were unanticipated, and the consolidation of knowledge can be expected to continue. Clearly, the isolation and characterization of each of the putatively distinct monokines will further clarify our understanding although the final conclusions may have to await the isolation of the structural genes and sequence determination, activities which are now under way.

Taken as a whole it would appear that IL-1 may play two distinctly different roles in physiology—one as an endocrine hormone and one as a paracrine or autocrine hormone (Sporn and Todaro, 1980). Its role as an endocrine hormone is now generally appreciated with respect to its role in triggering the systemic defense reactions against infection, i.e., fever, acute-phase changes, neutrophilia, and immune stimulation. Its role as a paracrine (acting between neighboring cells of the same tissue) or autocrine hormone (acting on the producing cell) is less widely appreciated but is becoming increasingly apparent. For example, the mesangial cells reportedly both produce and respond to IL-1 (Lovett *et al.*, 1983; Melcion *et al.*, 1982) as do human monocytes which are now reported to respond to IL-1 with the secretion of PG (Dinarello *et al.*, 1983). On the other hand, both the brain and liver appear to use IL-1 as a paracrine hormone. In the first case, IL-1 is produced by glial cells and affects the temperature-sensitive neurons; in the second, it is secreted by Kupffer cells and affects the hepatocyte. Finally, although both the synovium and the cornea are reported to make and respond to IL-1, the identity of the respective cell types is unknown. In view of the recent observations that more conventional hormones such as insulin or somatostatin can also act as autocrine or paracrine hormones, these observations seem less bizarre (Roth *et al.*, 1982). Nevertheless, they emphasize the necessity for future research to distinguish between those effects of IL-1 which can be mediated by physiological concentrations of circulating IL-1 and those mediated only by locally high concentrations.

Future research will also be directed toward interfering with the action of IL-1. Today, for example, the only clinically useful inhibitors of IL-1 secretion are the corticosteroids (Stosic-Grujicic and Simic, 1982; Snyder and Unanue, 1982); more selective agents are needed. Once a receptor assay and a sequence becomes available, it may also be possible to design receptor inhibitors. Finally, as the understanding of the mechanism of IL-1 action improves, tissue-specific inhibitors may be possible.

In summary, it appears that the monokines and lymphokines are the hormones of the inflammatory response. As in classical endocrinology, these "hormones" must be regulated by complex feedback loops. Is CSF the macrophage "tropic hormone" and IL-1 the "IL-2-releasing hormone"? Obviously, we all have a lot to learn.

ACKNOWLEDGMENTS. I would like to thank Eileen M. Frees for her help with the preparation of this review and my family for supporting me through the piles of papers and the weekends of writing. Special thanks also goes to the Merck, Sharp, and Dohme Research Laboratories which sponsored my research while this review was being prepared.

REFERENCES

Aarden, L. A., *et al.*, 1979, Revised nomenclature for antigen non-specific T cell proliferation and helper factors, *J. Immunol.* **123:**2928.

Abbott, J., Doyle, P. J., Ngiam, K., and Olson, C. L., 1981, Ontogeny of murine T lymphocytes. 1. Maturation of thymocytes induced *in vitro* by tumor necrosis factor-positive serum (TNF+), *Cell Immunol.* **57:**237.

Amento, E. P., Kurnick, J. T., Epstein, A., and Krane, S. M., 1982a, Modulation of synovial cell products by a factor from a human cell line: T lymphocyte induction of a mononuclear cell factor, *Proc. Natl. Acad. Sci. USA* **79:**5307.

Amento, E. P., Kurnick, J. T., and Krane, S. M., 1982b, Interleukin-1 production by a human monocyte cell line is induced by a T lymphocyte product, *Immunobiology* **163:**276.

Atkins, E., and Francis, L., 1978, Pathogenesis of fever in delayed hypersensitivity: Factors influencing release of pyrogen-inducing lymphokines, *Infect. Immun.* **21:**806.

Atkins, E., Bodel, P., and Francis, L., 1967, Release of an endogenous pyrogen *in vitro* from rabbit mononuclear cells, *J. Exp. Med.* **126:**357.

Atkins, E., Feldman, J. D., Francis, L., and Hursh, E., 1972, Studies on the mechanism of fever accompanying delayed hypersensitivity: The role of the sensitized lymphocyte, *J. Exp. Med.* **135:**1113.

Atkins, E., Francis, L., and Bernheim, H. A., 1978, Pathogenesis of fever in delayed hypersensitivity: Role of monocytes, *Infect. Immun.* **21:**813.

Atkins, E., Askenase, P. W., Francis, L., and Bernheim, H. A., 1980, Release of an endogenous pyrogen from guinea pig leukocytes, *J. Immunol.* **125:**2069.

Bach, F. H., Alter, B. J., Solliday, S., Zoschke, D. C., and Janis, M., 1970, Lymphocyte reactivity *in vitro*. II. Soluble reconstituting factor permitting response of purified lymphocytes, *Cell. Immunol.* **1:**219.

Balow, J. E., and Rosenthal, A. S., 1973, Glucocorticoid suppression of macrophage migration inhibitory factor, *J. Exp. Med.* **137:**1031.

Baracos, V., Rodemann, H. P., Dinarello, C. A., and Goldberg, A. L., 1983, Stimulation of muscle protein degradation and prostaglandin E_2 release by leukocytic pyrogen (interleukin-1). *N. Engl. J. Med.* **308:**553.

Beeson, P. B., 1948, Temperature-elevating effects of a substance obtained from polymorphonuclear leukocytes, *J. Clin. Invest.* **27:**524.

Beller, D. I., and Unanue, E. R., 1977, Thymic maturation *in vitro* by a secretory product from macrophages, *J. Immunol.* **118:**1780.

Beller, D. I., and Unanue, E. R., 1978, Thymic macrophages modulate one stage of T cell differentiation *in vitro*, *J. Immunol.* **121:**1861.

Beller, D. I., and Unanue, E. R., 1979, Evidence that thymocytes require at least two distinct signals to proliferate, *J. Immunol.* **123:**2890.

Ben-Ezra, D., and Gery, I., 1979, Stimulation of keratoycte metabolism by products of lymphoid cells, *Invest. Ophthalmol. Vis. Sci.* **18:**317.

Bendtzen, K., 1981, Induction of antigen-specific immunological unresponsiveness by inhibitors of human lymphocyte-activating factor, *Scand. J. Immunol.* **14:**427.

Benson, M. D., and Aldo-Benson, M., 1979, Effect of purified protein SAA on immune response *in vitro:* Mechanisms of suppression, *J. Immunol.* **122:**2077.
Benson, M. D., and Kleiner, E., 1980, Synthesis and secretion of serum amyloid protein A (SAA) by hepatocytes in mice treated with casein, *J. Immunol.* **124:**495.
Benson, M. D., Scheinberg, M. A., Shirahama, T., Cathcart, E. S., and Skinner, M., 1977, Kinetics of serum amyloid protein A in casein-induced murine amyloidosis, *J. Clin. Invest.* **59:**412.
Ben-Zvi, A., Mizel, S. B., and Oppenheim, J. J., 1981, Generation of human peripheral blood stable E-rosette-forming T cells by interleukin 1, *Clin. Immunol. Immunopathol.* **19:**330.
Bernheim, H. A., and Kluger, M. J., 1976, Effect of drug-induced antipyresis on survival, *Science* **16:**237.
Bernheim, H. A., Block, L. H., and Atkins, E., 1979, Fever: Pathogenesis, pathophysiology, and purpose, *Ann. Intern. Med.* **91:**261.
Bernheim, H. A., Block, L. H., Francis, L., and Atkins, E., 1980, Release of endogenous pyrogen-activating factor from concanavalin A-stimulated human lymphocytes, *J. Exp. Med.* **152:**1811.
Biozzi, G., Benacerraf, B., and Halpern, B. N., 1955, The effect of *Salmonella typhimurium* and its endotoxin on the phagocytic activity of the reticuloendothelial system in mice, *Br. J. Exp. Pathol.* **36:**226.
Block, L. H., Georgopoulos, A., Mayer, P., and Drews, J., 1978, Nonspecific resistance to bacterial infection: Enhancement by ubiquinone-8, *J. Exp. Med.* **148:**1228.
Blomgren, H., 1974, Steroid sensitivity of the response of human lymphocytes to phytohemagglutinin and pokeweed mitogen: Role of phagocytic cells, *Scand. J. Immunol.* **3:**655.
Blyden, G., and Handschumacher, R. E., 1977, Purification and properties of human lymphocyte activating factor (LAF), *J. Immunol.* **118:**1631.
Bodel, P., 1970, Studies on the mechanism of endogenous pyrogen production. I. Investigation of new protein synthesis in stimulated human blood leukocytes, *Yale J. Biol. Med.* **43:**145.
Bodel, P., 1974, Studies on the mechanism of endogenous pyrogen production. III. Human blood monocytes, *J. Exp. Med.* **140:**954.
Bodel, P., 1975, Colchicine stimulation of pyrogen production by human blood monocytes, *J. Exp. Med.* **143:**1015.
Bodel, P., 1978, Spontaneous pyrogen production by mouse histiocytic and myelomonocytic tumor cell lines *in vitro, J. Exp. Med.* **147:**1503.
Bodel, P., and Hollingsworth, J. W., 1968, Pyrogen release from human synovial exudate cells, *Br. J. Exp. Pathol.* **49:**11.
Bodel, P., and Miller, H., 1977, Differences in pyrogen production of mononuclear phagocytes and by fibroblasts or HeLa cells, *J. Exp. Med.* **145:**607.
Bornstein, D. L., and Walsh, E. C., 1978, Endogenous mediators of the acute-phase reaction. I. Rabbit granulocytic pyrogen and its chromatographic subfractions, *J. Lab. Clin. Med.* **91:**236.
Bradley, L. M., and Mishell, R. I., 1981, Differential effects of glucocorticosteroids on the functions of helper and suppressor T lymphocytes, *Proc. Natl. Acad. Sci. USA* **78:**3155.
Braun, W., and Nakano, M., 1967, Antibody formation: Stimulation by polyadenylic and polycytidylic acids, *Science* **157:**819.
Broxmeyer, H. E., Smithyman, A., Eger, R. R., Meyers, P. A., and de Sousa, M., 1978, Identification of lactoferrin as the granulocyte-derived inhibitor of colony-stimulating activity production, *J. Exp. Med.* **148:**1052.
Cabanac, M., Stolwijk, J. A. J., and Hardy, J. D., 1968, Effect of temperature and pyrogens on single-unit activity in the rabbit's brain stem, *J. Appl. Physiol.* **24:**645.
Calderon, J., Kiely, J. M., Lefko, J. L., and Unanue, E. R., 1975, The modulation of lymphocyte functions by molecules secreted by macrophages. I. Description and partial biochemical analysis, *J. Exp. Med.* **142:**151.
Cameron, P. M., and Wood, D. D., 1978, Response of CBA/N mice to human B cell activating factor, *Cell. Immunol.* **38:**176.
Cebula, T. A., Hanson, D. F., Moore, D. M., and Murphy, P. A., 1979, Synthesis of four pyrogens by rabbit macrophages, *J. Lab. Clin. Med.* **94:**95.
Chao, P., Francis, L., and Atkins, E., 1977, The release of endogenous pyrogen from guinea pig leukocytes *in vitro, J. Exp. Med.* **145:**1288.

Charon, J. A., Luger, T. A., Mergenhagen, S. E., and Oppenheim, J. J., 1982, Increased thymocyte-activating factor in human gingival fluid during gingival inflammation, *Infect. Immun.* **38:**1190.

Chedid, L., Audibert, F., Bona, C., Damais, C., Parant, F., and Parant, M., 1975, Biological activities of endotoxins detoxified by alkylation, *Infect. Immun.* **12:**714.

Chen, C., and Hirsch, J. G., 1972, The effects of mercaptoethanol and of peritoneal macrophages on the antibody forming capacity of nonadherent mouse spleen cells *in vitro*, *J. Exp. Med.* **136:**604.

Chen, D.-M., and DiSabato, G., 1976, Further studies on the thymocyte stimulating factor, *Cell. Immunol.* **22:**211.

Chvapil, M., 1976, Effect of zinc on cells and biomembranes, *Med. Clin. North Am.* **60:**799.

Chvapil, M., Stankova, L., Zukoski, C., and Zukoski, C., 1977, Inhibition of some functions of polymorphonuclear leukocytes by *in vitro* zinc, *J. Lab. Clin. Med.* **89:**135.

Claesson, M. H., Whittingham, S., Rodger, M. B., and Burgess, A. W., 1977, Colony growth of human T lymphocytes in agar: Effect of a soluble factor from adherent cells, *Eur. J. Immunol.* **7:**608.

Clark, I. A., Virelizier, J.-L., Carswell, E. A., and Wood, P. R., 1981, Possible importance of macrophage-derived mediators in acute malaria, *Infect. Immun.* **32:**1058.

Cohen, A. S., Gross, E., and Shirahama, I., 1965, The light and electron microscopic autoradiographic demonstration of local amyloid formation in spleen explants, *Am. J. Pathol.* **47:**1079.

Cohen, J. J., and Claman, H. N., 1971, Thymus–marrow immunocompetence. V. Hydrocortisone-resistant cells and processes in the hemolytic antibody response of mice, *J. Exp. Med.* **133:**1026.

Cone, R. E., and Johnson, A. G., 1972, Regulation of the immune system by synthetic polynucleotides. IV. Amplification of proliferation of thymus-influenced lymphocytes, *Cell. Immunol.* **3:**283.

Conlon, P. J., Henney, C. S., and Gillis, S., 1982, Cytokine-dependent thymocyte responses: Characterization of IL-1 and IL-2 target subpopulations and mechanisms of action, *J. Immunol.* **128:**797.

Cooper, K. E., Cranston, W. I., and Snell, E. S., 1964, Temperature regulation during fever in man, *Clin. Sci.* **27:**345.

Cooper, K. E., Cranston, W. I., and Honour, J., 1967, Observations on the site and mode of action of pyrogens in the rabbit brain, *J. Physiol. (London)* **191:**325.

Covert, J. B., and Reynolds, W. W., 1977, Survival value of fever in fish, *Nature (London)* **267:**43.

Crabtree, G. R., Gillis, S., Smith, K. A., and Munck, A., 1980, Mechanisms of glucocorticoid-induced immunosuppression: Inhibitory effects on expression of Fc receptors and production of T-cell growth factor, *J. Steroid Biochem.* **12:**445.

Damais, C., Riveau, G., Parant, M., Gerota, J., and Chedid, J., 1982, Production of lymphocyte activating factor in the absence of endogenous pyrogen by rabbit or human leukocytes stimulated by a muramyl dipeptide derivative, *Int. J. Immunopharmacol.* **4:**451.

Dayer, J. M., Krane, S. M., Russell, R. G. G., and Robinson, D. R., 1976, Production of collagenase and prostaglandins by isolated adherent rheumatoid synovial cells, *Proc. Natl. Acad. Sci. USA* **73:**945.

Dayer, J. M., Robinson, D. R., and Krane, S. M., 1977a, Prostaglandin production by rheumatoid synovial cells: Stimulation by a factor from human mononuclear cells, *J. Exp. Med.* **145:**1399.

Dayer, J. M., Russell, R. G. G., and Krane, S. M., 1977b, Collagenase production by rheumatoid synovial cells: Stimulation by a human lymphocyte factor, *Science* **195:**181.

Dayer, J. M., Bread, J., Chess, L., and Krane, S. M., 1979, Participation of monocyte-macrophages and lymphocytes in the production of a factor that stimulates collagenase and prostaglandin release by rheumatoid synovial cells, *J. Clin. Invest.* **64:**1386.

Dayer, J. M., Goldring, S. R., Robinson, D. R., and Krane, S. M., 1980a, Cell–cell interactions and collagenase production, in: *Collagenase in Normal and Pathological Connective Tissues* (D. E. Woolley and J. M. Evanson, eds.), pp. 83–104, Wiley, New York.

Dayer, J. M., Passwell, J. H., Schneeberger, E. E., and Krane, S. M., 1980b, Interactions among rheumatoid synovial cells and monocyte-macrophages: Production of collagenase-stimulating factor by human monocytes exposed to concanavalin A or immunoglobulin F_c fragments, *J. Immunol.* **124:**1712.

Dayer, J. M., Stephenson, M. L., Schmidt, E., Karge, W., and Krane, S. M., 1981, Purification of a factor from human blood monocyte-macrophages which stimulates the production of collagenase and prostaglandin E_2 by cells cultured from rheumatoid synovial tissues, *FEBS Lett.* **124**:253.

Dempsey, R. A., Dinarello, C. A., Mier, J. W., Rosenwasser, L. J., Allegretta, M., Brown, T. E., and Parkinson, D. R., 1982, The differential effects of human leukocytic pyrogen/lymphocyte-activating factor, T cell growth factor, and interferon on human natural killer activity, *J. Immunol.* **129**:2504.

Deshmukh-Phadke, K., Lawrence, M., and Nanda, S., 1978, Synthesis of collagenase and neutral proteases by articular chondrocytes: Stimulation by a macrophage-derived factor, *Biochem. Biophys. Res. Commun.* **85**:490.

Deshmukh-Phadke, K., Nanda, S., and Lee, K., 1980, Macrophage factor that induces neutral protease secretion by normal rabbit chondrocytes, *Eur. J. Biochem.* **104**:175.

Diamantstein, T., and Ulmer, A., 1976, Two distinct lymphocyte-stimulating soluble factors (LAF) released from murine peritoneal cells. I. The cellular source and the effect of cGMP on their release, *Immunology* **30**:741.

Dimitriu, A., and Fauci, A. S., 1978, Activation of human B lymphocytes. IX. Modulation of antibody by products of activated macrophages, *J. Immunol.* **120**:1818.

Dinarello, C. A., 1979, Production of endogenous pyrogen, *Fed. Proc.* **38**:52.

Dinarello, C. A., 1981, Demonstration of a human pyrogen-inducing factor during mixed leukocyte reactions, *J. Exp. Med.* **153**:1215.

Dinarello, C. A., and Wolff, S. M., 1977, Partial purification of human leukocytic pyrogen, *Inflammation (N.Y.)* **2**:179.

Dinarello, C. A., and Wolff, S. M., 1979, Mechanisms in the production of fever in humans, *Semin. Infect. Dis.* **2**:173.

Dinarello, C. A., Bodel. P., and Atkins, E., 1968, The role of the liver in the production of fever and in pyrogenic tolerance, *Trans. Assoc. Am. Physicians* **81**:334.

Dinarello, C. A., Goldin, N. P., and Wolff, S. M., 1974, Demonstration and characterization of two distinct human leukocytic pyrogens, *J. Exp. Med.* **139**:1369.

Dinarello, C. A., Renfer, L., and Wolff, S. M., 1977, The production of antibody against human leukocytic pyrogen, *J. Clin. Invest.* **60**:465.

Dinarello, C. A., Rosenwasser, L. J., and Wolff, S. M., 1981, Demonstration of a circulating suppressor factor of thymocyte proliferation during endotoxin fever in humans, *J. Immunol.* **127**:2517.

Dinarello, C. A., Bendtzen, K., and Wolff, S. M., 1982, Studies on the active site of human leukocytic pyrogen, *Inflammation* **6**:63.

Dinarello, C. A., Marnoy, S. O., and Rosenwasser, L. J., 1983, Role of arachidonate metabolism in the immunoregulatory function of human leukocytic pyrogen/lymphocyte-activating factor/interleukin-1, *J. Immunol.* **130**:890.

Dingle, J. T., Saklatvala, J., Hembry, R., Tyler, J., Fell, H. B., and Jubb, R., 1979, A cartilage catabolic factor from synovium, *Biochem. J.* **184**:177.

DiSabato, G., Chen, D.-M., and Erickson, J. W., 1975, Production by murine spleen cells of activity stimulating the PHA-responsiveness of thymus lymphocytes, *Cell. Immunol.* **17**:495.

DiSabato, G., Moraes, E. K., and Altin, M., 1979, Effect of thymocyte-stimulating factor-containing supernatants on the surface antigens of murine thymocytes, *Cell. Immunol.* **44**:252.

Duff, G. W., and Durum, S., 1983, Fever and immunoregulation. II. Are the pyrogenic and mitogenic actions of interleukin-1 related? *Nature (London)* **304**:449.

Duncan, R. L., Jr., and McArthur, W. P., 1981, Lactoferrin-mediated modulation of mononuclear cell activities. 1. Suppression of the murine *in vitro* primary antibody response, *Cell. Immunol.* **63**:308.

Durum, S. K., and Gershon, R. K., 1982, Interleukin-1 can replace the requirement for I-A-positive cells in the proliferation of antigen-primed T cells, *Proc. Natl. Acad. Sci. USA* **79**:4747.

Economou, J. S., and Shin, H. S., 1978, Lymphocyte-activating factor. I. Generation and physicochemical characterization, *J. Immunol.* **21**:1446.

Eddington, C. L., Upchurch, H. F., and Kampschmidt, R. F., 1972, Quantitation of plasma α_2-AP globulin before and after stimulation with leukocyte extracts, *Proc. Soc. Exp. Biol. Med.* **139:**565.

Efremov, O. M., Sorokin, A. V., and El'kina, O. A., 1978, Formation of endogenous pyrogen by bone marrow cells, *Byull. Eksp. Biol. Med.* **85:**17.

Eisenman, J. S., and Jackson, D. C., 1967, Thermal response patterns of septal and preoptic neurons in cats, *Exp. Neurol.* **19:**33.

Erb, P., and Feldmann, M., 1975a, The role of macrophages in the generation of T-helper cells. I. The requirement for macrophages in helper cell induction and characteristics of the macrophage T-cell interaction, *Cell. Immunol.* **19:**356.

Erb, P., and Feldmann, M., 1975b, The role of macrophages in the generation of T-helper cells. III. Influence of macrophage-derived factors in helper cell induction, *Eur. J. Immunol.* **5:**759.

Erb, P., Vogt, P., Meier, B., and Feldmann, M., 1977, The role of macrophages in the generation of T helper cells. V. Evidence for differential activation of short-lived T_1 and long-lived T_2 lymphocytes by the macrophage factors GRF and NMF, *J. Immunol.* **119:**206.

Farr, A. G., Dorf, M. E., and Unanue, E. R., 1977, Secretion of mediators following T lymphocyte–macrophage interaction is regulated by the major histocompatibility complex, *Proc. Natl. Acad. Sci. USA* **74:**3542.

Farrar, J. J., 1974, *In vitro* reconstitution of T cell deficient mouse spleen cells by cocultivation with human lymphocytes, *J. Immunol.* **112:**1613.

Farrar, J. J., 1975, The xenogeneic effect. I. Antigen and mitogen-stimulated human lymphocytes produce a non-antigen-specific factor which reconstitutes the antibody response of T-cell deficient mouse spleen cells, *J. Immunol.* **115:**1295.

Farrar, J. J., Mizel, S. B., Fuller-Bonar, J., Hilfiker, M. L., and Farrar, W. L., 1980, Lipopolysaccharide mediated adjuvanticity: Effect of lipopolysaccharide on the production of thymus derived growth factor (interleukin 2), in: *Microbiology—1980* (D. Schlessinger, ed.), p. 36, American Society of Microbiology, Washington, D.C.

Farrar, W. L., Mizel, S. B., and Farrar, J. J., 1980, Participation of lymphocyte activating factor (interleukin 1) in the induction of cytotoxic T cell responses, *J. Immunol.* **124:**1371.

Farrar, W. L., Johnson, H. M., and Farrar, J. J., 1981, Regulation of the production of immune interferon and cytotoxic T lymphocyte by interleukin-2, *J. Immunol.* **126:**1125.

Finelt, M., and Hoffmann, M. K., 1979, A human monocyte function test: Release of B cell differentiation factor, *Clin. Immunol. Immunopathol.* **12:**281.

Finke, J. H., Sharma, S. D., and Scott, J. W., 1981, Generation of alloreactive cytotoxic T lymphocytes: Production of T cell and Mϕ helper factors in addition to IL-1 and IL-2 by peritoneal cells from mice immunized to *Listeria monocytogenes*, *J. Immunol.* **127:**2354.

Fontana, A., Hengartner, H., Weber, E., Fehr, K., Grob, P. J., and Cohen, G., 1982a, Interleukin-1 activity in the synovial fluid of patients with rheumatoid arthritis, *Rheumatol. Int.* **2:**49.

Fontana, A., Kristensen, F., Dubs, R., Gemsa, D., and Weber, E., 1982b, Production of prostaglandin E and interleukin-1-like factor by cultured astrocytes and C_6 glioma cells, *J. Immunol.* **129:**2413.

Galili, U., Rosenthal, L., and Klein, E., 1981, Activated T cells in the synovial fluid of arthritic patients. II. *In vitro* activation of the autologous blood lymphocytes, *J. Immunol.* **127:**430.

Gery, I., 1982, Production and assay of interleukin-1 (IL-1) in: *Isolation, Characterization, and Utilization of T Lymphocyte Clones* (C. G. Fathman and F. Fitch, eds.), pp.41–56, Academic Press, New York.

Gery, I., and Handschumacher, R. E., 1974, Potentiation of the T lymphocyte response to mitogens. III. Properties of the mediator(s) from adherent cells, *Cell. Immunol.* **11:**162.

Gery, I., and Waksman, B. H., 1972, Potentiation of the T-lymphocyte response to mitogens. II. The cellular source of potentiating mediator(s), *J. Exp. Med.* **136:**143.

Gery, I., Gershon, R. K., and Waksman, B. H., 1972, Potentiation of the T-lymphocyte response to mitogens. I. The responding cell, *J. Exp. Med.* **136:**128.

Gery, I., Davies, P., Derr, J., Krett, N., and Barranger, J. A., 1981a, Relation between production and release of lymphocyte activating factor (interleukin-1) by murine macrophages. I. Effects of various agents, *Cell. Immunol.* **64:**293.

Gery, I., Seminara, D., Derr, J., and Barranger, J. A., 1981b, Production and release of lymphocyte activating factor (interleukin-1) by human monocytes and their derived macrophages, in: *Mecha-*

nisms of Lymphocyte Activation (K. Resch and H. Kirchner, eds.), pp. 541–543, Elsevier/North-Holland, Amsterdam.

Gillis, S., and Mizel, S. B., 1981, T cell lymphoma model for the analysis of interleukin-1 mediated T cell activation, *Proc. Natl. Acad. Sci. USA* **78:**113.

Gillis, S., Smith, K. A., and Watson, J., 1980, Biochemical characterization of lymphocyte regulatory molecules. II. Purification of a class of rat and human lymphokines, *J. Immunol.* **124:**1954.

Glaser, M., and Nelken, D., 1972, Inhibitory effect of α-globulin on the second set allograft reaction, *Proc. Soc. Exp. Biol. Med.* **140:**996.

Goodman, M. G., Chenoweth, D. E., and Weigle, W. O., 1982, Induction of interleukin-1 secretion and enhancement of humoral immunity by binding of human C5a to macrophage surface C5a receptors, *J. Exp. Med.* **156:**912.

Goodrum, K. J., and Berry, L. J., 1979, The use of Reuber hepatoma cells for the study of a lipopolysaccharide-induced macrophage factor, *Lab. Invest.* **41:**174.

Gorczynski, R. M., 1977, Role of macrophage-derived factors in generation of cytotoxic and antibody responses, *Scand. J. Immunol.* **6:**665.

Gorczynski, R. M., and Price, G. B., 1979, The role of macrophages in stimulation of immune induction and myelopoiesis. II. Analysis of genetic restrictions involved in the stimulation of granulocyte colony precursors or mature lymphocytes using factors prepared from different recombinant inbred strains of mice, *Immunopharmacology.* **1:**187.

Gowen, M., Wood, D. D., Ihrie, E. J., Meats, J. E., and Russell, R. G. G., 1985a, Stimulation by human interleukin-1 of cartilage breakdown and production of collagenase and proteoglycanase by human chondrocytes but not by human osteoblasts *in vitro, Biochim. Biophys. Acta,* in press.

Gowen, M., Wood, D. D., Ihrie, E. J., McGuire, M. K. B., and Russell, R. G. G., 1985b, An interleukin-1-like factor stimulates bone resorption *in vitro, Nature (London),* in press.

Grabner, G., Luer, T. A., Smolin, G., and Oppenheim, J. J., 1982, Corneal epithelial cell-derived thymocyte-activating factor (CETAF), *Invest. Ophthalmol. Vis. Sci.* **23:**757.

Grieger, T. A., and Kluger, M. J., 1978, Fever and survival: The role of serum iron, *J. Physiol. (London)* **279:**187.

Haeseler, F., Bodel, P., and Atkins, E., 1977, Characteristics of pyrogen production by isolated rabbit Kupffer cells *in vitro, J. Reticuloendothelial Soc.* **22:**569.

Hanson, D. F., Murphy, P. A., and Windle, B. E., 1980, Failure of rabbit neutrophils to secrete endogenous pyrogen when stimulated with staphylococci, *J. Exp. Med.* **151:**1360.

Hanson, D. F., Murphy, P. A., Silicano, R., and Shin, H. S., 1983, The effect of temperature on the activation of thymocytes by interleukin-I and II, *J. Immunol.* **130:**216.

Hardy, J. D., Hellon, R. F., and Sutherland, K., 1964, Temperature-sensitive neurons in the dog's hypothalamus, *J. Physiol. (London)* **173:**242.

Harwell, L., Kappler, J. W., and Marrack, P., 1976, Antigen-specific and nonspecific mediator(s) of T cell/B cell cooperation. III. Characterization of the nonspecific mediator(s) from different sources, *J. Immunol.* **116:**1379.

Hoffeld, J. T., and Oppenheim, J. J., 1980, Enhancement of the primary antibody response by 2-mercaptoethanol is mediated by its action on glutathione in the serum, *Eur. J. Immunol.* **10:**391.

Hoffmann, M. K., 1980, Macrophages and T cells control distinct phases of B cell differentiation in the humoral immune response *in vitro, J. Immunol.* **125:**2076.

Hoffmann, M. K., and Watson, J., 1979, Helper T cell-replacing factors secreted by thymus-derived cells and macrophages: Cellular requirements for B cell activation and synergistic properties, *J. Immunol.* **122:**1371.

Hoffmann, M. K., Hammerling, U., Simon, M., and Oettgen, H. F., 1976, Macrophage requirements of CR^- and CR^+ B lymphocytes for antibody production *in vitro, J. Immunol.* **116:**1447.

Hoffmann, M. K., Oettgen, H. F., Old, L. J., Chin, A. F., and Hammerling, U., 1977, Endotoxin-induced serum factor controlling differentiation of bone marrow derived lymphocytes, *Proc. Natl. Acad. Sci. USA* **74:**1200.

Hoffmann, M. K., Oettgen, H. F., Old, L. J., Mittler, R. S., and Hammerling, U., 1978, Induction and immunological properties of tumor necrosis factor, *J. Reticuloendothelial Soc.* **23:**307.

Hoffmann, M. K., Koenig, S., Mittler, R. S., Oettgen, H. F., Ralph, P., Galanos, C., and Hammerling, U., 1979, Macrophage factor controlling differentiation of bone marrow derived cells, *J. Immunol.* **122:**497.

Huybrechts-Godin, G., Hauser, P., and Vaes, G., 1979, Macrophage–fibroblast interactions in collagenase production and cartilage destruction, *Biochem. J.* **184:**643.

Igarashi, T., Okada, M., Kishimoto, T., and Yamamura, Y., 1977, *In vitro* induction of polyclonal killer T cells with 2-mercaptoethanol and the essential role of macrophages in this process, *J. Immunol.* **118:**1697.

Igarashi, T., Rodrigues, D., and Ting, C., 1979, Studies of the mechanisms for the induction of *in vitro* tumor immunity. IV. Enhancement of the *in vitro* generation of secondary cell-mediated cytotoxic response by normal peritoneal macrophages and their culture supernatants, *J. Immunol.* **122:**1519.

Ihrie, E. J., and Wood, D. D., 1984, Heterogeneity of human interleukin-1. I. Biochemical characterization, submitted to *J. Immunol.*

Iribe, H., Koga, T., Onoue, K., Kotani, S., Kusumoto, S., and Shiba, T., 1981, Macrophage-stimulating effect of a synthetic muramyl dipeptide and its adjuvant-active and -inactive analogs for the production of T-cell activating monokines, *Cell Immunol.* **64:**73.

Iribe, H., Koga, T., and Onoue, K., 1982, Production of T-cell activating monokine of guinea pig macrophages induced by MDP and partial characterization of the monokine, *J. Immunol.* **129:**1029.

Ise, K., Nakamura, S., Ohkawara, S., and Yoshinaga, M., 1982, DNA synthesis-potentiating activity on mouse thymocytes of synovial fluid of rheumatoid arthritis patients, *Acta Pathol. Jpn.* **32:**491.

Jalkanen, M., 1981, Connective tissue activating macromolecules in macrophage culture medium, *Connect. Tissue Res.* **9:**19.

Jasin, H. E., and Dingle, J. T., 1981, Human mononuclear cell factors mediate cartilage matrix degradation through chondrocyte activation, *J. Clin. Invest.* **68:**571.

Kammer, G. M., and Unanue, E. R., 1980, Accessory cell requirement in the proliferative response of T lymphocytes to hemocyanin, *Clin. Immunol. Immunopathol.* **15:**434.

Kampschmidt, R. F., 1979, Role of RES and leukocytic endogenous mediator in iron, zinc and copper metabolism, in: *Macrophages and Lymphocytes: Nature, Functions and Interaction* (M. R. Escobar and H. Friedmann, eds.), pp. 402–411, Plenum Press, New York.

Kampschmidt, R. F., 1982, Leukocytic endogenous mediator/endogenous pyrogen, in: *Infection: The Physiologic and Metabolic Responses of the Host* (M. C. Powanda and P. G. Canonics, eds.), pp. 505–541, Elsevier, New York.

Kampschmidt, R. F., and Pulliam, L. A., 1975, Stimulation of antimicrobial activity in the rat with leukocytic endogenous mediator, *J. Reticuloendothelial Soc.* **17:**162.

Kampschmidt, R. F., and Upchurch, H. F., 1969a, Lowering of plasma iron concentration in the rat with leukocytic extracts, *Am. J. Physiol.* **216:**1287.

Kampschmidt, R. F., and Upchurch, H. F., 1969b, Some effects of endotoxin and leukocytic pyrogen on the body temperature of rats, *Proc. Soc. Exp. Biol. Med.* **131:**864.

Kampschmidt, R. F., and Upchurch, H. F., 1974, Effect of leukocytic endogenous mediator on plasma fibrinogen and haptoglobin, *Proc. Soc. Exp. Biol. Med.* **146:**904.

Kampschmidt, R. F., and Upchurch, H. F., 1980a, Neutrophil release after injections of endotoxin or leukocytic endogenous mediator into rats, *J. Reticuloendothelial Soc.* **28:**191.

Kampschmidt, R. F., and Upchurch, H. F., 1980b, Rate of clearance of circulating leukocytic endogenous mediator in the rat, *Proc. Soc. Exp. Biol. Med.* **164:**537.

Kampschmidt, R. F., Pulliam, L. A., and Upchurch, H. F., 1973a, Sources of leukocytic endogenous mediator in the rat, *Proc. Soc. Exp. Biol. Med.* **144:**882.

Kampschmidt, R. A., Upchurch, H. F., Eddington, C. L., and Pulliam, L. A., 1973b, Multiple biological activities of a partially purified leukocytic endogenous mediator, *Am. J. Physiol.* **224:**530.

Kampschmidt, R. F., Pulliam, L. A., and Upchurch, H. F., 1980, The activity of partially purified leukocytic endogenous mediator in endotoxin-resistant C3H/HeJ mice, *J. Lab. Clin. Med.* **95:**616.

Katz, S. P., Shimamura, T., Dessaint, J.-P., Braverman, D., and Waksman, B. H., 1980, Mechanisms of action of "lymphocyte activating factor" (LAF). IV. Differential stimulation of T lymphocyte by individual macrophage enzymes (catheptic carboxypeptidase B and serine proteases), *Cell. Immunol.* **56:**68.

Kierszenbaum, F., and Waksman, B. H., 1977, Mechanism of action of "lymphocyte activating factor" (LAF). I. Association of lymphocyte activating factor action with early DNA synthesis in PHA-stimulated lymphocytes, *Immunology* **33:**663.

Klempner, M. S., Dinarello, C. A., and Gallin, J. I., 1978, Human leukocytic pyrogen induces release of specific granule contents from human neutrophils, *J. Clin. Invest.* **61:**1330.

Klempner, M. S., Dinarello, C. A., Henderson, W. R., and Gallin, J. I., 1979, Stimulation of neutrophil oxygen-dependent metabolism by human leukocytic pyrogen, *J. Clin. Invest.* **64:**996.

Klimpel, G. R., 1980, Soluble factor(s) from LPS-activated macrophages induce cytotoxic T cell differentiation from alloantigen-primed spleen cells, *J. Immunol.* **125:**1243.

Kluger, M. J., Ringler, D. H., and Anver, M. R., 1975, Fever and survival, *Science* **188:**166.

Koopman, W. J., Farrar, J. J., Oppenheim, J. J., Fuller-Bonar, J., and Dougherty, S., 1977, Association of a low molecular weight helper factor(s) with thymocyte proliferative activity, *J. Immunol.* **119:**55.

Koopman, W. J., Farrar, J. J., and Fuller-Bonar, J., 1978, Evidence for the identification of lymphocyte activating factor as the adherent cell-derived mediator responsible for enhanced antibody synthesis by nude mouse spleen cells, *Cell. Immunol.* **35:**92.

Korn, J. H., Halushka, P. V., and LeRoy, E. C., 1980, Mononuclear cell modulation of connective tissue function: Suppression of fibroblast growth by stimulation of endogenous prostaglandin production, *J. Clin. Invest.* **65:**543.

Kotani, S., Watanabe, Y., Shimono, T., Narita, T., Kato, K., Stewart-Tull, D. E. S., Kinoshita, F., Yokogawa, K., Kawata, S., Shiba, T., Kusumoto, S., and Tarumi, Y., 1975, Immunoadjuvant activities of cell walls, their water-soluble fractions and peptidoglycan subunits, prepared from various gram-positive bacteria, and of synthetic *N*-acetylmuramyl peptides, *Z. Immunitaetsforsch. Bd.* **149:**S302.

Kotani, S., Watanabe, Y., Shimono, T., Harada, K., Shiba, T., Kusumoto, S., Yokogawa, K., and Taniguchi, M., 1976, Correlation between the immunoadjuvant activities and pyrogenicities of synthetic *N*-acetylmuramyl-peptides or amino acids, *Biken J.* **19:**9.

Krakauer, T., Mizel, D., and Oppenheim, J. J., 1982, Independent and synergistic thymocyte proliferative activities of PMA and IL-1, *J. Immunol.* **129:**939.

Kurland, J. I., Kincade, P. W., and Moore, M. A. S., 1977, Regulation of B-lymphocyte clonal proliferation by stimulatory and inhibitory macrophage-derived factors, *J. Exp. Med.* **146:**1420.

Lachman, L. B., and Metzgar, R. S., 1980a, Characterization of high and low molecular weight lymphocyte-activating factor (interleukin I) from P388D1 and J774.1 mouse macrophage cell lines, *J. Reticuloendothelial Soc.* **27:**621.

Lachman, L. B., and Metzgar, R. S., 1980b, Purification and characterization of human lymphocyte activating factor, in: *Biochemical Characterization of Lymphokines* (A. L. DeWeck, F. Kristensen, and M. Landy, eds.), 405–409, Academic Press, New York.

Lachman, L. B., Hacker, M. P., Blyden, G. T., and Handschumacher, R. E., 1977a, Preparation of lymphocyte-activating factor from continuous murine macrophage cell lines, *Cell. Immunol.* **34:**416.

Lachman, L. B., Hacker, M. P., and Handschumacher, R. E., 1977b, Partial purification of human lymphocyte-activating factor (LAF) by ultrafiltration and electrophoretic techniques, *J. Immunol.* **199:**2019.

Lachman, L. B., Moore, J. O., and Metzgar, R. S., 1978, Preparation and characterization of lymphocyte-activating factor (LAF) from acute monocytic and myelomonocytic leukemia cells, *Cell. Immunol.* **41:**199.

Lachman, L. B., Page, S. O., and Metzgar, R. S., 1980, Purification of human interleukin-1, *J. Supramol. Struct.* **13:**457.

Larsson, E. L., Iscove, N. N., and Coutinho, A., 1980, Two distinct factors are required for induction of T-cell growth, *Nature (London)* **283:**664.

Le, P., Muller, M. T., and Mortensen, R. F., 1982, Acute phase reactants of mice. I. Isolation of serum amyloid P-component (SAP) and its induction by a monokine, *J. Immunol.* **129:**665.

Lee, K., Langman, R. E., Paetku, V. H., and Deiner, E., 1975, The cellular basis of cortisone-induced immunosuppression of the antibody response studied by its reversal *in vitro*, *Cell. Immunol.* **17:**405.

Lee, K. C., Wong, M., and McIntyre, D., 1981, Characterization of macrophage subpopulations responsive to activation by endotoxin and lymphokines, *J. Immunol.* **126:**2474.

Lin, H.-S., Medoff, G., and Kobayashi, G. S., 1977, Effects of amphotericin B on macrophages and their precursor cells, *Antimicrob. Agents Chemother.* **11:**154.

Lindsay, H. L., Trown, P. W., Brandt, J., and Forbes, M., 1969, Pyrogenicity of poly I: poly C in rabbits, *Nature (London)* **223:**717.

Linker-Israeli, M., Bakke, A. C., Kitridou, R. C., Gendler, S., Gillis, S., and Horwitz, D. A., 1983, Defective production of interleukin-1 and interleukin-2 in patients with systemic lupus erythematosis (SLE), *J. Immunol.* **130:**2651.

Lipsky, P. E., Thompson, P. A., Rossenwasser, L. J., and Dinarello, C. A., 1983, The role of interleukin-1 in human B cell activation: Inhibition of B cell proliferation and the generation of immunoglobulin-secreting cells by an antibody against human leukocytic pyrogen, *J. Immunol.* **130:**2708.

Lonai, P., and Steinman, L., 1977, Physiological regulation of antigen binding to T cells: Role of a soluble macrophage factor and of interferon, *Proc. Natl. Acad. Sci. USA* **74:**5662.

Lorber, D., Tenenbaum, M., Thurston, S., Gander, G. W., and Goodale, F., 1971, The fate of circulating leukocytic pyrogen in the rabbit, *Proc. Soc. Exp. Biol. Med.* **137:**896.

Lovett, D. H., Ryan, J. L., and Sterzel, R. B., 1983, A thymocyte activating factor derived from glomerular mesangial cells, *J. Immunol.* **130:**1796.

Lowy, I., Bona, C., and Chedid, L., 1977, Target cells for the activity of a synthetic adjuvant: Muramyl dipeptide, *Cell Immunol.* **29:**195.

Luger, T. A., Stadler, B. M., Katz, S. I., and Oppenheim, J. J., 1981, Epidermal cell (keratinocyte)-derived thymocyte-activating factor (ETAF), *J. Immunol.* **127:**1493.

Luger, T. A., Stadler, B. M., Luger, B. M., Mathieson, B. J., Mage, M., Schmidt, J. A., and Oppenheim, J. J., 1982, Murine epidermal cell derived thymocyte-activating factor resembles murine interleukin-I, *J. Immunol.* **128:**2147.

Lutz, C. T., Glasebrook, A. L., and Fitch, F. W., 1981, Alloreactive cloned T cell lines. III Accessory cell requirement for the growth of cloned cytologic T lymphocytes, *J. Immunol.* **126:**1404.

McAdam, K. P. W. J., and Dinarello, C. A., 1981, Induction of serum amyloid A synthesis by human leukocytic pyrogen, in: *Bacterial Endotoxins and Host Response* (M. K. Agarwal, ed.), pp. 167–178, Elsevier/North-Holland, Amsterdam.

McAdam, K. P. W. J., and Ryan, J. L., 1978, C57BL/10/CR mice: Nonresponders to activation by the lipid A moiety of bacterial lipopolysaccharide, *J. Immunol.* **120:**249.

McAdam, K. P. W. J., Westermark, P., Anders, R. F., and Voller, A., 1979, Juvenile amyloidosis in the Anga peoples of Papua New Guinea, in: *Proceedings, 3rd International Symposium on Amyloidosis* (C. G. Glenner, P. Pinho e Costa, and A. Falcao de Freitas, eds.), pp. 207–210, Excerpta Medica, Amsterdam.

McGuire, M. K. B., Meats, J. E., and Russell, R. G. G., 1980, Cell–cell interactions in the rheumatoid joint, *Agents Actions* **10:**486.

McGuire-Goldring, M. K. B., Meats, J. E., Wood, D. D., Ihrie, E. J., Ebsworth, N. M., and Russell, R. G. G. 1984, Activation of human chondrocytes and synoviocytes *in vitro* by human interleukin-1, submitted to *Arth. Rheum.*

MacPherson, R. K., 1959, The effect of fever on temperature regulation in man, *Clin. Sci.* **18:**281.

Maizel, A. L., Mehta, S. R., Ford, R. J., and Lachman, L. B., 1981a, Effect of interleukin-1 on human thymocytes and purified human T cells, *J. Exp. Med.* **153:**470.

Maizel, A. L., Mehta, S. R., Hauft, S., Franzini, D., Lachman, L. B., and Ford, R. J., 1981b, Human T lymphocyte/monocyte interaction in response to lectin: Kinetics of entry into the S phase, *J. Immunol.* **127:**1058.

Mannel, D. N., Farrar, J. J., and Mergenhagen, S. E., 1980, Separation of a serum-derived tumoricidal factor from a helper factor for plaque-forming cells, *J. Immunol.* **124:**1106.

Martin, B. M., Gimbrone, M. A., Jr., Unanue, E. R., and Cotran, R. S., 1981, Stimulation of nonlymphoid mesenchymal cell proliferation by a macrophage-derived growth factor, *J. Immunol.* **126**:1510.

Meats, J. E., McGuire, M. B., and Russell, R. G. G., 1980, Human synovium releases a factor which stimulates chondrocyte production of PGE and plasminogen activator, *Nature (London)* **286**:891.

Melcion, C., Lachman, L., Killen, P. D., Morel-Maroger, L., and Striker, G. E., 1982, Mesangial cells, effects of monocyte products on proliferation and matrix synthesis, *Transplant. Proc.* **14**:559.

Meltzer, M. S., and Oppenheim, J. J., 1977, Bidirectional amplification of macrophage–lymphocyte interactions: Enhanced lymphocyte activation factor production by activated adherent mouse peritoneal cells, *J. Immunol.* **118**:77.

Merrill, W. W., Naegel, G. P., Matthay, R. A., and Reynolds, H. Y., 1980, Alveolar macrophage-derived chemotactic factor, *J. Clin. Invest.* **65**:268.

Merriman, C. R., Pulliam, L. A., and Kampschmidt, R. F., 1975, Effect of leukocytic endogenous mediator on C-reactive protein in rabbits, *Proc. Soc. Exp. Biol. Med.* **149**:782.

Merriman, C. R., Pulliam, L. A., and Kampschmidt, R. F., 1977, Comparison of leukocytic pyrogen and leukocytic endogenous mediator, *Proc. Soc. Exp. Biol. Med.* **154**:224.

Mickenberg, I. D., Root, R. K., and Wolff, S. M., 1972, Bactericidal and metabolic properties of human eosinophils, *Blood* **39**:67.

Mishell, R. I., Bradley, L. M., Chen, Y.-H. U., Grabstein, K. H., and Shiigi, S. M., 1979, Glucocorticosteroid response-modifying factors derived from accessory cells, *Ann. N.Y. Acad. Sci.* **332**:433.

Mishell, R. I., Bradley, L. M., Chen, Y.-H. U., Grabstein, K. H., and Shiigi, S. M., 1980a, Protection of helper thymus derived cells from glucocorticosteroids by mediators from adjuvant activated monocytes, in: *Microbiology—1980* (D. Schlessinger, ed.), pp. 82–86, American Society of Microbiology, Washington, D.C.

Mishell, R. I., Shiigi, J. M., Mishell, B. B., Grabstein, K. H., and Shiigi, S. M., 1980b, Prevention of the immunosuppressive effects of glucocorticosteroids by cell-free factors from adjuvant-activated accessory cells, *Immunopharmacology* **2**:233.

Mishell, R. I., Chen, Y. U., Clark, G. C., Gold, M. R., Hill, J. L., Kwan, E., and Lee, D. A., 1981, Induction of murine lymphocytes and macrophages by components of bacterial cell walls and membranes, in: *Chemistry and Biological Activities of Bacterial Surface Amphiphiles* (G. D. Shockman and A. J. Wickin, eds.), p. 376–388, Academic Press, New York.

Mishell, R. I., Lee, D. A., Grabstein, K. H., and Lachman, L. B., 1982, Prevention of the *in vitro* myelosuppressive effects of glucocorticosteroids by interleukin-1 (IL-1), *J. Immunol.* **128**:1614.

Mizel, S. B., 1979a, Biochemical and biological characterization of lymphocyte-activating factor (LAF) produced by the murine macrophage cell line, P388D_1, *Ann. N.Y. Acad. Sci.* **332**:539.

Mizel, S. B., 1979b, Biochemical characteristics of macrophage-derived immunostimulatory factors, in: *Molecular Mediators of Cellular Immunity: Characterizations and Actions* (J. W. Hadden and W. E. Stewart, eds.), p. 365–382, Humana Press, Clifton, N.J.

Mizel, S. B., 1979c, Physicochemical characterization of lymphocyte-activating factor (LAF), *J. Immunol.* **122**:2167.

Mizel, S. B., 1980, Studies on the purification and structure function relationships of lymphocyte activating factor (interleukin-1), *Mol. Immunol.* **17**:571.

Mizel, S. B., and Ben-Zvi, A., 1980, Studies on the role of lymphocyte-activating factor (interleukin-1) in antigen-induced lymph node lymphocyte proliferation, *Cell. Immunol.* **54**:382.

Mizel, S. B., and Mizel, D., 1981, Purification to apparent homogeneity of murine interleukin-1, *J. Immunol.* **126**:834.

Mizel, S. B., and Rosenstreich, D. L., 1979, Regulation of lymphocyte activating factor (LAF) production and secretion in P388D_1 cells: Identification of high molecular weight precursors of LAF, *J. Immunol.* **122**:2173.

Mizel, S. B., Oppenheim, J. J., and Rosenstreich, D. L., 1978a, Characterization of lymphocyte-activating factor (LAF) produced by the macrophage line P388D_1. I. Enhancement of LAF production by activated T lymphocytes, *J. Immunol.* **120**:1497.

Mizel, S. B., Oppenheim, J. J., and Rosenstreich, D. L., 1978b, Characterization of lymphocyte-activating factor (LAF) produced a macrophage cell line, P388D_1. II. Biochemical characterization of LAF induced by activated T cells and LPS, *J. Immunol.* **120**:1504.

Mizel, S. B., Rosenstreich, D. L., and Oppenheim, J. J., 1978c, Phorbol myristic acetate stimulates LAF production by the macrophage cell lines, P388D$_1$, *Cell. Immunol.* **40:**230.

Mizel, S. B., Dayer, J. M., Krane, S. M., and Mergenhagen, S. E., 1981, Stimulation of rheumatoid synovial cell collagenase and prostaglandin production by partially purified lymphocyte activating factor (interleukin-1), *Proc. Natl. Acad. Sci. USA* **78:**2474.

Moore, D. M., Murphy, P. A., Chesney, P. W., and Wood, W. B., Jr., 1973, Synthesis of endogenous pyrogen by rabbit leukocytes, *J. Exp. Med.* **137:**1263.

Moore, R. N., Goodrum, K. J., Couch, R. E., Jr., and Berry, L. J., 1978, Elicitation of endotoxemic effects in C3H/HeJ mice with glucocorticoid antagonizing factor and partial characterization of the factor, *Infect. Immun.* **19:**79.

Moore, R. N., Oppenheim, J. J., Farrar, J. J., Carter, C. S., Jr., Waheed, A., and Shadduck, R. K., 1980, Production of lymphocyte-activating factor (interleukin-I) by macrophages activated with colony-stimulating factors, *J. Immunol.* **125:**1302.

Morgan, E. L., and Weigle, W. O., 1980, Polyclonal activation of murine B lymphocytes by F$_c$ fragments. I. The requirement for two signals in the generation of polyclonal antibody response induced by F$_c$ fragments, *J. Immunol.* **124:**1330.

Morgan, E. L., Hugli, T. E., and Weigle, W. O., 1982, Isolation and identification of a biologically active peptide derived from the CH3 domain of human IgG$_1$, *Proc. Natl. Acad. Sci., USA,* **79:**5388.

Mosier, D. E., 1967, A requirement for two cell types for antibody formation *in vitro, Science,* **158:**1573.

Murphy, P. A., Simon, P. L., and Willoughby, W. F., 1980, Endogenous pyrogens made by rabbit peritoneal exudate cells are identical with lymphocyte-activating factors made by rabbit alveolar macrophages, *J. Immunol.* **124:**2498.

Murphy, P. A., Cebula, T. A., Levin, J., and Windle, B. E., 1981a, Rabbit macrophages secrete two biochemically and immunologically distinct endogenous pyrogens, *Infect. Immun.* **34:**177.

Murphy, P. A., Cebula, T. A., and Windle, B. E., 1981b, Heterogeneity of rabbit endogenous pyrogens is not attributable to glycosylated variants of a single polypeptide chain, *Infect. Immun.* **34:**184.

Nakayama, T., and Hori, T., 1973, Effect of anaesthetic and pyrogen on thermally sensitive neurons in the brain stem, *J. Appl. Physiol.* **34:**351.

Nakayama, T., Hammel, H. T., Hardy, J. D., and Eisenman, J. S., 1963, Thermal stimulation of electrical activity of single units of the preoptic region, *Am. J. Physiol.* **204:**1122.

Newsome, D. A., and Gross, J., 1979, Regulation of corneal collagenase production: Stimulation of serially passaged stromal cells by blood mononuclear cells, *Cell* **16:**895.

Nordlund, J. J., Root, R. K., and Wolff, S. M., 1970, Studies on the origin of human leukocytic pyrogen, *J. Exp. Med.* **131:**727.

Okada, M., Kishimoto, T., Igarashi, T., Teranishi, T., and Yamamura, Y., 1978, LPS- or 8 Br-cyclic AMP-induced production of T cell-activating factor(s) in macrophage tumor cell line J774.1, *J. Immunol.* **120:**1097.

Ooi, Y. M., Weiss, M. A., Hsu, A., and Ooi, B. S., 1983, Mechanisms of suppression of mouse mesangial cell proliferation by macrophage supernatants, *J Immunol.* **130:**1790.

Opitz, H. G., Opitz, U., Lenke, H., Flad, H. D., Hewlett, G., and Schlumberger, H. D., 1977, Humoral primary immune response *in vitro* in a homologous mouse system: Replacement of fetal calf serum by a 2-mercaptoethanol or macrophage-activated fraction of mouse serum, *J. Immunol.* **119:**1089.

Oppenheim, J. J., and Gery, I., 1982, Interleukin-1 is more than an interleukin, *Immunol. Today.* **3:**113.

Oppenheim, J. J., Leventhal, B. G., and Hersh, E. M., 1968, The transformation of column-purified lymphocytes with nonspecific and specific antigenic stimuli, *J. Immunol.* **101:**262.

Oppenheim, J. J., Shneyour, A., and Kook, A. I., 1976, Enhancement of DNA synthesis and cAMP content of mouse thymocytes by mediator(s) derived from adherent cells, *J. Immunol.* **116:**1466.

Oppenheim, J. J., Mizel, S. B., and Meltzer, M. S., 1979a, Biological effects of lymphocyte and macrophage-derived mitogenic "amplification" factors, in: *Biology of Lymphokines* (S. Cohen, E. Pick, and J. J. Oppenheim, eds.), pp. 291–323, Academic Press, New York.

Oppenheim, J. J., Moore, R., Gmelig-Meyling, F., Togawa, A., Wahl, S., Mathieson, B. J., Dougherty, S., and Carter, C., 1980a, Role of cytokine- and endotoxin-induced monokines in lymphocyte proliferation, differentiation, and immunoglobulin production, in: *Macrophage Regulation of Immunity* (E. R. Unanue and A. S. Rosenthal, eds.), pp. 379–398, Academic Press, New York.

Oppenheim, J. J., Northoff, H., Greenhill, A., Mathieson, B. J., Smith, K., and Gillis, S., 1980b, Properties of human monocyte derived lymphocyte activating factor (LAF) and lymphocyte derived mitogenic factor (LMF), in: *Biochemical Characterization of Lymphokines* (A. L. DeWeck, F. Kristensen, and M. Landy, eds.), pp. 399–404, Academic Press, New York.

Oppenheim, J. J., Togawa, A., Chedid, L., and Mizel, S., 1980c, Components of mycobacteria and muramyl dipeptide with adjuvant activity induce lymphocyte activity factor, *Cell. Immunol.* **50**:71.

Otterness, I. G., Lachman, L. B., and Bliven, M. L., 1980, Effects of levamisole on the proliferation of thymic lymphocyte subpopulations, *Immunopharmacology* **3**:61.

Palacios, R., amd Moller, G., 1981, HLA-DR antigens render resting T cells sensitive to interleukin-2 and induce production of the growth factor in the autologous mixed lymphocyte reaction, *Cell. Immunol.* **63**:143.

Palacios, R., Ivhed, I., Sideras, P., Nilsson, K., Sugawara, I., and Fernandez, C., 1982, Accessory function of human tumor cell lines. I. Production of interleukin-1 by the human histiocytic lymphoma cell line U-937, *Eur. J. Immunol.* **12**:895.

Pekarek, R. S., Powanda, M. C., and Wannemacher, R. W., Jr., 1972a, The effect of leukocyte endogenous mediator (LEM) on serum copper and ceruloplasmin concentrations in the rat, *Proc. Soc. Exp. Biol. Med.* **141**:1029.

Pekarek, R. S., Wannemacher, R. W., Jr., and Beisel, W. R., 1972b, The effect of leukocytic endogenous mediator (LEM) on the tissue distribution of zinc and iron, *Proc. Soc. Exp. Biol. Med.* **140**:685.

Phadke, K., Nanda, S., Marder, P., and Carlson, D. G., 1981, Release of chondrocyte-stimulating factor by rabbit peritoneal macrophages, *Clin. Exp. Immunol.* **43**:408.

Piantelli, M., Lauriola, L., Maggiano, N., Ranelletti, F. O., and Musiani, P., 1981, Role of interleukin-1 and 2 on human thymocyte mitogen activation, *Cell. Immunol.* **64**:337.

Postlethwaite, A. E., Lachman, L. B., Mainardi, C. L., and Kang, A. H., 1983, Interleukin-1 stimulation of collagenase production by cultured fibroblasts, *J. Exp. Med.* **157**:801.

Price, G. B., and Gorczynski, R. M., 1979, The role of macrophages in stimulation of immune induction and myelopoiesis. I. Comparison of activity of macrophage-derived factors in granulopoiesis and immunostimulation, *Immunopharmacology* **1**:175.

Pryor, D. S., 1967, Tropical splenomegaly in New Guinea, *Q. J. Med.* **36**:321.

Puri, J., and Lonai, P., 1980, Mechanism of antigen binding by T cells: H-2 (I-A)-restricted binding of antigen plus Ia by helper cells, *Eur. J. Immunol.* **10**:273.

Puri, J., Shinitzky, M., and Lonai, P., 1980, Concomitant increase in antigen binding and in T cell membrane lipid viscosity induced by the lymphocyte-activating factor, LAF, *J. Immunol.* **124**:1937.

Ramic, Z., Lukic, M. L., and Simic, M. M., 1979a, Macrophage production of lymphoregulatory factors in BCG infected guinea pigs, *Yugoslav. Physiol. Pharmacol. Acta* **15**:**444**.

Ramic, Z., Stosic-Grujicic, S., Pavlovic, Z., Ejdus, L., and Simic, M. M., 1979b, Carrageenan potentiates the helper activity of macrophages in the response of T lymphocytes to mitogens, *Period. Biol.* **81**:167.

Rao, A., Mizel, S. B., and Cantor, H., 1983, Disparate functional properties of two interleukin-1 responsive Ly-1^+2^- T cell clones: Distinction of T cell growth factor and T cell-replacing factor activities, *J. Immunol.* **130**:1743.

Raviola, E., 1975, Thymus, in: *A Textbook of Histology* (W. Bloom and D. Fawcett, eds.), p. 457, Saunders, Philadelphia.

Ridge, S. C., Oronsky, A. L., and Kerwar, S. S., 1980, Induction of the synthesis of latent collagenase and latent neutral protease in chondrocytes by a factor synthesized by activated macrophages, *Arthritis Rheum.* **23**:448.

Roberts, D. W., and Weidanz, W. P., 1978, Splenomegaly, enhanced phagocytosis, and anemia are thymus dependent responses to malaria, *Infect. Immun.* **20**:728.

Rollinghoff, M., Pfizenmaier, K., and Wagner, H., 1982, T–T cell interactions during cytotoxic T-cell responses. IV. Murine lymphoid dendritic cells are powerful stimulators for helper T lymphocytes. *Eur. J. Immunol.* **12:**337.

Root, R. K., Nordlund, J. J., and Wolff, S. M., 1970, Factors affecting the quantitative production and assay of human leukocytic pyrogen, *J. Lab. Clin. Med.* **75:**679.

Rosenberg, S. A., and Lipsky, P. E., 1980, The role of monocyte factors in the differentiation of immunoglobulin secreting cells from human peripheral blood B cells, *J. Immunol.* **125:**232.

Rosenberg, S. A., and Lipsky, P. E., 1981, The role of monocytes in pokeweed mitogen-stimulated human B cell activation: Separate requirements for intact monocytes and a soluble monocyte factor, *J. Immunol.* **126:**1341.

Rosenstreich, D. L., and Mizel, S. B., 1978, The participation of macrophages and macrophage cell lines in the activation of T lymphocytes by mitogens, *Immunol. Rev.* **40:**102.

Rosenstreich, D. L., and Wilton, J. M., 1975, The mechanism of action of macrophages in the activation of T lymphocytes *in vitro* by antigens and mitogens, in: *Immune Recognition* (A. S. Rosenthal, ed.), pp. 113–132, Academic Press, New York.

Rosenstreich, D. L., Farrar, J. J., and Dougherty, S., 1976, Absolute macrophage dependency of T lymphocyte activation by mitogens, *J. Immunol.* **116:**131.

Rosenthal, C. J., and Sullivan, L., 1978, Serum amyloid A: Evidence for its origin in polymorphonuclear leukocytes, *J. Clin. Invest.* **62:**1181.

Rosenwasser, L. J., and Dinarello, C. A., 1981, Ability of human leukocytic pyrogen to enhance phytohemagglutinin induced murine thymocyte proliferation, *Cell. Immunol.* **63:**134.

Rosenwasser, J., and Rosenthal, A. S., 1978a, Adherent cell function in murine T lymphocyte antigen recognition. I. A macrophage-dependent T cell proliferation assay in the mouse, *J. Immunol.* **120:**1991.

Rosenwasser, L. J., and Rosenthal, A. S., 1978b, Adherent cell function in murine T lymphocyte antigen recognition. II. Definition of genetically restricted and nonrestricted macrophage functions in T cell proliferation, *J. Immunol.* **121:**2497.

Rosenwasser, L. J., Dinarello, C. A., and Rosenthal, A. S., 1979, Adherent cell function in murine thymus derived lymphocyte antigen recognition. IV. Enhancement of murine thymus derived cell antigen recognition by human leukocytic pyrogen, *J. Exp. Med.* **150:**709.

Roth, J., Le Roith, D., Shiloach, J., Rosenzweig, J. L., Lesniak, M. A., and Havrankova, J., 1982, The evolutionary origin of hormones, neurotransmitters, and other extracellular chemical messengers: Implications for mammalian biology, *N. Engl. J. Med.* **306:**523.

Rupp, R. G., and Fuller, G. M., 1979, Comparison of albumin and fibrinogen biosynthesis in stimulated rats and cultured fetal rat hepatocytes, *Biochem. Biophys. Res. Commun.* **88:**327.

Sakata, Y., Morimoto, A., Takase, Y., and Murakami, N., 1981, Direct effect of endogenous pyrogen on medullary temperature-responsive neurons in rabbits, *Jpn. J. Physiol.* **31:**247.

Saklatvala, J., and Dingle, J. T., 1980, Identification of catabolin, a protein from synovium which induces degradation of cartilage in organ culture, *Biochem. Biophys. Res. Commun.* **96:**1225.

Saunder, D. N., Carter, C. S., Katz, S. I., and Oppenheim, J. J., 1982, Epidermal cell production of thymocyte activating factor (ETAF), *J. Invest. Dermatol.* **79:**34.

Saunder, D. N., Mounessa, N. L., Katz, S. I., Dinarello, C. A., and Gallin, J. I., 1983, Chemotactic properties of human ETAF/LP/IL-1, *Fed. Proc.* **42:**449.

Schenck, J. R., Hargie, M. P., Brown, M. S., Ebert, D. S., Yoo, A. L., and McIntire, F. C., 1969, The enhancement of antibody formation by *Escherichia coli* lipopolysaccharide and detoxified derivative, *J. Immunol.* **102:**1411.

Schmidt, J. A., Mizel, S. B., Cohen, D., and Green, I., 1982, Interleukin-1, a potential regulator of fibroblast proliferation, *J. Immunol.* **128:**2177.

Schrader, J. W., 1973, Mechanism of activation of the bone marrow-derived lymphocyte. III. A distinction between a macrophage-produced triggering signal and the amplifying effect on triggered B lymphocytes of allogeneic interactions, *J. Exp. Med.* **138:**1466.

Selinger, M. J., McAdam, K. P. W. J., Kaplan, M. M., Sipe, J. D., Vogel, S. N., and Rosenstreich, D. L., 1980, Monokine-induced synthesis of serum amyloid A protein by hepatocytes, *Nature (London)* **285:**498.

Shaw, J., Caplan, B., Paetkau, V., Pilarsky, L. M., Delovitch, T. L., and McKenzie, I. F. C., 1980,

Cellular origin of co-stimulator (1L-2) and its activity in cytotoxic T lymphocyte responses, *J. Immunol* **124:**2231.

Shiozawa, C., Longenecker, M. B., and Diener, E., 1980, *In vitro* cooperation of antigen-specific T cell-derived helper factor, B cells, and adherent cells or their secretory product in a primary IgM response to chicken MHC antigens, *J. Immunol.* **125:**68.

Shirley, S. F., and Little, J. R., 1979, Immunopotentiating effects of amphotericin B. I. Enhanced contact sensitivity in mice, *J. Immunol.* **123:**2878.

Simon, P. L., and Willoughby, W. F., 1981, The role of subcellular fractions in pulmonary immune function: Physiochemical characterization of two distinct species of lymphocyte activating factor produced by rabbit alveolar macrophages, *J. Immunol.* **126:**1534.

Sipe, J. D., McAdam, K. P. W. J., and Uchino, F., 1978, Biochemical evidence for the biphasic development of experimental amyloidosis, *Lab. Invest.* **38:**110.

Sipe, J. D., Vogel, S. N., Ryan, J. L., McAdam, K. P. W. J., and Rosenstreich, D. L., 1979, Detection of a mediator derived from endotoxin-stimulated macrophages that induces the acute phase serum amyloid A response in mice, *J. Exp. Med.* **150:**597.

Skopinska, E., 1972, Some effects of *Escherichia coli* endotoxin on the graft-versus-host reaction in mice, *Transplantation* **14:**432.

Smith, K. A., Gillis, S., Baker, P. E., and McKenzie, D., 1979, T cell growth factor-mediated T cell proliferation, *Ann. N.Y. Acad. Sci.* **332:**423.

Smith, K. A., Gilbride, K. J., and Favata, M. F., 1980a, Lymphocyte activating factor promotes T cell growth factor production by cloned murine lymphoma cells, *Nature (London)* **287:**853.

Smith, K. A., Lachman, L. B., Oppenheim, J. J., and Favata, M. F., 1980b, The functional relationship of the interleukins, *J. Exp. Med.* **151:**1551.

Snyder, D. S., and Unanue, E. R., 1982, Corticosteroids inhibit murine macrophage Ia expression and interleukin-1 production, *J. Immunol.* **129:**1803.

Solomons, N. W., Elson, C. O., Pekarek, R. S., Jacob, R. A., Sandstead, H. H., and Rosenberg, I. H., 1978, Leukocytic endogenous mediator in Crohn's disease, *Infect. Immun.* **22:**637.

Sporn, M. B., and Todaro, G. J., 1980, Autocrine secretion and malignant transformation of cells, *N. Engl. J. Med.* **303:**878.

Sredni, B., Michlin, H., Kalechman, Y., and Rozenszajn, L. A., 1978, Regulatory effects of macrophage-secreted factors on T lymphocyte colony growth, *Cell. Immunol.* **36:**15.

Stamenkovic, M., and Simic, M. M., 1979, Partial biochemical characterization of carrageenan-induced T cell activating factor (TAF), *Yugoslav. Physiol. Pharmacol. Acta* **15:**469.

Staruch, M.-J., and Wood, D. D., 1983, The adjuvanticity of interleukin-1 *in vivo*, *J. Immunol.* **130:**2191.

Stevenson, R. D., 1976, Studies on the production and action of polymorph migration stimulator, *Clin. Exp. Immunol.* **24:**527.

Stevenson, R. D., and Gray, A. C., 1976, Studies on the physiochemical characteristics of polymorph migration stimulator, *Clin. Exp. Immunol.* **26:**457.

Stosic-Grujicic, S., and Simic, M. M., 1979, Factors affecting the secretion of TAF by carrageenan-pretreated macrophages: The effects of mitogen-activated T cells and of hydrocortisone, *Yugoslav. Physiol. Pharmacol. Acta* **15:**488.

Stosic-Grujicic, S., and Simic, M. M., 1982, Modulation of interleukin-1 production by activated macrophages: *In vitro* action of hydrocortisone, colchicine, and cytochalasin B, *Cell. Immunol.* **69:**235.

Sugimoto, M., Germain, R. N., Chedid, L., and Benacerraf, B., 1978, Enhancement of carrier-specific helper T cell function by the synthetic adjuvant, *N*-acetyl muramyl-L-alanyl-D-isoglutamine (MDP), *J. Immunol.* **120:**980.

Sztein, M. B., Vogel, S. N., Sipe, J. D., Murphy, P. A., Mizel, S. B., Oppenheim, J. J., and Rosenstreich, D. L., 1981, The role of macrophages in the acute-phase response: SAA inducer is closely related to lymphocyte activating factor and endogenous pyrogen, *Cell. Immunol.* **63:**164.

Sztein, M. B., Luger, T. A., and Oppenheim, J. J., 1982, An epidermal cell-derived cytokine triggers the *in vivo* synthesis of serum amyloid A by hepatocytes, *J. Immunol.* **129:**87.

Tanabe, M. J., Tsurumi, Y., and Nakano, M., 1977, An endotoxin induced serum factor that causes enhancement of antibody response to heterologous erythrocytes, *Microbiol. Immunol.* **21:**653.

Tanaka, A., Nagao, S., Nagao, R., Kotani, S., Shiba, T., and Kusumoto, S., 1979, Stimulation of the reticuloendothelial system of mice by muramyl dipeptide, *Infect. Immun.* **24:**302.

Taniyama, T., and Holden, H. T., 1979, Requirement of histocompatible macrophages for the induction of a secondary cytotoxic response to syngeneic tumor cells *in vitro, J. Immunol.* **123:**43.

Taub, R. N., Krantz, A. R., and Dresser, D. W., 1970, The effect of localized injection of adjuvant material on the draining lymph node, *Immunology* **18:**171.

Tenu, J.-P., Lederer, E., and Petit, J.-F., 1980, Stimulation of thymocyte mitogenic protein secretion and of cytostatic activity of mouse peritoneal macrophages by trehalose dimycolate and muramyl-dipeptide, *Eur. J. Immunol.* **10:**647.

Thoman, M. L., Morgan, E. L., and Weigle, W. O., 1980, Polyclonal activation of murine B lymphocytes by F_c fragments. II. Replacement of T cells by a soluble helper T cell-replacing factor (TRF), *J. Immunol.* **125:**1630.

Thompson, W. L., Abeles, F. B., Beall, F. A., Dinterman, R. E., and Wannemacher, R. W., Jr., 1975, LEM-induced synthesis of hepatic RNA and acute phase serum globulins, *Fed. Proc.* **34:**620.

Thompson, W. L., Abeles, F. B., Beall, F. A., Dinterman, R. E., and Wannemacher, R. W., Jr., 1976, Influence of the adrenal glucocorticoids on the stimulation of synthesis of hepatic ribonucleic acid and plasma acute-phase globulins by leukocytic endogenous mediator, *Biochem. J.* **156:**23.

Tocco, R. J., Kahn, L. L., Kluger, M. J., and Vander, A. J., 1983, Relationship of trace metals to fever during infection: Are prostaglandins involved?, *Am. J. Physiol.* **244:**R368.

Togawa, A., Oppenheim, J. J., and Mizel, S. B., 1979, Characterization of lymphocyte activating factor (LAF) produced by human mononuclear cells: Biochemical relationship of high and low molecular weight forms of LAF, *J. Immunol.* **122:**2112.

Triglia, D., and Rothenberg, E., 1981, "Mature" thymocytes are not glucocorticoid-resistant *in vitro, J. Immunol.* **127:**64.

Tubbs, H., 1980, Endotoxin in human and murine malaria, *Trans. R. Soc. Trop. Med. Hyg.* **74:**121.

Turchik, J. B., and Bornstein, D. L., 1980, Role of the central nervous system in acute-phase responses to leukocytic pyrogen, *Infect. Immun.* **30:**439.

Ulrich, F., 1977, Studies of lymphocyte activating factor from alveolar macrophages, *J. Reticuloendothelial Soc.* **21:**33.

Unanue, E. R., and Kiely, J.-M., 1977, Synthesis and secretion of a mitogenic protein by macrophages: Description of a superinduction phenomenon, *J. Immunol.* **119:**925.

Unanue, E. R., Kiely, J.-M., and Calderon, J., 1976, The modulation of lymphocyte function by molecules secreted by macrophages. II. Conditions leading to increased secretion, *J. Exp. Med.* **144:**155.

Vaes, G., 1980, Cellular secretions and tissue breakdown: Cell-to-cell interactions in the secretion of enzymes of connective tissue breakdown, collagenase and proteoglycan-degrading neutral proteases, *Agents Actions* **10:**474.

Wagner, H., Feldmann, M., Boyle, W., and Schrader, J. W., 1972, Cell-mediated immune response *in vitro*. III. The requirement for macrophages in cytotoxic reactions against cell-bound and subcellular alloantigens, *J. Exp. Med.* **136:**331.

Wahl, S. M., Wahl, L. M., McCarthy, J. B., Chedid, L., and Mergenhagen, S. E., 1979, Macrophage activation by mycobacterial water soluble compounds and synthetic muramyl dipeptide, *J. Immunol.* **122:**2226.

Wannemacher, R. W., Jr., DuPont, H. L., Pekarek, R. S., Powanda, M. C., Schwartz, A., Hornic, R. B., and Beisel, W. R., 1972, An endogenous mediator of depression of amino acids and trace metals in serum during typhoid fever, *J. Infect. Dis.* **126:**77.

Wannemacher, R. W., Jr., Pekarek, R. S., Thompson, W. L., Curnow, R. T., Beall, F. A., Zenser, T. V., DeRubertis, F. R., and Beisel, W. R., 1975, Protein from polymorphonuclear leukocytes (LEM) which affects rate of hepatic amino-acid transport and synthesis of acute-phase globulins, *Endocrinology* **96:**651.

Watson, J., Gillis, S., and Smith, K., 1980, Molecular characterization of lymphokines that enhance immune responses, in: *Biochemical Characterization of Lymphokines* (A. L. DeWeck, F. Kristensen, and M. Landy, eds.), pp. 463–470, Academic Press, New York.

Weinberg, E. D., 1978, Iron and infection, *Microbiol. Rev.* **42:**45.

Weinberg, J. B., Chapman, H. A., and Hibbs, J. B., Jr., 1978, Characterization of the effects of endotoxin on macrophage tumor cell killing, *J. Immunol.* **121**:72.

Wharton, W., Gillespie, G. Y., Russell, S. W., and Pledger, W. J., 1982, Mitogenic activity elaborated by macrophage-like cell lines acts as competence factor(s) for Balb/c 3T3 cells, *J. Cell Physiol.* **110**:93.

Wood, D. D., 1977, Role of adherent cell products in the immune response, in: *Regulatory Mechanisms in Lymphocyte Activation* (D. Lucas, ed.), pp. 117–134, Academic Press, New York.

Wood, D. D., 1979a, Purification and properties of human B cell activating factor, *J. Immunol.* **123**:2395.

Wood, D. D., 1979b, Mechanism of action of human B cell activating factor. I. Comparison of the plaque stimulating activity with thymocyte stimulating activity, *J. Immunol.* **123**:2400.

Wood, D. D., 1979c, Comparison of the plaque stimulating and thymocyte stimulating activities derived from human monocytes, *Ann. N.Y. Acad. Sci.* **332**:491.

Wood, D. D., and Cameron, P. M., 1975, Studies on the mechanism of stimulation of the humoral response of murine spleen cultures by culture fluids from human moncytes, *J. Immunol.* **114**:1094.

Wood, D. D., and Cameron, P. M., 1976, Stimulation of the release of a B cell activating factor from human monocytes, *Cell. Immunol.* **21**:133.

Wood, D. D., and Cameron, P. M., 1978, Relationship between bacterial endotoxin and human B cell activating factor, *J. Immunol.* **121**:53.

Wood, D. D., and Gaul, S. L., 1974, Enhancement of the humoral response of T cell depleted murine spleens by a factor derived from human monocytes *in vitro*, *J. Immunol.* **113**:925.

Wood, D. D., and Staruch, M.-J., 1980, Biochemical properties and cellular requirements of BAF, in: *Biochemical Characterization of Lymphokines* (A. L. DeWeck, F. Kristensen, and M. Landy, eds.), pp. 423–425, Academic Press, New York.

Wood, D. D., Cameron, P. M., Poe, M. T., and Morris, C. A., 1976, Resolution of a factor which enhances the antibody response of T cell depleted murine splenocytes from other monocyte products, *Cell. Immunol.* **21**:88.

Wood, D. D., Hamerman, D., Ihrie, E. J., and Papovitch, L., 1983a, Stimulation of synoviocyte glucosaminoglycan production by synoviocyte-derived interleukin-1, *Fed. Proc.* **42**:1200.

Wood, D. D., Ihrie, E. J., Dinarello, C. A., and Cohen, P. L., 1983b, Isolation of an interleukin-1-like factor from human joint effusions, *Arthritis Rheum.* **26**:975.

Wood, D. D., Ihrie, E. J., and Hamerman, D., 1984, Production of interleukin-1 by human synovial tissue, submitted to *J. Clin. Invest.*

Woolley, D. E., Harris, E. D., Jr., Mainardi, C. L., and Brinckerhoff, C. E., 1978, Collagenase immunolocalization in cultures of rheumatoid synovial cells, *Science* **200**:773.

Wyler, D.-J., Oppenheim, J. J., and Koonty, L. C., 1979, Influence of malaria infection of the elaboration of soluble mediators by adherent mononuclear cells, *Infect. Immun.* **24**:151.

Yamamoto, Y., and Onoue, K., 1979, Functional activation of immune lymphocyte by antigenic stimulation in cell-mediated immunity. IV. Role of macrophage and its soluble factor in antigen-induced MIF production of immune T lymphocytes, *J. Immunol.* **122**:924.

Yamamoto, Y., Onoue, K., and Ohishi, M., 1977, Functional activation of immune lymphocytes by antigenic stimulation in cell-mediated immunity. III. A soluble factor released from LPS-stimulated peritoneal adherent cells effective in antigenic activation of sensitized lymphocytes, *Cell. Immunol.* **37**:432.

13

Lymphocyte Mediators That Modulate the Behavior of Macrophages

ROSS ROCKLIN

1. INTRODUCTION

T lymphocytes mediate a number of cellular-immune reactions including cutaneous delayed hypersensitivity of the tuberculin or contact types, resistance to infection by intracellular facultative microorganisms, host versus graft and graft versus host rejection phenomena, and tumor surveillance. These reactions result from complex cellular interactions between subpopulations of T lymphocytes and T lymphocytes and macrophages. The T cell may function directly as an effector cell or indirectly by orchestrating interactions between lymphocytes and macrophages. As a result of these activation signals, the macrophage may then develop into a more efficient phagocytic "killer cell" or in turn transmit signals that modulate T-cell functions in either a positive or a negative way.

Both cutaneous delayed hypersensitivity and resistance to infection usually develop in parallel following exposure to a variety of microorganisms. These reactions are thought to be distinct manifestations of the same general phenomenon and differ primarily in the way in which they are measured. Based on data obtained in animal studies, it has been demonstrated that over 95% of the mononuclear cells found infiltrating cutaneous delayed hypersensitivity reactions have been nonspecifically recruited to the site of inflammation. That is, only a small number of cells are present at the site specifically sensitized to the antigen that initiated the reaction. This has led to the hypothesis that these few sensitized cells are responsible for elaborating substances that bring about the recruitment of the other cells and thus amplify the inflammatory response. The factors that are presumed to play a major role in the expression of these reactions have been collectively termed mediators of cellular immunity and include sub-

ROSS ROCKLIN • Allergy Division, Department of Medicine, New England Medical Center, Tufts University School of Medicine, Boston, Massachusetts 02111.

stances produced by lymphocytes (lymphokines) and monocytes (monokines). Despite the fact that these substances are produced in very minute quantities, they have marked biologic effects on a variety of cell types including T and B lymphocytes, macrophages, eosinophils, basophils, and neutrophils. This chapter will focus upon the lymphokines that influence the behavior of macrophages and thus may be involved in the expression of various cellular-immune phenomena.

2. EFFECTS OF LYMPHOKINES ON MACROPHAGE FUNCTION

The experimental data described in this chapter were derived using macrophages from a variety of species (guinea pig, mouse, rabbit, human) and from a variety of sources (peritoneal exudate, alveolar macrophage, blood monocyte, and bone marrow). In addition, the macrophages were studied under different initial levels of activation; e.g., unstimulated "resident" washout cells with low-basal-activity as well as those that were recruited to sites of inflammation by a stimulant and were at a higher level of activity. It should also be pointed out that the term "activation," which is used to describe the altered behavior of lymphokine-treated macrophages, is difficult to define because the level of activation achieved in a given population under study will vary depending upon the stimulus used, the source of the cell population, and the initial state of maturation of the cells. For example, some stimuli induce certain changes in macrophage function but not others and whether one decides the cells are "activated" or not may depend upon the choice of the assay system employed. Changes in either structure, metabolism, or cell function of lymphokine-treated macrophages are described in this chapter. These changes are categorized in Table 1.

2.1. STRUCTURE

2.1.1. Morphology

The incubation of "normal" macrophages with lymphokine-containing supernatants generated in response to antigen or mitogen induces profound effects in cellular morphology at the light microscope level. During the first hour of incubation, inhibition of macrophage spreading onto glass or plastic surfaces is commonly reported and by 24 hr the cells have rounded up, lost their pseudopodia, and are not very motile (David, 1966). Following 48 hr of incubation with lymphokine-containing supernatants, macrophages exhibit increased spreading with the formation of long pseudopodia; cellular aggregates are also noted (Lolekha *et al.*, 1970; Dvorak *et al.*, 1972). By 72 hr of incubation, the macrophages are enlarged, exhibit enhanced adherence to surfaces, and demonstrate increased membrane ruffling and amoeboid movement (Nathan *et al.*, 1971). Such cells are also enriched in vacuoles and lysosomal granules.

Electron microscopic studies of macrophages that have been incubated with

TABLE 1. ENHANCEMENT OF MACROPHAGE BEHAVIOR BY LYMPHOKINES

Structure
Ruffled membrane
Electron-dense surface membrane material
Complement receptors
Cell fusion
Ia
Metabolism
Glucose oxidation
Glucosamine incorporation
Protein synthesis
Phospholipid synthesis—prostaglandins
DNA synthesis and proliferation
Oxygen consumption
Adenylate cyclase
Functions
Cell migration—inhibition and stimulation
Aggregation
Chemotaxis
Pinocytosis
Surface tension
Phagocytosis
Bacteriostatic-cidal activity
Parasitocidal activity
Tumoricidal activity
Secretion—lysosomal enzymes
C2
Plasminogen activator
Tissue factor
Collagenase
Interleukin 1

lymphokine-containing supernatants also show alterations, particularly in the plasma membrane. Such cells tend to form aggregates characterized by intensive intercellular contact and the loss of normal extramembranous electron-dense material (Dvorak *et al.*, 1972). These aggregated cells also exhibit increased amounts of microvilli (Smyth and Weiss, 1970). The development of cell aggregation may be the initial step in a process that leads to the induction of macrophage fusion. The latter reaction may proceed to the formation of giant cells *in vitro* as has been documented to occur by incubating macrophages with cell-free supernatants obtained from BCG-stimulated lymphocyte cultures (Galindo, 1972; Galindo *et al.*, 1974). The ability of macrophages to form giant cells and epithelioid sheets *in vitro* in a manner similar to that observed in granuloma formation *in vivo* is very intriguing and is a subject of intense investigation.

2.1.2. Receptors

The macrophage possesses a number of receptors in common with other cells such as B lymphocytes; very little information is available concerning the ability of lymphokines to modulate these receptors. Recent studies carried out in a murine macrophage system indicate that a low-molecular-weight factor derived from lymphocytes increases complement receptors (Griffin and Griffin, 1979). In these latter studies, BCG-immune lymphocytes were stimulated with tuberculin PPD and elaborated a lymphokine that induced murine macrophages to increase their complement receptors as measured by a phagocytic assay that utilized IgG-coated immune complexes. This factor was found to have a molecular weight of less than 10,000 and appeared to act directly on contact with the macrophages (Griffin and Griffin, 1980). The mechanism of action of this factor was explored and several possibilities were suggested by the authors. They found that the lymphokine does not cause increased phagocytic activity at the plasma membrane or cause increased synthesis of complement receptors. The lymphokine may, however, either induce an increased insertion of complement receptors into the membrane, a rearrangement of the existing numbers of complement receptors, or their function.

2.1.3. Expression of Ia Antigen

Scher *et al.* (1980) have demonstrated that mouse peritoneal macrophages express increased Ia antigen when exposed to supernatants derived from *Listeria monocytogenes*-immune lymphocytes stimulated by specific antigen. Following the intraperitoneal injection of such supernatants, a progressive increase in the number of Ia-positive cells was noted with a minimum of 2 days being required. The lymphokine is not genetically restricted in its action since it will induce the expression of Ia antigen on macrophages from a number of murine species. Of particular interest, peritoneal exudate cells generated by an inflammatory stimulus such as oil or proteose peptone have little Ia antigen on their surface. It is only during an immune response that most of the macrophages develop Ia antigen. The presence of Ia and specific antigen on macrophages is thought to be required for the activation of T cells.

2.2. METABOLIC EFFECTS

2.2.1. Metabolism

The metabolic activities of macrophages following incubation with lymphokine-containing preparations are considerably altered, and changes in carbohydrate, protein, and lipid metabolism are noted. For example, guinea pig peritoneal macrophages or human blood monocytes incubated with lymphokine-containing supernatants for several days exhibit increased glucose oxidation through the hexose monophosphate shunt pathway as illustrated in Fig. 1 (Nathan *et al.*, 1971; Rocklin *et al.*, 1974). The latter activity is normally accompanied by increases in phagocytic activity and may be a major step in preparing macrophages for bactericidal activity since the hexose monophosphate shunt pathway is indirectly involved in the generation of oxygen radicals. Block *et al.*

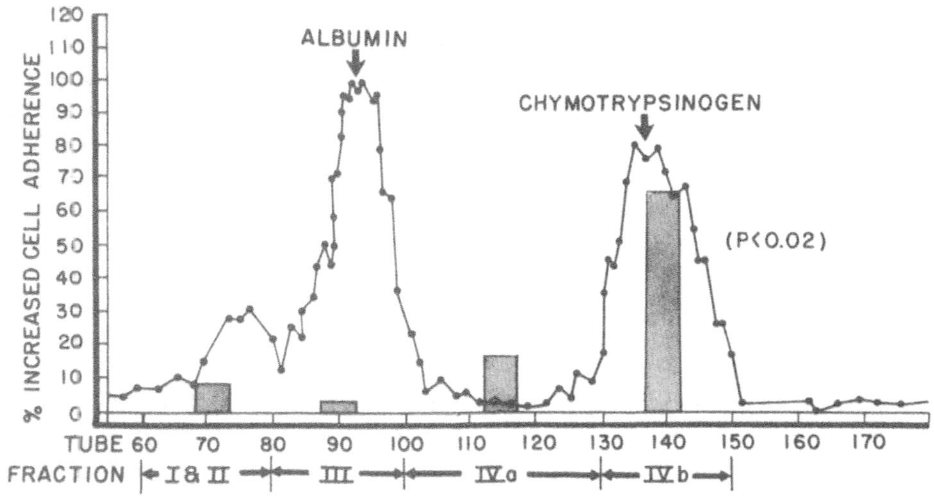

FIGURE 1. Elution pattern of adherence-promoting activity from Sephadex G-100 columns. Percent increase in cell adherence of monocytes incubated for 3 days in fractions from supernatants of antigen-stimulated lymphocyte cultures compared to control fraction is plotted as bars. Note that only the fraction (IVb) eluting at position of the chymotrypsinogen marker is active.

(1980) showed that human monocytes incubated for 14 hr with highly purified human MIF preparations exhibit a fourfold increase in their oxygen consumption. In addition, lymphokine-treated guinea pig macrophages exhibit enhanced uptake of radiolabeled glucosamine into membrane-associated materials (Hammond and Dvorak, 1972; Hammond *et al.*, 1975; Wilton *et al.*, 1975). The latter observation may reflect membrane repair of coat glycoproteins lost during activation or an increase in active membrane transport. Lymphokine-treated macrophages exhibit increased protein synthesis and phospholipid metabolism (Nathan *et al.*, 1971, 1973; Bray *et al.*, 1978). That a lymphokine can stimulate phospholipid metabolism is of particular interest because increased prostaglandin E synthesis has been shown to be involved in the expression of suppressor activity of monocytes/macrophages. It should also be noted that some investigators have reported the occurrence of proliferation of mature macrophages after incubation with lymphokine supernatants for 2–8 days (Godal *et al.*, 1971; Hadden *et al.*, 1975). The latter factor may be implicated in the proliferation of macrophages that is normally observed at the site of delayed hypersensitivity reactions.

2.2.2. Secretory Products

Lysosomal enzyme levels are influenced following incubation of macrophages with lymphokine preparations. At present, however, the data are somewhat conflicting on this aspect of macrophage activation. Some investigators (Pantalone and Page, 1975, 1977) reported that a 72-hr incubation of normal mouse peritoneal macrophages with supernatants from mitogen-stimulated human peripheral blood lymphocytes significantly enhanced the selective production and secretion of hydrolytic enyzmes by these cells. In other species, Poulter and Turk (1975) also observed an increase in lysosomal enzyme activity following a 72-hr incubation of guinea pig macrophages with lymphokine preparations. These findings are in contrast to those of Remold and Mednis (1975) who reported that guinea pig peritoneal exudate cells incubated with partially purified MIF fractions exhibited a consistent decrease in lysosomal enzyme content measured after 48 hr. The reduction in hydrolysis observed in their experiments was not the result of enzyme secretion. The differences in results obtained by various investigators again may reflect the use of macrophages in different stages of maturation or differences in lymphokine preparations or experimental conditions.

Remold-O'Donnell and Remold (1974) reported that guinea pig macrophages exposed to MIF-rich fractions had increased adenylate cyclase activity. However, the actual changes in cAMP levels in macrophages varied tremendously depending upon the time after incubation that such determinations were made. Most studies failed to show any increase in cAMP levels in whole cell preparations at any time during a 72-hr incubation (Remold-O'Donnell and Remold, 1974).

Additional metabolic studies have demonstrated that lymphokine-treated macrophages secrete biologically active molecules that could be of considerable importance at sites of inflammation. For example, lymphokine-treated macrophages secrete collagenase into the local milieu (Wahl *et al.*, 1975; Pantalone and Page, 1977). The latter enzyme may have importance in lesions mediated by immunologic mechanisms that result in collagen damage. Furthermore, a number of investigators have reported that lymphokines induced the synthesis of plasminogen activator by unstimulated macrophages (Wahl *et al.*, 1975; Vassalli and Reich, 1977; Klimentzek and Sorg, 1977; Greineder *et al.*, 1979). The latter studies have utilized either murine, guinea pig, or human monocytes and have shown that maximum synthesis of plasminogen activator occurs following a 48- to 72-hr incubation. The secretion of plasminogen activator by lymphokine-treated macrophages could be augmented by latex ingestion, although the ingestion of latex beads in the absence of lymphokine did not induce secretion (Klimentzek and Sorg, 1977). The release of plasminogen activator by activated macrophages could provide an important link between cell-mediated immune reactions and other inflammatory components such as the fibrinolytic, complement, and kinin systems.

Littman and Ruddy (1977) reported that human monocytes treated with lymphokine preparations synthesized increased amounts of the second component of complement. The synthesis of C2 could be partially blocked by the addition of α-L-fucose, a sugar known to inhibit the response of macrophages to MIF (see Section 4.1). Other studies have shown that a lymphokine is responsible for the production of endogenous pyrogen (interleukin 1) from guinea pig macrophages or human monocytes (Chao *et al.*, 1977; Dinarello and Rosenwasser, 1981). The release of endogenous leukocytic pyrogen by activated macrophages could explain the association between delayed hypersensitivity and fever. These studies also imply that activated monocytes/macrophages can modulate T-cell functions since it has been shown that interleukin 1 induces thymocyte proliferation, stimulates lymphocytes to produce a factor that enhances the synthesis of serum amyloid A protein, and is capable of triggering T-suppressor cells in response to signals by histamine or Con A (Rosenwasser *et al.*, 1979; Beer *et al.*, 1982; McAdam and Dinarello, 1981).

Monocytes stimulated by activated lymphocytes or lymphokine-containing preparations have been shown to produce a procoagulant activity that has been identified as tissue factor (Edwards and Rickles, 1978). At least two pathways of tissue factor generation by monocytes have been identified (Edwards and Rickles, 1980). One pathway is T-cell independent, and endotoxin or tuberculin PPD may serve as stimulants. The other pathway is T-cell dependent, and phytohemagglutinin has been used as a stimulant. In related studies, Geczy and Hopper (1981) observed that the induction of this tissue factor activity in macrophages caused a decreased chemotactic response of these cells as well as decreased cell migration as measured in the capillary tube assay. Separation of the macrophages by sedimentation velocity revealed a fraction of large macrophages producing the highest amount of procoagulant activities. They also noted that the additon of heparin *in vitro* prevented macrophages from responding to MIF in the migration assay. The latter finding may help explain the clinical observation that anticoagulation prevents the expression of cutaneous delayed hypersensitivity (Colvin *et al.*, 1973; Edwards and Rickles, 1980).

2.3. MACROPHAGE FUNCTIONS

2.3.1. Cell Migration

The first lymphokine described that affected macrophage function was the migration inhibitory factor (MIF) (David, 1966). This factor was shown to alter the random migration of macrophages from a number of sources including the peritoneum and alveolar cavity as well as monocytes isolated from peripheral blood or bone marrow. In addition to MIF, whose primary effect is to inhibit migration, stimulation or enhanced macrophage migration as measured in the conventional MIF assay is occasionally observed (David, 1966; Fox *et al.*, 1974; Svejcar and Johanovsky, 1961). This enhancement in cell migration has been attributed to a lymphokine(s) that is apparently separable from MIF. Several investigators have termed this factor "macrophage enhancement factor" or "macrophage stimulation factor" (Weisbart *et al.*, 1974). The occurrence of at least two factors in lymphokine-containing supernatants having opposite effects on migration points out the difficulties in dealing with crude preparations and bioassays.

In addition to affecting the random movement, a lymphokine which can alter the directed movement or chemotactic response of macrophages has also been described. This factor, first reported by Ward *et al.* (1969), was found in the culture fluid obtained from stimulated guinea pig lymphocytes, and increased the directed movement of macrophages in the direction of an increasing concentration gradient of the macrophage chemotactic factor. Macrophage chemotactic systems have been described in human, murine, rat, and chicken as reviewed by Altman (1978).

2.3.2. Pinocytosis

Lymphokine treatment of guinea pig macrophages lead to enhanced pinocytosis using colloidal gold (Meade *et al.*, 1974) or horseradish peroxidase as particles (Shubert *et al.*, 1980). For this process to occur to its fullest extent, anaerobic glycolysis is a critical metabolic requirement, whereas submaximal stimulation can occur in the absence of aerobic respiration (Shubert *et al.*, 1980). In addition, protein synthesis is required but neither microtubule nor microfilament function is necessary. Bacterial LPS also increases pinocytosis of horseradish peroxidase by guinea pig macrophages. This appears to be a direct effect of LPS on the macrophages and does not appear to be T cell or B cell dependent (Shubert and David, 1980).

2.3.3. Phagocytosis

Exposure of macrophages to lymphokines can either result in enhanced or depressed phagocytosis depending upon the nature of the particle. For example, Nathan *et al.* (1971) demonstrated that killed mycobacteria are readily engulfed by MIF-activated guinea pig macrophages. Similarly, human monocytes demonstrate a rapid increase in phagocytosis of latex beads following activation. In contrast, Remold and Mednis (1975) reported a decreased uptake of aggregated, denatured hemoglobin even though the protein was adherent to the macrophage surface. Similarly, Neta and Salvin (1971) found a reduction in the ingestion of *Candida albicans* by lymphokine-treated guinea pig macrophages; in another study, phagocytosis of radiolabeled *C. albicans* was increased following exposure of human monocytes to lymphokine preparations (Unsgaard, 1979). In related studies, Thrasher *et al.* (1973) demonstrated that lymphokine preparations alter the surface tension of the macrophage membrane. This apparently is a concomitant of phagocytosis and is required if the macrophage is to ingest the particle. This physical property is a reflection of the molecular composition and configuration of the membrane and any surface coats associated with it, indicating that membrane remodeling is an early event in the macrophage-activating process *in vitro*.

2.3.4. Bactericidal/Parasitocidal Activity

Lymphokines can augment another important aspect of macrophage function and that is how they cope with microorganisms. Incubation of macrophages from a variety of sources and species with lymphokine-containing supernatants enhances the bacteriostatic and bactericidal properties of these cells (Patterson and Youmans, 1970; Godal *et al.*, 1971; Krahenbuhl and Remington, 1971;

Fowles *et al.*, 1973; Anderson and Remington, 1974). This activity has been documented for a number of microorganisms including bacteria (*Listeria monocytogenes*), *Rickettsia* (*R. tsu tsu gamushi*), and protozoa (*Toxoplasma gondii*). Of particular importance, the activated macrophages exhibit enhanced abilities to deal with the specific organisms, i.e., predominantly those used to stimulate the sensitized lymphocytes (Borgis and Johnson, 1974; Anderson *et al.*, 1976). However, in most instances the antigenicity of the microorganism is irrelevant, indicating the nonspecific nature of the macrophage activity (Patterson and Youmans, 1970). A recent study has investigated a possible mechanism by which macrophages exert their bactericidal activity (Sharma *et al.*, 1980). These workers observed that guinea pig macrophages infected with mycobacteria produce a supernatant factor that has bactericidal activity and which is not lysozyme.

2.3.5 Tumoricidal Activity

Due to the potentially important role played by macrophages as an effector cell involved in the destruction of neoplastic tissue, many investigators have sought to delineate the mechanism of this reaction *in vitro*. Initial studies revealed that lymphokine-rich supernatants may substitute for an immune response *in vivo* and render the macrophage tumoricidal *in vitro* (Krahenbuhl *et al.*, 1973; Churchill *et al.*, 1975; Fidler *et al.*, 1977). The specificity of the cytotoxic response by activated macrophages on tumor cells has become the subject of controversy. In some *in vitro* systems, the cytotoxic response is very specific in that only tumor cells that are identical to the neoplastic cells used to activate sensitized lymphocytes are destroyed (Evans and Alexander, 1976). In other systems, however, the activation seems to be nonspecific and all tumor cells, but not normal cells, are destroyed (Piessens *et al.*, 1975).

This controversy may be the result of the independent activity of two distinct lymphokines, the specific macrophage-arming factor (Evans and Alexander, 1976) and the macrophage-activating factor (Churchill *et al.*, 1975; Piessens *et al.*, 1975). The specific arming factor is a product of stimulated T lymphocytes that have interacted with tumor antigen and subsequently activates the macrophages to only kill that tumor (Evans and Alexander, 1976; Lohmann-Matthes *et al.*, 1973). The arming factor binds to the macrophage, i.e., it is cytophilic and can thus be absorbed by these cells. It can also be absorbed by the specific tumor used to induce it. The arming factor is thought to be a cytotoxic receptor shed into the culture medium by the activated lymphocytes (Lohmann-Matthes *et al.*, 1973) or a unique cytophilic antibody (Pels and Den-Otter, 1974). The macrophage-activating factor is also a product of antigen-activated lymphocytes, but unlike the arming factor, its tumoricidal activity is nonspecific (Piessens *et al.*, 1975; Churchill *et al.*, 1975). The latter factor is not cytophilic since activated macrophages can be trypsinized without affecting their tumoricidal activity. However, trypsinization of macrophages prior to incubation with the activating factor prevents their acquisition of a cytotoxic capability, suggesting that there may be a trypsin-sensitive receptor for the activating factor on the macrophage membrane (Hibbs *et al.*, 1977).

An analysis of the kinetic events of *in vitro* tumor killing has recently been presented (Poste and Kirsch, 1979). Macrophages induced by an inflammatory stimulus and isolated from C57BL/6 mice were tested at various times following the introduction of the stimulant and tested for their ability to kill various tumor cell lines including a melanoma and fibrosarcoma line. The results showed that macrophages stimulated for less than 4 days exhibited no spontaneous tumoricidal activity but were able to become cytotoxic for syngeneic and allogeneic tumors by incubation with lymphokines *in vitro*. If the cells were harvested between 4 and 7 days after stimulation, then these cells exhibited spontaneous cytotoxicity and were able to be induced to a cytotoxic state by lymphokines. If the cells were not harvested until 7 days after stimulation, then they lacked spontaneous cytotoxicity and were also not inducible by lymphokines *in vitro*. These alterations in cytotoxic activity were correlated with decreased numbers of peroxidase-positive-staining cells in the population and therefore appear to depend upon the fresh influx of macrophages into the inflammatory exudate.

In related studies, macrophages which appear to be refractory to lymphokines can be reactivated if the latter are presented bound to liposomes. Folger *et al.* (1980) tested alveolar and peritoneal macrophages harvested from mice that were incubated with lymphokines and encapsulated within liposomes. The latter cells were shown to be tumoricidal *in vitro* at lower concentrations of lymphokine than material not bound to liposomes. Furthermore, the liposome-bound lymphokines appear to act intracellularly following release from internalized liposomes. This *in vitro* tumoricidal activation of macrophages by lymphokines could be duplicated *in vivo* by the intraperitoneal injection of liposome-bound lymphokines and subsequent harvest of macrophages from that site and testing their tumoricidal activity *in vitro*. With alveolar macrophages, the intraperitoneal injection of liposome-bound lymphokines did not result in tumoricidal activity *in vivo* whereas the intravenous injection of the material did, suggesting that the route of administration was a critical factor.

The ability of macrophages to become triggered by lymphokine and/or LPS signals has recently been investigated (Taramelli *et al.*, 1981; Taffet *et al.*, 1981; Meltzer, 1981). Bacterial LPS in nanogram amounts together with low concentrations of lymphokines have a synergistic effect on the cytotoxic activity of macrophages (Meltzer, 1981). In addition, high concentrations of lymphokine alone will also activate macrophages for a cytotoxic response. In analyzing the synergistic effects of these signals, it was found that macrophages exposed to a low concentration of lymphokine first (no LPS contained in the preparation) became receptive to a subsequent signal by LPS. This initial permissive period was achieved by a 4-hr incubation with low concentrations of lymphokine or a 1-hr incubation with a high concentration of factor. The activation of macrophages by lymphokine required 4 hr of incubation but the triggering of the cells, once primed, only required a 20-min incubation.

It has also been shown in the above-described murine macrophage system that LPS treatment alone results in a rapid loss of cytotoxic activity. This hyporesponsiveness was thought to be due to the production of prostaglandins by LPS-stimulated macrophages. However, the combination of LPS and lymphokine treatment results in continued cytotoxic activity of the cells. The ability of two signals to preserve the cytotoxic response was interpreted to mean that the lymphokine treatment in some way reduced the sensitivity of activated macrophages to prostaglandin. The mechanism apparently did not involve a generalized inhibition of macrophage responsiveness to the hormone because lymphokine treatment itself did not reduce the cAMP response of macrophages exposed to prostaglandin E (Taffet *et al.*, 1981).

The lymphokine signals provided to macrophages to enable them to act as regulators of immune function were compared to those that influence their tumoricidal effector role (Taramelli *et al.*, 1981). Murine peritoneal exudate macrophages induced by proteose peptone and subsequently activated by lymphokines *in vitro* were shown to be capable of inhibiting the production of lymphokines such as MIF and MAF. The regulatory cells were found to be adherent, phagocytic, did not stain positively with an anti-T-cell marker, possessed macrophage morphology under light microscopy, and the requirement for LPS was minimal. In contrast, the ability to become cytotoxic against a lymphoma tumor line required the combined signals of lymphokine plus LPS for full tumoricidal activity. These results were interpreted to mean that lymphokine treatment alone is sufficient to induce macrophages to become suppressor or regulatory cells, whereas an additional signal is required to induce the cytolytic component. An alternative explanation could be that subpopulations of macrophages have different functions (similar to those described for T cells). The ability of macrophages to act as suppressor cells provides a negative feedback mechanism for the control of lymphokine production by T cells through the initial activation of the macrophages by lymphokine.

3. CHARACTERIZATION OF LYMPHOKINES AFFECTING MACROPHAGES

Because of the minute quantities in which lymphokines are produced *in vitro*, there has been great difficulty in purifying them and ascertaining their structural characteristics. Three of the factors that have effects on macrophages have been studied in detail. These include MIF and macrophage CF. Some of the other less well-characterized factors will be briefly mentioned.

3.1. BIOCHEMICAL PROPERTIES OF MIF

The physical-chemical characteristics of MIF from three species (guinea pig, mouse, and man) have been described in some detail. These findings are summarized in Table 2. In general, MIF from all species appear to be heterogeneous and include both protein and glycoprotein species with molecular weights less than immunoglobulins. However, based on their known physical-chemical properties, significant interspecies differences exist in the molecular structure of

TABLE 2. PHYSICOCHEMICAL PROPERTIES OF MIF

Property	Guinea pig	Mouse	Human
Molecular weight (Sephadex chromatography)	25,000–43,000 (pH 5 MIF) 65,000 (pH 3 MIF)	48,000–67,000	23,000–55,000
Chymotrypsin treatment	Sensitive	Sensitive	Sensitive
Neuraminidase treatment	Sensitive	—	Sensitive
Heat stability: 80°C	—	Sensitive	—
56°C	Stable	Stable	Stable
Isoelectric point	3–4.5 (pH 3 MIF) 5–5.5 (pH 5 MIF)	3–4.3 4.6–5.2	2.4–3.3 4.3–5.6
Polyacrylamide gel electrophoresis	Prealbumin	β-Globulin	Prealbumin
Buoyant density (CsCl)	Denser than protein	Denser than protein	Denser than protein
Salt precipitation, $(NH_4)_2SO_4$	50–80% saturation		

MIF. This is further evidenced by the fact that MIF from one animal may act as an immunogen when injected into animals of other species.

There appears to be heterogeneity of antigen-induced and particularly mitogen-induced MIF from guinea pigs since activity obtained after molecular sieve chromatography has sometimes been associated with a relatively high-molecular-weight fraction (approximately 56,000–82,000) as well as with a low-molecular-weight fraction (approximately 12,000–56,000) (Yoshida and Reisfeld, 1970; Dumonde *et al.*, 1972; Remold *et al.*, 1972; Sorg and Bloom, 1973). Remold and Mednis (1977) provided further evidence that MIF activity obtained from guinea pig lymphocytes can be separated into at least two distinct molecular species. Isoelectric focusing of partially purified MIF revealed the presence of a high-molecular-weight (55,000) MIF with an isoelectric point of 3–4.5 and low-molecular-weight (25,000) MIF having an isoelectric point of 5.5. Further experiments with polyacrylamide gels supported their view that two sizes of MIF exist. Recent experiments involving the purification of human MIF further support its heterogeneity (Weiser *et al.*, 1981). Using mitogen-generated MIF preparations, they demonstrated that within the first 24 hr of culture, one species of MIF was produced having a molecular weight of 23,000 and an isoelectric point of 4.3–5.2. The buoyant density of this MIF was shown to be that of a protein and was sensitive to trypsin but not neuraminidase. Analysis of the material generated during the second 24-hr incubation period identified two peaks of MIF. One peak had a 65,000 molecular weight and an isoelectric point of 2.4–3.3. The second peak revealed a lower-molecular-weight material (23,000–43,000) having a different isoelectric point (4.3–5.6). Both of these MIF activities were thought to be glycoproteins by virtue of their buoyant density, sensitivity to chymotrypsin and neuraminidase, and lack of sensitivity to trypsin. Therefore, both protein and glycoprotein forms of MIF are produced with the same stimulus and the exact role of these activities and their effects on macrophages remain to be defined.

Very little is known about the molecular structure of MIF except that human MIF may contain disulfide bonds as determined by the irreversible blocking of MIF activity by the reducing agent L-cysteine (Bartfeld and Atoynatan, 1971). Guinea pig MIF, on the other hand, is dissociated into fragments of lower molecular weight by treatment with agents such as mercaptoethanol and guanidine HCl, but the fragments reassociate to biologically active MIF molecules upon removal of the reducing and denaturing agents (Kotkes and Pick, 1977). However, if an alkylating agent such as iodoacetamide is added following reduction and denaturation, then MIF activity is irreversibly lost, suggesting that disulfide bonds are present in the molecule (Kotkes and Pick, 1979).

3.2. BIOCHEMICAL PROPERTIES OF MAF

The physical-chemical properties of MAF obtained from the guinea pig and man are indistinguishable from those of MIF. Guinea pig MAF, like MIF, elutes from Sephadex G-100 with molecules having molecular weights between 25,000 and 68,000. Both MAF and MIF activities are destroyed by neuraminidase and have a bouyant density slightly greater than that of albumin as determined by isopynic centrifugation in cesium chloride (Nathan *et al.*, 1973). Recent evidence indicates that MAF, like guinea pig MIF, is heterogeneous in that both pH 3 and pH 5 MIF activities also contain macrophage-activating properties (Churchill and Wong, 1980). A comparison of the properties of MIF and MAF in one species is shown in Table 3. In man, MAF and MIF cochromatograph on Sephadex G-100 (Rocklin *et al.*, 1974).

The lymphokines responsible for inducing other changes in function in macrophages may be the same as MIF/MAF. For example, the lymphokine

TABLE 3. COMPARISON OF MAF AND MIF[a]

	MAF		MIF	
	Guinea pig	Man	Guinea pig	Man
Receptors				
Fucose	+		+	+
Sialic acid	+	ND	+	
Enhancement of mediator by treatment with				
AT III	+	+	+	+?
STI	ND	+	+	
DSA	+	+	+	
Fractionation				
pH 3	+	+	+	+
pH 5	+	+	+	+

[a]From Churchill and Cameron (1980).

responsible for increasing pinocytosis has a molecular weight between 25,000 and 68,000, is sensitive to neuraminidase, and has a buoyant density similar to that of glycoprotein (Shubert *et al.*, 1980). Similarly, the guinea pig lymphokine responsible for increasing the production of tissue factor has a molecular weight between 35,000 and 50,000, although it has not been characterized further (Geczy and Hopper, 1981). In the mouse, the factor(s) responsible for tumoricidal activity or resistance to infection by microorganisms or that responsible for increasing complement receptors appear to be due to different activities. For example, the factor responsible for tumoricidal activity was reported to have a 45,000 molecular weight while that inducing macrophages to eliminate *Rickettsia* was heterogeneous having molecular weights of 115,000–125,000, 35,000, and less than 10,000 (Nacy *et al.*, 1981). In another study, it was reported that the factor responsible for tumoricidal activity could be separated from MIF by virtue of having a molecular weight (30,000) and two isoelectric points (7.4 and 8.4) which were different from MIF (Kniep *et al.*, 1981). Furthermore, this tumoricidal activity was not sensitive to treatment by trypsin and neuraminidase. The mouse lymphokine that is thought to increase the availability of complement receptors on macrophages has a molecular weight of less than 10,000 (Griffin and Griffin, 1980).

3.3. PHYSICAL-CHEMICAL PROPERTIES OF MACROPHAGE CHEMOTACTIC FACTOR

The macrophage chemotatic factor described in the guinea pig has an apparent molecular weight between 24,000 and 55,000, migrates with albumin on polyacrylamide gel electrophoresis, and has been separated from the chemotactic factor for polymorphonuclear leukocytes (Ward *et al.*, 1969; Altman *et al.*, 1973, 1975; Wahl *et al.*, 1974). The human macrophage chemotactic factor has a lower molecular weight (12,000), has isoelectric points of 10.1 and 5.6, and is sensitive to treatment by chymotrypsin while resistant to treatment by RNase and neuraminidase (Snyderman *et al.*, 1977; Ward and Rocklin, 1975). Both human and guinea pig macrophage chemotactic factors are heat stable and antigenically distinct from C3 and C5. These properties are summarized in Table 4.

3.4. MACROPHAGE GROWTH FACTORS

Lymphokines have been described in the guinea pig, mouse, and man that induce proliferation and colony formation *in vitro* (Hadden *et al.*, 1975). These factors have molecular weights between 35,000 and 70,000, an isoelectric point between 3.2 and 5.0, are heat stable to 70°C, and are adsorbed to Con A-Sepharose. Their mechanism of action may involve prostaglandin synthesis since indomethacin can antagonize their biologic effect. Furthermore, these factors increase cGMP levels within minutes after incubation with macrophages as

TABLE 4. PHYSICOCHEMICAL PROPERTIES OF LYMPHOKINE CHEMOTACTIC FACTOR[a]

Properties	Monocyte-macrophage	PMN leukocyte
Temperature (56°C, 30 min)	Stable[b]	Stable[c]
Sieve chromatography	24,000–55,000[c]; 12,000[b]	24,000–55,000[c]
Polyacrylamide gel electrophoresis	Albumin[b]	Prealbumin[c]
Isoelectric point	10.1 and 5.6[b]	—
Chymotrypsin	Sensitive[b]	Sensitive[c]
RNase	Resistant[b]	Resistant[c]
Neuraminidase	Resistant[b]	Resistant[c]

[a]From Churchill and Cameron (1980).
[b]Human.
[c]Guinea pig.

well as calcium influx. These factors are thought to not only induce a mitogenic signal in macrophages but also to influence their maturational state.

4. MECHANISMS OF LYMPHOKINE-MEDIATED ACTIVATION OF MACROPHAGES

4.1. MIF RECEPTOR

The interaction of MIF/MAF with the macrophage has been the subject of intense study and appears to occur at the cell surface (Leu *et al.*, 1972; Remold, 1973). Receptor models for MIF/MAF–macrophage interaction have been surmised from experiments showing that these activities are removed from supernatants following incubation with macrophages, whereas lymphocytes and PMN leukocytes have no such absorbing capacities. Furthermore, trypsin-treated macrophages do not respond to MIF, but this effect is reversible after removal of the enzyme and further culture for 24 hr. The restoration of responsiveness is presumably due to the regeneration of an MIF receptor (Leu *et al.*, 1972; Manheimer and Pick, 1973).

It has also been shown that the monosaccharide α-L-fucose specifically blocks the biologic activity of MIF-rich supernatants obtained from guinea pig lymphocyte cultures. Furthermore, guinea pig macrophages treated with fucosidase, an enzyme that cleaves terminal fucose residues from oligosaccharides, no longer respond to MIF (Remold, 1973). These findings suggest that α-L-fucose constitutes part of an MIF receptor that may be susceptible to the action of trypsin. Experiments using fucosidase suggest that α-L-fucose is also the terminal sugar on a receptor for human MIF on human blood monocytes (Rocklin, 1976).

The evidence for an MIF receptor is further strengthened by the observation that inhibition of macrophage migration does not require contact between the migrating cells and MIF for the entire assay period. Exposure of macrophages to MIF for 2 hr at 37°C, followed by washing of the cells, still results in marked migration inhibition (Manheimer and Pick, 1973). Furthermore, Higgins *et al.* (1978) and Liu *et al.* (1980) have suggested that fucogangliosides serve as MIF recognition units on macrophages. They showed that aqueous glycolipids obtained from guinea pig macrophages enhanced the responsiveness of untreated macrophages to MIF. Furthermore, this effect was abolished after either fucosidase or neuraminidase treatment of the active glycolipids, indicating that fucose and sialic acid may be important parts of the putative MIF receptor.

It should be noted that the interaction of MIF with macrophage receptors is complicated by the fact that one or several macrophage surface esterases are capable of inactivating MIF. Thus, guinea pig macrophages pretreated with diisopropylphosphofluorodate (DFP) or with soybean trypsin inhibitor demonstrate enhanced inhibition of migration when exposed to MIF. Serum pretreated with DFP and then freed of the inhibitor does not enhance MIF activity. The most likely explanation for these findings is that there is an active esterase(s) on the macrophage surface that destroys MIF activity. Moreover, physiological concentrations of the plasma esterase and proteinase inhibitors α_2-macroglobulin, α_1-antitrypsin, C1-esterase inhibitor, and antithrombin-heparin cofactor also enhance the response *in vitro* of macrophages to MIF (Remold and Rosenberg, 1975). This suggests a mechanism by which esterase inhibitors of normal plasma may play a regulatory role in cell-mediated immune reactions *in vivo*.

The mechanism by which the inhibitory signal reaches the interior of the macrophage is largely unknown. Altered membrane calcium transport and changes in the cellular levels of cAMP and cGMP appear to be involved. Furthermore, MIF increases microtubular density in macrophages and this may in fact be the primary event; alterations in cyclic nucleotide levels may be a consequence rather than a cause of the changes in cellular microtubular functions (Pick and Grunspan-Swirsky, 1977).

4.2. MIF/MAF CONTINUUM

Although MIF activity is detectable within 24 hr, this does not rule out the possibility that migration inhibition and activation of macrophages are different manifestations of the same lymphokine. Thus, it appears that macrophages cultured *in vitro* respond to the lymphokine with migration inhibition before they become sensitive to its activating influence. Moreover, if MIF-rich material is allowed to remain in contact with macrophages or monocytes, the cells escape inhibition and ultimately begin to migrate at rates faster than the control-treated cells. Activation by MAF is enhanced if the macrophages are pretreated with agents that also enhance MIF activity, such as esterase inhibitors or a surface-active agent, diazotized sulfanilic acid (Remold, 1977; Churchill and Cameron, 1980).

4.3. ROLE OF MEMBRANE-BOUND GLYCOPROTEINS

Recent evidence suggests that a transformation-sensitive glycoprotein of connective tissue cells, termed "fibronectin," may serve an important function in migration inhibition of macrophages. Fibronectin has been shown to have an important function in cell aggregation, adhesion, and motility. Remold *et al.* (1981) have shown that guinea pig peritoneal exudate cells release a factor which causes an increased response of normal macrophages to MIF and also restores the response of trypsinized macrophages to MIF. An antibody directed against fibronectin blocks the above-mentioned activities. Furthermore, addition of plasma fibronectin to macrophages before exposure to peritoneal extract reduces this enhanced response to MIF, presumably by competing for the binding site for fibronectin.

As mentioned previously, it appears that coagulation proteins may also be involved in the migration response as shown by Geczy and Hopper (1981). In their experiments, the induction of procoagulant activity by lymphokines results in a decreased chemotactic response of macrophages as well as decreased migration of these cells from capillary tubes.

4.4. PRODUCTS OF OXYGEN REDUCTION

A very novel hypothesis to explain the effects of MIF on macrophages has recently been presented by Keisari and Pick (1980). They proposed that MIF acts as a stimulant of the respiratory burst in macrophages and that unstable products of oxygen reduction (0_2^-, OH^- and O_2^-, or the more stable H_2O_2) formed during the MIF-induced respiratory burst are responsible for most if not all the effects of MIF. Furthermore, it was suggested that inhibition of migration, the most common of all MIF effects, is the result of oxidative damage by oxygen byproducts to membrane lipids, protein, or to cytoplasmic elements, possibly belonging to the cytoskeleton. Furthermore, MIF-mediated macrophage activation, as expressed by augmented bactericidal and cytotoxic capacity, is the functional expression of the enhanced ability of MIF-activated cells to produce H_2O_2 in response to phagocytic stimuli or other types of membrane perturbation.

5. MODULATION OF LYMPHOKINE PRODUCTION AND ACTION

5.1. MODULATION OF LYMPHOKINE PRODUCTION

There is abundant evidence that there may be natural regulation of lymphokine production. Antigen-stimulated lymphocytes release a mediator that, when incubated with B cells stimulated with the same antigens, prevents them from making MIF (Cohen and Yoshida, 1977). Although many explanations are possible, there is reason to believe that the MIF inhibitory factor acts directly on the B cells to prevent synthesis or release of MIF. The presence of a natural regulator mechanism that prevents excessive mediator production may also account for the previous observation that more MIF is produced if the cutlure medium is changed during lymphokine production than if no change is made.

Agents which block DNA synthesis and/or replication in general have little effect on the production of MIF (Bloom *et al.*, 1972; Rocklin, 1973; Mizoguchi *et al.*, 1973). However, blocking of DNA-dependent RNA synthesis with actinomycin D and protein synthesis with puromycin or cycloheximide results in a reduction in lymphokine production (David and David, 1972; Mizoguchi *et al.*, 1973; Pekarek *et al.*, 1976). The production of lymphokines is also dependent upon intact microfilament and microtubule function as evidenced by the fact that cytochalasin B (Pick, 1974) or colchicine (Henney *et al.*, 1974; Pick, 1974) inhibits MIF release.

The mechanism of lymphocyte triggering is not fully understood but measurable RNA, protein, and DNA synthesis is preceded by one or more steps initiated by the interaction of antigen or mitogen with the lymphocyte membrane. Cap formation and pinocytosis of antigen– or mitogen–receptor complex are recognized to be essential steps leading to lymphocyte activation. These steps depend upon intact microfilament function. On the other hand, agents that inhibit the formation of microtubules and interfere with the formation of mitotic spindles such as colchicine or vinblastine do not influence early mediator production by stimulated lymphocytes.

The production of lymphokines appears to be completely blocked by the addition of cAMP and by agents that increase the endogenous levels of cAMP (Pick, 1974). Thus, β-adrenergic drugs, prostaglandin E_1, and phosphodiesterase inhibitors all reduce MIF production. In contrast, agents that increase levels of cGMP such as cholinergic drugs lead to an enhancement of mediator production. Corticosteroids appear to have little effect on lymphokine production (Ballow and Rosenthal, 1973; Pekarek *et al.*, 1976).

5.2. MODULATION OF LYMPHOKINE ACTION

The influence on MIF action by agents that interfere with macrophage DNA replication, transcription, and/or translation appears to be limited. However, blocking protein synthesis with puromycin or cycloheximide leads to a reduction in the effects of MIF on macrophages (Manheimer and Pick, 1973). The requirement for intact microfilament and microtubule function has been demonstrated (Pick and Abrahamer, 1973).

It appears that drugs that raise intracellular levels of cAMP, or cAMP itself, counteract events occurring after exposure of macrophages to MIF. In order to prevent the action of these lymphokines, the agents must be present during the initial stage of the interaction between the lymphokine and the target cell (Pick, 1977). In addition, macrophages treated with MIF-containing supernatants exhibit prolonged (24 hr) but minimal decreases in cAMP concentrations compared to control-treated cells. However, the subtle cAMP lowering effect is similar to and only slightly more pronounced than the decrease seen when macrophages are treated with supernatants from unstimulated lymphocytes (Pick, 1977). The reduction in cAMP concentrations has been attributed to diminished cAMP synthesis rather than to increased cAMP degradation (Pick and Grunspan-Swirsky, 1977). Thus, direct inhibition of macrophage adenylate cyclase has not been demonstrated (Pick and Grunspan-Swirsky, 1977). In fact, a late (24–48 hr) serum-dependent increase in adenylate cyclase activity of intact macrophages exposed to MIF-rich supernatants has been reported (Remold-O'Donnell and Remold, 1974). It is therefore probable that MIF, if at all active in this system, interferes with the early signal transfer from the membrane receptors to the enzyme. The effect of MIF on the intracellular level of cGMP is minimal (Pick, 1977). It is of interest that while glucocorticoids have little effect on the production of MIF, they do inhibit the response of macrophages to preformed MIF (Balow and Rosenthal, 1973; Pekarek *et al.*, 1976; Wahl *et al.*, 1975).

6. CONCLUSION

A variety of soluble lymphokines that are prime candidates for mediating cell-mediated immune or delayed hypersensitivity phenomena have been discussed. As more and more information is uncovered relating to their *in vitro* effects, the exact extent of their role in these reactions will be more clearly defined. It should be pointed out, however, that the biological effects of lymphokines can be duplicated to varying degrees by other immunologic systems such as antigen–antibody complex effects on target cells and various components of the complement system. What still remains unique about this process, however, is the fact that the lymphocyte has evolved a special triggering mechanism, which the other systems lack.

By virtue of the nature of their biologic activity, a role for lymphokines in the expression of cell-mediated immunity had been suggested. After activation of T or B lymphocytes, the relevant factors would be produced to mobilize cells both by way of vessel permeability effects and by direct chemotactic activity on macrophages. In the classical delayed hypersensitivity reaction, the macrophage infiltration predominates. Once the inflammatory cells are recruited to the site, their random movement can be retarded by MIF so that they remain there. This may be followed by a state of increased activation. The latter would lead to enhanced phagocytosis and suppression of intracellular replication of a variety of bacterial, viral, and other pathogens and in some instances, an ability to kill them. The extracellular release of lysosomal hydrolases by activated macrophages could result in damage to both the target cells and normal tissue. With further advances in the biochemical characterization and purification of these factors, more insight will be provided as to their role in this process.

REFERENCES

Altman, L. C., 1978, Monocyte chemotactic factor, in: *Leukocyte Chemotaxis* (J. I. Gallin and P. G. Quie, eds.), p. 267, Raven Press, New York.

Altman, L. C., Snyderman, R., Oppenheim, J. J., and Mergenhagen, S. E., 1973, A human mononuclear leukocytic chemotactic factor: Characterization, specificity and kinetics of production by homologous leukocytes, *J. Immunol.* **110**:801.

Altman, L. C., Chassy, B., and Macklin, B. F., 1975, Physicochemical characterization of chemotactic lymphokines produced by human T and B lymphocytes, *J. Immunol.* **115**:18.

Anderson, S. E., and Remington, J. S., 1974, Effect of normal and activated human macrophages on *Toxoplasma gondii, J. Exp. Med.* **139:**1154.

Anderson, S. E., Bautista, S., and Remington, J. S., 1976, Induction of resistance to *Toxoplasma gondii* in human macrophages by soluble lymphocyte products, *J. Immunol.* **117:**381.

Balow, J. E., and Rosenthal, A. S., 1973, Glucocorticoid suppression of macrophage migration inhibitory factor, *J. Exp. Med.* **137:**1031.

Bartfeld, H., and Atoynatan, T., 1971, Activity and properties of macrophage migration inhibitory factor produced in MLC, *Nature (London)* **230:**246.

Beer, D. J., Dinarello, C. A., Rosenwasser, L. J., and Rocklin, R. E., 1982, Human monocyte-derived soluble product has an accessory function in the generation of histamine- and concanavalin A-induced suppressor T cells, *J. Clin. Invest.* **70:**393.

Block, L. H., Bernheim, H. A., and Jacksche, H., 1980, Purified human MIF: Effects on oxidative metabolism and surface architecture of effector cells, in: *Biochemical Characterization of Lymphokines* (A. deWeck, ed.), p. 79, Academic Press, New York.

Bloom, B. L., Gaffney, J., and Jimenez, L., 1972, Dissociation of MIF production and cell proliferation, *J. Immunol.* **109:**1395.

Borgis, J. S., and Johnson, W. D., 1974, Inhibition of multiplication of *Toxoplasma gondii* by human monocytes exposed to T-lymphocyte products, *J. Exp. Med.* **141:**483.

Bray, M. A., Gordon, D., and Morley, J., 1978, Prostaglandins as regulators in cellular immunity, *Prostaglandins Med.* **1:**183.

Chao, P., Francis, L., and Atkins, E., 1977, The release of an endogenous pyrogen from guinea pigs *in vitro, J. Exp. Med.* **145:**1288.

Churchill, W. H., and Cameron, D., 1980, Macrophage activating factor (MAF) induced cytotoxicity: Similarities in man and guinea pig, in: *Biochemical Characterization of Lymphokines* (A. de Weck, ed.), p. 137, Academic Press, New York.

Churchill, W. H., and Wong, C., 1980, Mediator-induced macrophage activation as shown by enhanced cytotoxicity for tumor, requires macrophages surface fucose and sialic acid, *Cell. Immunol.* **55:**490.

Churchill, W. H., Piessens, W. F., Sulis, C. A., and David, J. R., 1975, Macrophages activated as suspension cultures with lymphocyte mediators devoid of antigen become cytotoxic for tumor cells, *J. Immunol.* **115:**781.

Cohen, S., and Yoshida, T., 1977, Suppression of B cell MIF production by T cells and soluble T cell-derived factors, *J. Immunol.* **119:**719.

Colvin, R. B., Johnson, R. A., Mihm, M. C., and Dvorak, H. F., 1973, Role of the clotting system in cell-mediated hypersensitivity: Fibrin deposition in delayed skin reactions in man, *J. Exp. Med.* **138:**686.

David, J. R., 1966, Delayed hypersensitivity *in vitro:* Its mediation by cell-free substances formed by lymphoid cell–antigen interactions, *Proc. Natl. Acad. Sci. USA* **56:**72.

David, J. R., and David, R. A., 1972, Cellular hypersensitivity and immunity: Inhibition of macrophage migration and lymphocyte mediators, *Prog. Allergy* **16:**300.

Dinarello, C. A., and Rosenwasser, L. J., 1981, Lymphocyte activating property of human leukocytic pyrogen, in: *Advances in Immunopharmacology* (J. W. Hadden, L. Chedid, and P. Mullen, eds.), p. 419, Pergamon Press, Elmsford, N.Y.

Dumonde, D. C., Page, D. A., Matthew, M., and Wolstencroft, R. A., 1972, Role of lymphocyte activation products (LAP) in cell-mediated immunity, *Clin. Immunol. Immunopathol.* **10:**25.

Dvorak, A. M., Hammond, M. E., Dvorak, H. F., and Karnovsky, M. J., 1972, Loss of cell surface material from peritoneal exudate cells associated with MIF activity, *Lab. Invest.* **27:**561.

Edwards, R. L., and Rickles, F. R., 1978, Delayed hypersensitivity: Effect of systemic anticoagulation, *Science* **200:**541.

Edwards, R. L., and Rickles, F. R., 1980, The role of human T cells (and T cell products) for monocytic tissue factor generation, *J. Immunol.* **125:**606.

Evans, R., and Alexander, P., 1976, Mechanisms of extra-cellular killing of nucleated mammalian cells by macrophages, in: *Immunobiology of the Macrophage* (D. S. Nelson, ed.), p. 536, Academic Press, New York.

Fidler, I. J., Darnell, J. H., and Budmen, M. D., 1977, Tumoricidal properties of mouse macrophages activated with mediators from rat lymphocytes stimulated with Con A, *J. Immunol.* **117**:666.

Folger, W. E., Raz, A., and Fidler, I. J., 1980, *In situ* activation of murine macrophages by liposomes containing lymphokines, *Cell. Immunol.* **53**:214.

Fowles, R. W., Fajardo, I. M., Lebowitch, J. L., and David, J. R., 1973, The enhancement of macrophage bacteriostasis by products of activated lymphocytes, *J. Exp. Med.* **138**:952.

Fox, R. A., Gregory, D. S., and Feldman, J. D., 1974, Migration inhibition factor (MIF) and migration stimulation factor (MSF) in fetal calf serum, *J. Immunol.* **112**:1861.

Galindo, B., 1972, Antigen-mediated fusion of specifically sensitized rabbit alveolar macrophages, *Infect. Immun.* **5**:583.

Galindo, B., Lazdins, J., and Castillo, R., 1974, Fusion of normal rabbit alveolar macrophages induced by supernatants from BCG-sensitized lymph node cells after elicitation by antigens, *Infect. Immun.* **9**:212.

Geczy, C. L., and Hopper, K. E., 1981, A mechanism of migration inhibition in delayed-type hypersensitivity reactions. II. Lymphokines promote procoagulant activity of macrophages *in vitro*, *J. Immunol.* **126**:1059.

Godal, T., Rees, R. J. W., and Lamvick, J. O., 1971, Lymphocyte-mediated modification of blood-derived macrophage function *in vitro:* Inhibition of growth of intracellular mycobacteria with lymphokines, *Clin. Exp. Immunol.* **8**:625.

Greineder, D. K., Connorton, K. J., and David, J. R., 1979, Plasminogen activator production by human monocytes. I. Enhancement by activated lymphocytes and lymphocyte products, *J. Immunol.* **123**:2808.

Griffin, F. M., Jr., and Griffin, J. A., 1980, Augmentation of macrophage complement receptor function *in vitro.* II. Characterization of the effects of a unique lymphokine upon the phagocytic capabilities of macrophages, *J. Immunol.* **125**:844.

Griffin, J. A., and Griffin, F. M. Jr., 1979, Augmentation of macrophage complement receptor function *in vitro* I. Characterizations of the cellular interactions required for the generation of a T lymphocyte product which enhances macrophage complement receptor function. *J. Exp. Med.* **150**:653.

Hadden, J. W., Sadlik, J. R., and Hadden, E. M., 1975, Macrophage proliferation induced *in vitro* by a lymphocyte factor, *Nature (London)* **257**:483.

Hammond, M. E., and Dvorak, H. F., 1972, Antigen-induced stimulation of glucosamine incorporation by guinea pig peritoneal macrophages in delayed hypersensitivity, *J. Exp. Med.* **136**:1518.

Hammond, M. E., Sekvagguim, S. S., and Dvorak, H. F., 1975, Antigen-enhanced glucosamine incorporation by peritoneal macrophages in cell-mediated hypersensitivity, *J. Immunol.* **115**:914.

Henney, C. S., Gaffney, J., and Bloom, B. R., 1974, On the relation of products of activated lymphocytes to cell-mediated cytolysis, *J. Exp. Med.* **140**:837.

Hibbs, J. B., Taintor, R. R., Chapman, N. A., and Weinberg, J. B., 1977, Macrophage tumor killing influence of the local environment, *Science* **197**:279.

Higgins, T. J., Sabatino, A. P., Remold, H. F., and David, J. R., 1978, Possible role of macrophage glycolipids as receptors for migration inhibitory factor (MIF), *J. Immunol.* **121**:880.

Keisari, T., and Pick, E., 1980, Lymphokine mimicry by PMA and the ionophore A23187: A new hypothesis for explaining the action mechanism of migration inhibitory factor, in: *Biochemical Characterization of Lymphokines* (A. de Weck, ed.), p. 113, Academic Press, New York.

Klimentzek, V., and Sorg, C., 1977, Lymphokine-induced secretion of plasminogen activation by murine macrophages, *Eur. J. Immunol* **7**:185.

Kniep, E. M., Domzig, W., Lohmann-Matthes, M., and Kickhofen, B., 1981, Partial purification and chemical characterization of macrophage cytotoxicity factor (MCF, MAF) and its separation from migration inhibitory factor (MIF), *J. Immunol.* **127**:417.

Kotkes, P., and Pick, E., 1977, New approaches to the characterization of guinea pig macrophage migration inhibitory factor, *Isr. J. Med. Sci.* **13**:1045.

Kotkes, P., and Pick, E., 1979, Purification of MIF after treatment with reducing and denaturing agents, *Clin. Exp. Immunol.* **37**:540.

Krahenbuhl, J. L., and Remington, J. S., 1971, *In vitro* introduction of non-specific resistance in macrophages by specifically sensitized lymphocytes, *Infect. Immun.* **4**:337.

Krahenbuhl, J. L., Rosenberg, L. T., and Remington, J. S., 1973, Role of T lymphocytes in the *in vitro* activation of macrophages to kill *Listeria monocytogenes*, *J. Immunol.* **111**:992.

Leu, R. W., Eddeston, A., Hadden, J. W., and Good, R. A., 1972, Mechanism of action of migration inhibitory factor (MIF), *J. Exp. Med.* **136**:589.

Littman, B. H., and Ruddy, S., 1977, Production of the second component of complement by human monocytes: Stimulation by antigen-activated lymphocytes of lymphokines, *J. Exp. Med.* **145**:1344.

Liu, D. Y., Petschek, K. D., Remold, H. G., and David, J. R., 1980, Role of sialic acid in the macrophage glycolipid receptor for MIF, *J. Immunol.* **124**:2042.

Lohmann-Matthes, M. L., Ziegler, F. G., and Fisher, H., 1973, Macrophage toxicity factor: A product of *in vitro* sensitized thymus-dependent cells, *Eur. J. Immunol.* **3**:56.

Lolekha, S., Dray, S., and Gotoff, S. P., 1970, Macrophage aggregation *in vitro:* A correlation of delayed hypersensitivity, *J. Immunol.* **104**:296.

McAdam, K. P. W. J., and Dinarello, C. A., 1980, Induction of serum amyloid A-synthesis by human leukocyte pyrogen, in: *Bacterial Endotoxins and Host Response* (M. K. Agarwal, ed.), p. 167, Elsevier/North-Holland, Amsterdam.

Manheimer, S., and Pick, E., 1973, The mechanism of action of soluble lymphocytic mediators, *Immunology* **24**:1027.

Meade, C. J., Ladmann, P. J., and Brenner, S., 1974, A sensitive assay for cellular hypersensitivity based on the uptake of radioactive colloidal gold, *Immunology* **27**:227.

Meltzer, M. S., 1981, Macrophage activation for tumor cytotoxicity: Characterization of priming and trigger signals during lymphokine activation, *J. Immunol.* **127**:177.

Mizoguchi, Y., Yamamoto, S., and Morisawa, S., 1973, Studies on the biosynthesis of macrophage migration inhibitory factor in delayed hypersensitivity, *J. Biochem.* **73**:467.

Nacy, C. A., Leonard, E. J., and Meltzer, M. S., 1981, Macrophages in resistance to rickettsial infections: Characterization of lymphokines that induce rickettsiacidal activity in macrophages, *J. Immunol.* **126**:204.

Nathan, C. F., Karnovsky, M. L., and David, J. R., 1971, Alterations of macrophage functions by mediators from lymphocytes, *J. Exp. Med.* **133**:1356.

Nathan, C. F., Remold, H. G., and David, J. R., 1973, Characterization of a lymphocyte factor which alters macrophage functions, *J. Exp. Med.* **137**:275.

Neta, R., and Salvin, S. B., 1971, Cellular immunity *in vitro:* Migration inhibition and phagocytosis, *Infect. Immun.* **4**:697.

Pantalone, R. M., and Page, R. C., 1975, Lymphokine-induced production and release of lysosomal enzymes by macrophages, *Proc. Natl. Acad. Sci. USA* **72**:2091.

Pantalone, R. M., and Page, R. C., 1977, Enzyme production and secretion by lymphokine-activated macrophages, *J. Reticuloendothelial Soc.* **21**:343.

Patterson, R. J., and Youmans, G. P., 1970, Demonstration in tissue culture of lymphocyte mediated immunity to tuberculosis, *Infect. Immun.* **1**:600.

Pekarek, J., Svejcar, J., Monza, K., and Johanovsky, J., 1976, Effect of immunosuppressive drugs on an *in vitro* correlate of cell-mediated immunity, *Immunology* **31**:773.

Pels, E., and Den-Otter, W., 1974, The role of a cytophilic factor from challenged immune peritoneal lymphocytes in specific macrophage cytotoxicity, *Cancer Res.* **34**:3089.

Pick, E., 1974, Soluble lymphocytic mediators. I. Inhibition of macrophage migration inhibitory factor production by drugs, *Immunology* **26**:649.

Pick, E., 1977, Lymphokines: Physiologic control and pharmacological modulation of their production and action, in: *Immunopharmacology* (J. W. Hadden and R. G. Coffey, eds.), p. 163, Plenum Press, New York.

Pick, E., and Abrahamer, H., 1973, Blocking of macrophage migration inhibitory factor action by microtubular disruptive drugs, *Int. Arch. Allergy Appl. Immunol.* **45**:295.

Pick, E., and Grunspan-Swirsky, A., 1977, The mechanism of action of soluble lymphocyte mediators, *Cell. Immunol.* **32**:340.

Piessens, W. F., Churchill, W. H., and David, J. R., 1975, Macrophages activated *in vitro* with lymphocyte mediators kill neoplastic but not normal cells, *J. Immunol.* **114**:293.

Poste, G., and Kirsch, R., 1979, Rapid decay of tumoricidal activity and loss of responsiveness to lymphokines in inflammatory macrophages, *Cancer Res.* **39**:2582.

Poulter, L. W., and Turk, J. L., 1975, Studies on the effect of soluble lymphocyte products on macrophage physiology, *Cell. Immunol.* **20**:25.

Remold, H. G., 1973, Requirement for α-L-fucose on the macrophage membrane receptor for MIF, *J. Exp. Med.* **138**:1065.

Remold, H. G., 1977, Chemical treatment of macrophages increases their responses to migration inhibitory factor, *J. Immunol.* **118**:1.

Remold, H. G., and Mednis, A., 1975, Decrease of three lysosomal enzymes in guinea pig macrophages activated by lymphocyte mediators, *Inflammation* **1**:175.

Remold, H. G., and Mednis, A., 1977, Two migration inhibitory factors with different chromatographic behavior and isoelectric points, *J. Immunol.* **118**:2015.

Remold, H. G., and Rosenberg, R. D., 1975, Enhancement of migration inhibitory factor activity by plasma esterase inhibitors, *J. Biol. Chem.* **250**:6608.

Remold, H. G., David, R. A., and David, J. R., 1972, Characterization of migration inhibitory factor (MIF) from guinea pig lymphocytes stimulated with concanavalin A, *J. Immunol.* **109**:578.

Remold, H. G., Shaw, J. E., and David, J. R., 1981, A macrophage surface component related to fibronectin is involved in the response to migration inhibitory factor, *Cell. Immunol.* **58**:175.

Remold-O'Donnell, E., and Remold, H. G., 1974, The enhancement of macrophage adenylate cyclase by products of stimulated lymphocytes, *J. Biol. Chem.* **249**:3622.

Rocklin, R. E., 1973, Production of macrophage migration inhibitory factor by nondividing lymphocytes, J. Immunol. **110**:674.

Rocklin, R. E., 1976, Role of monosaccharides in the interaction of two lymphocyte mediators with their target cells, *J. Immunol.* **116**:816.

Rocklin, R. E., Winston, C. T., and David, J. R., 1974, Activation of human blood monocytes by products of sensitized lymphocytes, *J. Clin. Invest.* **53**:559.

Rosenwasser, L. J., Dinarello, C. A., and Rosenthal, A. S., 1979, Adherent cell function in murine T-lymphocyte antigen recognition. IV. Enhancement of murine T-cell antigen recognition by human leukocytic pyrogen, *J. Exp. Med.* **150**:709.

Scher, M. G., Beller, D. I., and Unanue, E. R., 1980, Demonstration of a soluble mediator that induces exudates rich in Ia-positive macrophages, *J. Exp. Med.* **152**:1684.

Sharma, S. D., Piessens, W. F., and Middlebrook, G., 1980, *In vitro* killing of tumor cells by soluble products of activated guinea pig peritoneal macrophages, *Cell. Immunol.* **49**:379.

Shubert, R. D., and David, J. R., 1980, Stimulation of guinea pig macrophage pinocytosis by lipopolysaccharides (LPS): Evidence that LPS acts directly on the macrophage, *Cell. Immunol.* **55**:166.

Shubert, R. D., Wong, J., and David, J. R., 1980, Stimulation of pinocytosis in the macrophage by lymphocyte mediators. II. Evidence that the stimulating factor is MAF, and studies on the cellular requirements for response to the mediator, *Cell. Immunol.* **55**:155.

Smyth, A. C., and Weiss, L., 1970, Electron microscopic study of inhibition of macrophage migration in delayed hypersensitivity, *J. Immunol.* **105**:1360.

Snyderman, R., Meadows, L., and Amos, D. B., 1977, Characterization of human chemotactic lymphokine production induced by mitogens and mixed leukocyte reactions using a new microassay, *Cell. Immunol.* **30**:225.

Sorg, C., and Bloom, B. R., 1973, Products of activated lymphocytes. I. The use or radiolabelling techniques in the characterization and partial purification of the migration inhibitory factor of the guinea pig, *J. Exp. Med.* **137**:148.

Svejcar, J., and Johanovsky, J., 1961, Demonstration of delayed type hypersensitivity *in vitro.* II. Specific reaction of hypersensitive cells with antigens, *Z. Immunitaetsforsch.* **122**:420.

Taffet, S. M., Pace, J. L., and Russell, S. W., 1981, Lymphokine maintains macrophage activation for tumor cell killing by interfering with the negative regulatory effect of prostaglandin E_2, *J. Immunol.* **127**:121.

Taramelli, D., Holden, H. T., and Varesio, L., 1981, *In vitro* induction of tumoricidal and suppressor macrophages by lymphokines: Possible feedback regulation, *J. Immunol.* **126:**2123.

Thrasher, S. G., Yoshida, T., van Oss, C. J., Cohen, S., and Rose, N. R., 1973, Alteration of macrophage interfacial tension by supernatants of antigen-activated lymphocytes, *J. Immunol.* **110:**321.

Unsgaard, G., 1979, Cytostatic and phagocytic capacity of lymphokine-activated human monocytes, *Acta Pathol. Microbiol. Scand. Sect. C* **87:**325.

Vassalli, J., and Reich, E., 1977, Macrophage plasminogen activation: Induction by products of activated lymphoid cells, *J. Exp. Med.* **145:**429.

Wahl, L. M., Wahl, S. M., Mergenhagen, S. E., and Martin, G. R., 1975, Collagenase production by lymphokine-activated macrophages, *Science* **187:**261.

Washl, S. M., Iverson, G. M., and Oppenheim, J. J., 1974, Induction of B cell guinea pig lymphokine synthesis by mitogenic and non-mitogenic signals, *J. Exp. Med.* **140:**1631.

Ward, P. A., and Rocklin, R. E., 1975, Production by antigen-stimulated human lymphoid cells of a monocyte chemotactic factor, in: *The Immune System and Infectious Disease* (E. Neter and F. Milgrom, eds.), p. 470, Karger, Basel.

Ward, P. A., Remold, H. G., and David, J. R., 1969, Leukotactic factor produced by sensitized lymphocytes, *Science* **163:**1079.

Weisbart, R. H., Bluestone, R., Goldberg, L. S., and Pearson, C. M., 1974, Migration enhancement factor: A new lymphokine, *Proc. Natl. Acad. Sci USA* **74:**875.

Weiser, W. Y., Greineder, D. K., Remold, H. G., and David, J. R., 1981, Studies on human migration inhibitory factor: Characterization of three molecular species, *J. Immunol.* **126:**1958.

Wilton, J. M., Rosenstreich, D. L., and Oppenheim, J. J., 1975, Activation of guinea pig macrophages by bacterial lipopolysaccharide requires bone-marrow derived lymphocytes, *J. Immunol.* **114:**388.

Yoshida, T., and Reisfeld, R., 1970, Two fractions with macrophage migration inhibitory activity from sensitized lymphocyte cultures, *Nature (London)* **226:**856.

14

Role of Prostaglandins in Macrophage Cell Function

STEVEN L. KUNKEL, STEPHEN W. CHENSUE, JOSEPH C. FANTONE, and PETER A. WARD

1. INTRODUCTION

Since their discovery in the 1930s as potent autacoids, and their subsequent isolation and characterization in the 1960s as derivatives of arachidonic acid, prostaglandins have been the topic of many symposia and the basis for exhaustive research. These ubiquitous fatty acid derivatives have proven to be extremely powerful chemicals synthesized by nearly every cell in the human body, except the erythrocyte. Their synthesis and release have shown to be dependent upon a wide variety of cell membrane perturbations ranging from slight mechanical or chemical disturbances to the binding of compounds to specific receptors. Increasing evidence supports the theory that prostaglandins of all types are "made on demand" and not stored, since the amount of prostaglandins released from specific cells, in response to an appropriate stimulus, is greater than the total prostaglandin content of the cells prior to stimulation (Horton, 1979).

As illustrated in Fig. 1, appropriate membrane stimulation can result in the synthesis of a number of different prostaglandins, which are chemically defined as 20-carbon unsaturated carboxylic acids containing a cyclopentane ring. Naturally occurring prostaglandins all have in common an α-hydroxyl group at carbon-15, a functionality extremely important for biological activity yet very susceptible to the action of 15-hydroxyprostaglandin dehydrogenase (Hansen, 1976). It is generally accepted that this dehydrogenase plays a major role in limiting the half-life of the 15-hydroxyprostaglandins *in vivo*, thus regulating the biological activities of these autacoids. The potent and diverse nature of the biological activities of the prostaglandins on numerous cell systems have been detailed in recent reviews (Higgs *et al.*, 1979; Ramwell, 1980). Much of the experimental evidence from both *in vitro* and *in vivo* studies cumulatively gives

STEVEN L. KUNKEL, STEPHEN W. CHENSUE, JOSEPH C. FANTONE, and PETER A. WARD
• Department of Pathology, University of Michigan Medical School, Ann Arbor, Michigan 48190.

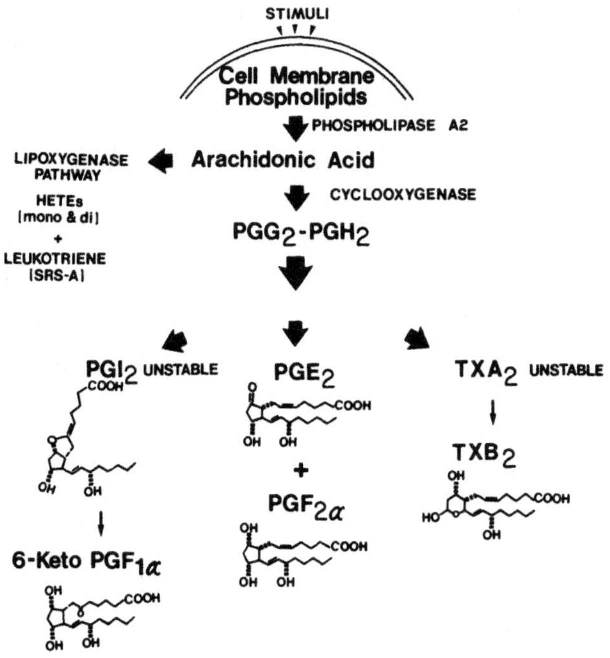

FIGURE 1. General metabolic pathway for the synthesis of cyclooxygenase products from arachidonic acid. Three major groups of biologically potent products comprise the cyclooxygenase family: the classical or stable prostaglandins, the prostacyclins, and the thromboxanes. The hydroxyl group at position 15 on all of the above structures is necessary for biological activity in many systems and is extremely susceptible to the 15-OH-prostaglandin dehydrogenase.

support to the involvement of the prostaglandins as a group of natural substances which mediate a key cell system, the inflammatory response.

2. PROSTAGLANDINS AND THE INFLAMMATORY RESPONSE

The experimental evidence which supports the view that prostaglandins influence the development and modulation of immune processes and inflammatory reactions is indeed voluminous (Parker, 1972; Vane, 1976; Goldyne, 1977; Pelu and Strausser, 1977; Kunkel *et al.*, 1981a). Although many prostaglandins, especially those of the E series, clearly are mediators of local inflammation, they also are able to immunoregulate diverse effector systems of the inflammatory response. Thus, prostaglandin E (PGE), possibly by increasing intracellular cAMP levels, inhibit lymphocyte-mediated cytotoxicity (Henney *et al.*, 1971), suppress IgE-induced release of histamine from basophils and mast cells (Lichtenstein and DiBernardo, 1971), and inhibit lysosomal enzyme release from polymorphonuclear leukocytes (Zurier *et al.*, 1974). In addition, pharmacological doses of PGE have been shown to suppress acute and chronic inflammation elicited in experimental animal models (Kunkel *et al.*, 1979, 1981b). PGE compounds can both suppress and enhance humoral and cell-mediated immunity *in vitro* and appear to regulate the character and intensity of immune response *in vivo*. The latter is exemplified by treatment of NZB/NZW mice (a murine model for human systemic lupus erythematosus) with PGE_1, resulting in both retardation of the progressive immune complex-induced glomerulonephritis and prolongation of animal survival (Zurier *et al.*, 1978). Although the role of prostaglandins in many immune/inflammatory reactions appears complex, these ubiquitous fatty acids are extremely important in regulating cell functions and host defenses.

3. PROSTAGLANDIN PRODUCTION BY MONONUCLEAR PHAGOCYTES

With regard to the involvement of prostaglandins and specific inflammatory cells, the macrophage takes precedence as a major prostaglandin-producing entity. Recent investigations have demonstrated this to be especially true in the case of resident macrophages (Bonney *et al.*, 1978), which can respond to a specific immune stimulus with the production of large amounts of both PGE_2 and prostacyclin (PGI_2). The latter is quantitated by measuring immunoreactive 6-keto-$PGF_{1\alpha}$, the stable metabolite of PGI_2. Cultured resident macrophages were shown to release approximately 80 ng PGE/10^6 cells per 4 hr when exposed to 50 μg/ml of zymosan. This accounted for an approximately 50-fold increase in the basal levels of PGE production (Bonney *et al.*, 1978). A similar increase in PGI_2 production above baseline levels was also observed, again using zymosan as the stimulus (Davies *et al.*, 1980). An interesting observation in the above experiments showed only basal levels of PGF in either nonstimulated or zymosan-stimulated resident macrophages. The synthesis and release of both PGE_2 and PGI_2 from zymosan-stimulated resident macrophages was demonstrated to be both a time-dependent and a dose-dependent phenomenon; with the production and release of either prostaglandin occurring prior to 30 min poststimulation and lasting for over 24 hr (Humes *et al.*, 1977). Although the release of either prostaglandin was linear with regard to time, the zymosan dose–response curve quickly reached a plateau using 50–100 μg of zymosan per culture plate.

In addition to a phagocytic stimulus, as in the case of zymosan-treated macrophage, other particulate and soluble stimuli have been examined for the ability to induce prostaglandin release from macrophages. Soluble agents such as phorbol myristate acetate (PMA) and lipopolysaccharide (LPS) have been shown to be potent stimulators of prostaglandin synthesis. The effects of endotoxic LPS on the production of PGE by mouse peritoneal macrophages were demonstrated to occur in a dose-dependent manner; progressive increase in PGE production was observed over a range of 0.1–20 μg LPS/ml (Kurtland *et al.*, 1978). Although LPS is an active soluble stimulus, its prostaglandin-stimulating activity is not as potent as is PMA. This stimulus, at nanomolar concentrations, has been shown to significantly increase the synthesis and release of both PGE and 6-keto-$PGF_{1\alpha}$ (Humes *et al.*, 1978).

As discussed previously, unopsonized zymosan can provide a phagocytic stimulus for the synthesis and release of large amounts of PGE_2 and 6-keto-$PGF_{1\alpha}$ from resident macrophages. Although this observation is of scientific merit, it may not be as important as the release of prostaglandins from immune complex-treated macrophages. Recent evidence has demonstrated antigen-antibody complexes formed at equivalence can stimulate the release of arachidonic acid and the synthesis of both PGe_2 and 6-keto-$PGF_{1\alpha}$ from mouse resident macrophages (Bonney *et al.*, 1979). The release of both prostaglandins is stimulated by as little as 2 μg/ml of immune complexes and the production increases in a dose-dependent manner. As with the other stimuli which increase prostaglandin synthesis and release, the immune complex-induced release occurs in a time-dependent manner. Also, the synthesis of prostaglandins by all of the above inflammatory stimuli can be inhibited by either indomethacin or physiological levels of glucocorticoids.

While the above discussion has been restricted to resident macrophages, it must be pointed out that activated macrophages can also synthesize prostaglandins (Farzod *et al.*, 1977). A fundamental difference between resident and activated macrophages appears to lie in the basal level of prostaglandin synthesis. Resident macrophages synthesize very low basal levels of prostaglandins and can respond to a specific stimulus by synthesizing and releasing prostaglandins many fold above their baseline. Recruited macrophages appear to produce a higher basal level of prostaglandins, but do not produce an excess amount upon stimulation. Investigations concerning the quantitation and characterization of prostaglandin synthetase products from resident, elicited, and other mononuclear phagocyte populations can be found in recent reviews (Davies *et al.*, 1980; Bockman, 1981).

4. MODULATION OF *IN VITRO* MACROPHAGE CELL FUNCTION BY PROSTAGLANDINS

A clear understanding of the control mechanisms which regulate the physiological changes in various macrophage populations would have its obvious benefits in the comprehension of inflammatory responses. This is especially true since various macrophage populations are involved in diverse immune/ inflammatory functions. Since many of the prostaglandins possess potent cell-regulating activity, these polyoxygenated fatty acids have been implicated in modulating the physiological function of macrophage populations and altering immune responsiveness. The ability of prostaglandins to immunoregulate macrophage function could constitute a natural means to limit inflammatory tissue damage due to a number of phlogistic products. Recent experimental evidence has demonstrated that toxic oxygen by-products, including superoxide anion, hydrogen peroxide, and hydroxyl radicals, can be generated by various macrophage populations and are extremely reactive to both invasive organisms and host tissue (Klebanoff and Hansen, 1975; Babior, 1978; Johnson *et al.*, 1981). Interestingly, the release of these reactive oxygen products can be modulated *in vitro* by exogenous prostaglandins, especially of the E series. The release of superoxide anion from elicited mouse peritoneal macrophages was shown to be significantly inhibited by PGE_1 (Smith and Weidemann, 1980; Weidemann *et al.*, 1978). In the previous studies, inhibition of chemiluminescence was detected by PGE_1 treatment of macrophages challenged with either a particulate stimulus, zymosan, or a soluble stimulus, the calcium ionophore A23187 (Table 1). However, equal molar concentrations of PGE_1 had no significant effect on chemiluminescence induced by the mono hydroperoxy fatty acid, 15-hydroperoxyeicosatetraenoic acid (15-HPETE) (Smith and Weidemann, 1980). This is an important observation suggesting that the inhibition of reactive oxygen products by PGE_1 treatment is somewhat specific. Suppression of specific superoxide anion production by macrophages has also been demonstrated by both PGE_1 and PGE_2 (Lehmeyer and Johnson, 1978). In this set of experiments superoxide anion levels were determined spectrophotometrically as the superoxide dismutase-inhibitable reduction of ferricytochrome C, which measures only the extracellular superoxide, that which would be available for tissue damage. Inhibition of O_2^- production by mononuclear phagocytes was observed consistently at both 10^{-5} and 10^{-6} M PGE_1 or PGF_2. If theophylline is added in addition to PGE in the above system, an even further, additive reduction was observed with regard to the release of this toxic oxygen species.

The evidence that theophylline, an inhibitor of phosphodiesterase activity, can enhance the suppressive effect of PGE compounds implicates the cAMP system as a mode of prostaglandin inhibitor action. Although the actual cellular site where PGE/cAMP exerts this inhibitory response is not clear, evidence suggests that increases in intracellular cAMP by the addition of dibutyryl derivatives also can reduce the chemiluminescence response.

TABLE 1. SUMMARY OF THE INHIBITION OF REACTIVE OXYGEN PRODUCTS RELEASED FROM MONONUCLEAR PHAGOCYTES BY VARIOUS PROSTAGLANDINS

Macrophage	Prostaglandin (concn)	Stimulus	Percent inhibition of reactive oxygen release[a]	Reference
Bone marrow-derived (mouse)	PGE_1 (2.8 μM)	Zymosan	39	Weidemann *et al.* (1978)
	PGE_2 (2.8 μM)	Zymosan	29	Weidemann *et al.* (1978)
	$PGF_{2\alpha}$ (2.8 μM)	Zymosan	7	Weidemann *et al.* (1978)
Thioglycollate-elicited, peritoneal-derived (mouse)	PGE_1 (20 μM)	Zymosan	37	Smith and Weidemann (1980)
	PGE_1 (20 μM)	A23187	80	Smith and Weidemann (1980)
	PGE_1 (20 μM)	15-HPETE[b]	4	Smith and Weidemann (1980)
Blood monocytes (human)	PGE_1 (1 μM) PGE_2 (1 μM)	IgG-coated filters	41	Lehmeyer and Johnson (1978)

[a]Inhibition based on reduction in chemiluminescence as compared to nontreated controls.
[b]15-Hydroperoxyeicosatetraenoic acid.

In addition to modulating the release of phlogistic mediators, prostaglandins have also been implicated in controlling macrophage cellular movement and phagocytosis (Oropeza-Rendon *et al.*, 1979). PGE_1, but not $PGF_{2\alpha}$, was demonstrated to reduce the phagocytosis of zymosan particles in a dose-dependent manner. Even at the lowest dose of PGE_1 examined, 10^{-9} M, there was still a 60% reduction in the phagocytic index compared to non-PGE_1-treated macrophages. Inhibition of phagocytosis, a paramount functional feature of the macrophage, by PGE_1 may again be due to increasing intracellular levels of cAMP, since both phagocytosis and unidirectional cell movement in other granulocyte systems have been shown to be under the control of intracellular cAMP levels (Rivikin *et al.*, 1975).

It is interesting to note that the ability to down-regulate inflammatory cell (i.e., macrophage) functions appears to be a feature characteristic of prostaglandins of the E series. This phenomenon is not observed with F-type prostaglandins. (Although PGI_2 may suppress inflammatory cell functions, an in-depth study remains to verify the exact role for this prostaglandin in the inflammatory response.) What may prove to be an important regulating system is the actual ratio of PGE : PGF in the inflammatory environment surrounding the various inflammatory cells, including the macrophage. As the ratio of PGE : PGF fluctuates, so may the inflammatory cell responsiveness.

As discussed in the previous section, various macrophage populations can synthesize prostaglandins in response to a given stimulus. It is generally accepted that prostaglandins released by macrophages *in vivo* can influence the activity of other immune cells. This is especially true in the regulation of lymphocyte function, where mononuclear phagocytes can suppress T-cell mitogenic activity through the production of PGE (Goodwin *et al.*, 1977; Goodwin and Webb, 1980). There is also evidence that the prostaglandins produced by macrophages can affect the activity of the macrophage itself. Prostaglandins of the E series can inhibit proliferation of the committed macrophage stem cell; therefore, macrophages may inhibit the proliferation of their own progenitor by the production of prostaglandins (Kurtland *et al.*, 1978). Thus, it appears the macrophage, through prostaglandin production, may greatly influence its own destiny.

5. MODULATION OF MACROPHAGE-DEPENDENT GRANULOMATOUS REACTIONS BY PROSTAGLANDINS: ANIMAL MODELS OF GRANULOMATOUS INFLAMMATION

The proliferative lesions found in chronic granulomatous diseases have generally been characterized as proliferative-necrotic/fibrotic or proliferative-nonecrotic (Oort and Scheper, 1977). With regard to animal models, the former is exemplified by true immune granulomas, BCG-induced granulomas, and schistosome egg-induced granulomas, while the latter is characterized by foreign body granulomas such as carrageenan sponge implants and Sephadex beads. Both foreign body and true immune granulomas have been used to examine the *in vivo* interactions between macrophages and prostaglandins. In the following discussion we will examine the ability of exogenous prostaglandins to regulate the above animal models of granuloma formation and scrutinize *in vivo* and *in vitro* interactions between prostaglandins and macrophages.

5.1. PROSTAGLANDIN SYNTHESIS AND RELEASE DURING GRANULOMA FORMATION

Although PGE_2 is generally accepted as the major prostaglandin found in granulomas, different laboratories have published quantitatively varied results concerning PGE_2 levels from granulomatous tissue (Bonta and Parnham, 1978b). Albeit PGE_2 is produced in high levels, significant amounts of thromboxane B_2 (TXB_2) and $PGF_{2\alpha}$ have also been observed during the early phase of the carrageenan sponge granuloma in the rat, while levels of the PGI_2 metabolite, 6-keto-$PGF_{1\alpha}$, remained unchanged (Tsurufuji *et al.*, 1978). The temporal sequence of PGE_2 production in the carrageenan granuloma was shown to progressively increase as the granulomatous reaction matured (Brogt and Bonta, 1979). Upon radioimmunoassay of tissue isolated from schistosome egg-induced granulomas, extremely high levels of PGE_2, $PGF_{2\alpha}$, and TXB_2 were also observed. Conversely, macrophages isolated from nonsynchronous schistosome egg-induced liver granulomas were shown to respond to opsonized zymosan by producing only a 1.7-fold increase above basal granuloma macrophage levels. Since the macrophages isolated from an active granulomatous lesion are in an activated state, the data described above corroborate those findings concerning PGE_2 production by thioglycollate-elicited macrophages (Humes *et al.*, 1977). Thus, elicited macrophages do not respond to a specific challenge with a large increase in cycloxygenase products.

5.2. REGULATION OF EXPERIMENTAL GRANULOMA FORMATION BY PROSTAGLANDINS

In chronic granulomatous inflammatory conditions there is considerable confusion over the exact role the prostaglandins play in the modulation of this chronic response. Since many experimental and clinical granulomas are self-abating, it is interesting to speculate that the macrophage–prostaglandin system may comprise a potent modulating entity. The ability of exogenous prostaglandin to regulate a nonimmune granuloma model (sponge implants) was examined by directly increasing PGE levels at the inflammatory site (Bonta and Parnham, 1979). The local administration of a single dose of PGE_1, during the early inflammatory phase, was demonstrated to stimulate granulomatous tissue formation. On the contrary, repeated local administration of PGE_1, after the appearance of inflammatory cells, inhibited the formation of additional granulomatous tissue (Bonta and Parnham, 1978a). This inhibitory dose of PGE_1 was of a comparable order of magnitude as has been reported in certain inflammatory exudates (Trang, 1977). When given under the same experimental conditions as outlined above, PGE_2, but not PGI_2, was observed to suppress the sponge implant-induced granuloma. Further investigations have demonstrated that a deficiency in PGE_1 production (through dietary manipulations) can lead to a diminished infiltration of inflammatory cells while enhancing the proliferative components of the granulomatous response (Bonta *et al.*, 1977). The latter observation can be reversed by the addition of exogenous PGE. It is becoming more evident that the presence of PGE_2 in a granulomatous inflammatory reaction may play a homeostatic role by inhibiting the proliferative events characteristic of inflammatory disorders.

Recent experimental evidence has demonstrated that *in vivo* treatment of a true immune granuloma with various prostaglandins can drastically alter the course of the granulomatous response. Specifically, we have shown that PGE_1 treatment can suppress the schistosome egg-induced liver and lung granulomatous response. As shown in Fig. 2, treatment of experimental animals from day 1 of egg challenge with a stable analog of PGE_1 (15-S-15-methyl PGE_1) (15M-PGE_1) significantly inhibited the lung granuloma development at days 4, 8, and 16. On the other hand, $PGF_{2\alpha}$ treatment actually enhanced the developing granuloma at each of the above time points. There is no significant difference between the area of a 16-day granuloma from a PGE_1-treated animal, as compared to the area of a 4-day granuloma from a nontreated animal. Also, the granuloma size from 15M-PGE_1-treated animals peaks at day 8 and, at this time point, represents a 50% suppression of the normal granulomatous response. By day 16 the 15M-PGE-treated animals exhibit a 75% reduction in the size of the schistome egg-induced lung granuloma, as compared to controls. The enhancement of lung granuloma formation by $PGF_{2\alpha}$ treatment can particularly be noted

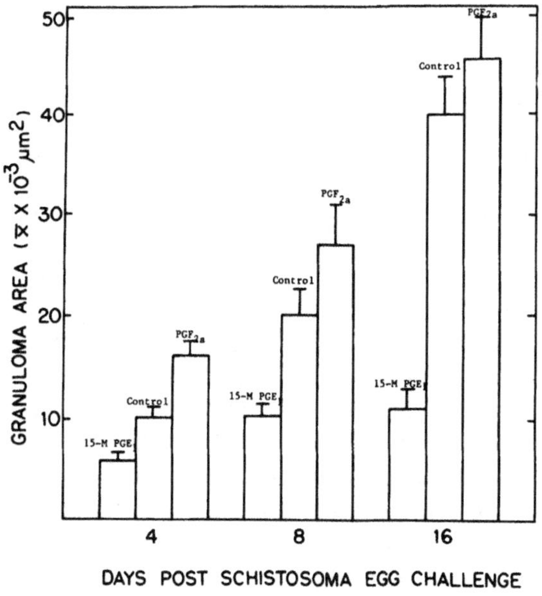

FIGURE 2. Modulation of schistosome egg-induced lung granuloma formation by prostaglandins. CBA-J mice were treated from day 1 of egg challenge with 1 μg prostaglandin/g body weight.

at day 4. At this early time point there is a 40% increase in lung granuloma size, above control values. Although by day 16 the control and $PGF_{2\alpha}$-treated granulomas approach the same size, the granulomas contained in the $PGF_{2\alpha}$-treated animals still are statistically larger than the controls. From this initial observation it appears that $PGF_{2\alpha}$ may be accelerating the immune granulomatous response and thus may be an extremely significant inflammatory mediator with regard to "turning on" certain granulomatous responses. The vast differences in the granulomatous response between $PGF_{2\alpha}$- and 15M-PGE_1-treated animals again may reflect the importance of the PGE : PGF ratio in a given inflammatory environment. Or, the PGE : PGF ratio in the inflammatory milieu may dictate the concentration of intracellular second messengers, cAMP and cGMP, both of which have profound effects on the individual inflammatory cells comprising a lesion. For example, cholera toxin, a potent β-adrenergic agent, can suppress both primary lung granulomas (induced by egg embolization) and the secondary granulomatous response, induced by egg embolization plus exogenous sensitized lymphocytes (Warren *et al.*, 1974). It is well established that the molecular target of both prostaglandins of the E series and cholera toxin is the membrane-bound adenylate cyclase system (Rivikin *et al.*, 1975).

Histologically at day 16, there is a striking difference between the lung granulomas of prostaglandin E- and F-treated animals and the non-prostaglandin-treated controls. As shown in Fig. 3, granuloma size and histology vary considerably depending upon the treatment regimen. The granulomas from the 15M-PGE_1-treated animals are obviously suppressed and appear to be of the same size and cellular composition as many nonspecific foreign body granulomas. Thus, PGE compounds may be important in modulating the recruit-

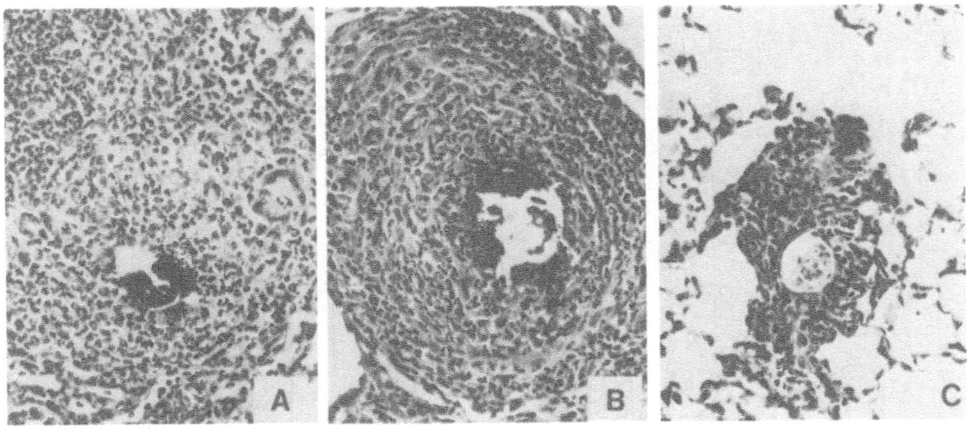

FIGURE 3. Modulation of egg granulomas by $PGF_{2\alpha}$ and 15M-PGE_1. (A) 16-day lung granuloma from animal treated with 1 μg $PGF_{2\alpha}$/g body weight; note the large number of giant macrophages and the enhancement of granuloma size. (B) 16-day lung granuloma from nontreated mice. (C) 16-day lung granuloma from 15M-PGE_1-treated mice (1 μg/g body weight); significant suppression of granuloma size can be easily observed. All animals were treated daily post egg challenge. Photographs are representative lesions of each group (200×).

ment of specific cells in a given granuloma. An observation which appears more subtle than the size of the granuloma from PGE-treated animals, is the number of large multinucleated giant macrophages which are seen in the lung granulomas from the $PGF_{2\alpha}$-treated animals. Although this point may seem trivial, these giant macrophages may play an extremely important role with respect to the production and release of inflammatory mediators and the suppression of these products by prostaglandins.

5.3. *IN VITRO* MODULATION OF GRANULOMA MACROPHAGE FUNCTION BY PROSTAGLANDINS

It has been well established that the macrophage is by far the basic constituent of both hypersensitivity (e.g., schistosome egg-induced granulomas) and foreign body (e.g., sponge/carrageenan implants) granulomatous reactions (Boros, 1978). The capacity of macrophages to multiply and become epithelioid or giant cells, their longevity, and their ability to secrete lysosomal enzymes and toxic oxygen products provide for a powerful array of armaments to contain an inflammatory stimuli. In examining one of the above parameters, we have shown that macrophages isolated from synchronous lung granulomas possess the ability to synthesize significant levels of superoxide anion (O_2^-). Superoxide anion production by phorbol myristate acetate-stimulated macrophages was demonstrated to increase as the lung granulomatous lesion matured. In assays of 1×10^6 granuloma macrophages, we observed a linear increase in O_2^- production ranging from 4 nmoles/10^6 cells per 2 hr from day 4 granulomas to 26 nmoles/10^6 cells per 2 hr from day 16 granulomas. An observation of special

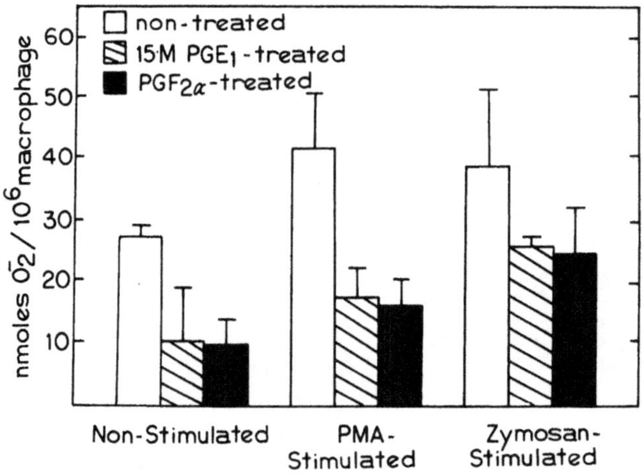

FIGURE 4. Suppression of superoxide anion (O_2^-) release from nonsynchronous 8-week hepatic granuloma macrophages by prostaglandins. Animals were treated with the various prostaglandins (1 μg/g body weight) 5 days prior to sacrifice. Macrophages were treated *in vivo* with the particular prostaglandin and challenge stimulated *in vitro* with 50 μg/ml PMA or 1 mg/ml zymosan.

importance here is the large number of giant cells from the day 16 granulomas as compared to day 4. The production of O_2^- from macrophages isolated from those granulomas which are naturally resolving is presently not known.

The ability of exogenous prostaglandins to act as a "down-modulating" mediator of O_2^- production by granuloma macrophages is shown in Fig. 4. The macrophages from hepatic granulomas were treated *in vivo* with the prostaglandins and challenged with either PMA or opsonized zymosan *in vitro*. Both the $PGF_{2\alpha}$ and the PGE_1 treatment were shown to decrease the amount of O_2^- released from the granuloma macrophages challenged with either of the stimuli. Although there were no statistical differences between the two prostaglandin groups, there was an obvious reduction in the O_2^- released between the macrophages from non-prostaglandin- and prostaglandin-treated animals. Therefore, it appears that certain prostaglandins can exert a profound influence on macrophage cellular function in both *in vitro* and *in vivo* experiments.

6. CONCLUDING REMARKS

Chronic granulomatous inflammatory reactions are predominantly the host macrophage reactions to persisting tissue irritants. The duration, intensity, and final resolution of the granuloma depend mainly on the chemical and biological activity of the irritant as well as the resulting host immune response. The key element of the latter is the extent and degree of macrophage activation. Minimal macrophage activation may result in a quiescent granulomatous lesion with minor fibrosis and negligible tissue damage. Conversely, highly activated macrophages may result in extensive fibrosis and significant tissue damage. As discussed above and described elsewhere (Davies and Allison, 1976), macrophages examined from various sites can release phlogistic mediators and regulate (enhance or suppress) inflammatory lesions. It is very possible that the prostaglandins, especially those of the E series, represent an arm of these mediators and play an important role in the modulation of macrophage-dependent inflammatory reactions; conceivably by down-regulating various inflammatory cells, including the macrophage itself, which make up the granulomatous lesion. A plethora of basic questions remain to be answered concerning macrophage–prostaglandin interactions in a granulomatous lesion. Of particular interest in the true immune hypersensitivity granuloma is the role of prostaglandins as modulators of macrophage–lymphocyte, macrophage–fibroblast, and macrophage–macrophage interactions. The observations supporting the role of prostaglandins as suppressors of tissue destruction and possible regulators of fibrotic reactions, should provide the kindling for an in-depth examination of the interactions between prostaglandins and macrophages in chronic granulomatous lesions.

ACKNOWLEDGMENTS. The authors' research reported herein was supported by NIH Grants HL-23192, HL-26809, HL-07517, HL-00889, and GM-28499.

REFERENCES

Babior, B. M., 1978, Oxygen-dependent microbial killing by phagocytes, *N. Engl. J. Med.* **298:**659.

Bockman, R. S., 1981, Prostaglandin production by human blood monocytes and mouse peritoneal macrophages: Synthesis dependent on *in vitro* culture conditions, *Prostaglandins* **21:**9.

Bonney, R. J., Wightman, P. D., Davies, P., Kuehl, F. A., and Humes, J. L., 1978, Regulation of prostaglandin synthesis and of selective release of lysosomal hydrolases by mouse peritoneal macrophage, *Biochem. J.* **176:**433.

Bonney, R. J., Naruns, P., Davies, P., and Humes, J. L., 1979, Antigen–antibody complexes stimulate the synthesis and release of prostaglandins by mouse peritoneal macrophages, *Prostaglandins* **18:**605.

Bonta, I. L., and Parnham, M. J., 1978a, Prostaglandins and chronic inflammation, *Biochem. Pharmacol.* **27:**1611.

Bonta, I. L., and Parnham, M. J., 1978b, Time-dependent pro and anti-inflammatory effects of prostaglandin (PG) E_1 on experimental granulomata in rats, *Br. J. Pharmacol.* **62:** 417.

Bonta, I. L., and Parnham, M. J., 1979, Cannulated sponge implants in rats for the study of time-dependent pharmacological influences on inflammatory granulomatous. *J. Pharmacol. Methods* **2:**1.

Bonta, I. L., Parnham, M. J., and Adolfs, M. J. P., 1977, Reduced exudation and increased tissue proliferation during chronic inflammation in rats deprived of endogenous prostaglandin precursors, *Prostaglandins* **14:**295.

Boros, D. L., 1978, Granulomatous inflammations, *Prog. Allergy* **24:**183.

Brogt, P. C., and Bonta, I. L., 1979, *In vivo* metabolism of [1-^{14}C]arachidonic acid during different phases of granuloma development in the rat, *Biochem. Pharmacol.* **28:**1581.

Davies, P., and Allison, A. C., 1976, The macrophage as a secretory cell in chronic inflammation, *Agents Actions* **6:**60.

Davies, P., Bonney, R. J., Humes, J. L., and Kuehl, F. A. 1980, The synthesis of arachidonic acid oxygenation products by various mononuclear phagocyte populations, in: *Mononuclear Phagocytes* (R. van Furth, ed.), pp. 1317–1350, Nijhoff, The Hague.

Farzod, A., Penneys, N. S., Ghaffar, A., Zibah, V. A., and Schlassberg, J., 1977, PGE_2 and $PGF_{2\alpha}$ biosynthesis in stimulated and nonstimulated peritoneal preparations containing macrophages, *Prostaglandins* **14:**829.

Goldyne, M. E., 1977, Prostaglandins and the modulation of immunological responses, *Int. J. Dermatol.* **16:**701.

Goodwin, J. S., and Webb, D. R., 1980, Regulation of the immune response by prostaglandins, *Clin. Immunol. Immunopathol.* **15:**106.

Goodwin, J. S., Bankhurst, A. D., and Messner, R. P., 1977, Suppression of human T-cell mitogenesis by prostaglandin: Existence of a prostaglandin-producing suppressor cell, *J. Exp. Med.* **146:**1719.

Hansen, H. S., 1976, 15-Hydroxyprostaglandin dehydrogenase: A review, *Prostaglandins* **12:**647.

Henney, C. S., Bourne, H. R., and Lichtenstein, L. M., 1971, The role of cyclic AMP in the specific cytolytic activity of lymphocytes, *J. Immunol.* **108:**1526.

Higgs, G. A., Higgs, E. A., and Solman, J. A., 1979, Prostacyclin and inflammation, in: Prostacyclin (J. R. Vane and S. Bergstrom, eds.), pp. 187–193, Raven Press, New York.

Horton, E. W., 1979, Prostanoids in health and disease, in: *Chemistry, Biochemistry, and Pharmacological Activity of Prostanoids* (S. M. Roberts and F. Scheinmann, eds.), pp. 1–16, Pergamon Press, Elmsford, N.Y.

Humes, J. L., Bonney, R. J., Pelus, L., Dahlgron, M. E., Kuehl, F. A., and Davies, P., 1977, Macrophages synthesize and release prostaglandins in response to inflammatory stimuli, *Nature (London)* **269:**149.

Humes, J. L., Davies, P., Bonney, R. J., and Kuehl, F. A., 1978, Phorbol myristate acetate (PMA) stimulates the release of arachidonic acid and its cyclooxygenation products by macrophages, *Fed. Proc.* **37:**1318.

Johnson, K. J., Fantone, J. C., Kaplan, J., and Ward, P. A., 1981, *In vivo* damage of rat lungs by oxygen metabolites, *J. Clin. Invest.* **67:**983.

Klebanoff, S. J., and Hansen, C. B., 1975, Antimicrobial systems of mononuclear phagocytes, in: *Mononuclear Phagocytes in Immunity, Infection and Pathology* (R. van Furth, ed.), pp. 507–517, Blackwell, Oxford.

Kunkel, S. L., Thrall, R. S., Kunkel, R. G., Ward, P. A., and Zurier, R. B., 1979, Suppression of immune complex vasculitis in rats by prostaglandins, *J. Clin. Invest.* **64**:1525.

Kunkel, S. L., Fantone, J. C., Ward, P. A., and Zurier, R. B., 1981a, Modulation of inflammatory reactions by prostaglandins, *Prog. Lipid Res.* **20**:249.

Kunkel, S. L., Ogawa, H., Conran, P., Ward, P. W., and Zurier, R. B., 1981b, Suppression of acute and chronic inflammation by orally administered prostaglandins, *Arthritis Rheum.* **24**:1151.

Kurtland, J. I., Broxmeyer, H. E., Pelus, L. M., Bickman, R. S., Moore, M. A. S., 1978, Role for monocyte-macrophage-derived colony-stimulating factor and prostaglandin E in the positive and negative feedback control of myeloid stem cell proliferation, *Blood* **52**:388.

Lehmeyer, J. E., and Johnson, R. B., 1978, Effects of anti-inflammatory drugs and agents that elevate intracellular cyclic AMP on the release of toxic oxygen metabolites by phagocytes: Studies in a model of tissue-bound IgG, *Clin. Immunol. Immunopathol.* **9**:482.

Lichtenstein, L. M., and DiBernardo, R., 1971, The immediate allergic response: *In vitro* action of cyclic AMP and other drugs on the two stages of histamine release, *J. Immunol.* **107**:1131.

Oort, J., and Scheper, R. J., 1977, Histopathology of acute and chronic inflammation, *Agents Actions Suppl.* **3**:25.

Oropeza-Rendon, R. L., Speth, V., Hiller, G., Weber, K., and Fischer, H., 1979, Prostaglandin E_1 reversibly induces morphological changes in macrophages and inhibits phagocytosis, *Exp. Cell Res.* **119**:365.

Parker, C. W., 1972, The role of prostaglandins in the immune response, in: *Prostaglandins in Cellular Biology* (P. W. Ramwell and B. B. Pharriss, eds.), pp. 173–190, Academic Press, New York.

Pelus, L. M., and Strausser, H. R., 1977, Prostaglandins and the immune response, *Life Sci.* **20**:903.

Ramwell, P., 1980, General introduction to clinical implications of prostaglandin synthetase inhibition, in: *Prostaglandin Synthetase Inhibitors: New Clinical Applications* (P. Ramwell, ed.), p. 5, Liss, New York.

Rivikin, I., Rosenblatt, J., and Becker, E. L., 1975, The role of cyclic AMP in the chemotactic responsiveness and spontaneous motility of rabbit peritoneal neutrophils, *J. Immunol.* **115**:1126.

Smith, R. L., and Weidemann, M. J., 1980, Reactive oxygen production associated with arachidonic acid metabolism by peritoneal macrophages, *Biochem. Biophys. Res. Commun.* **97**:973.

Trang, L. E., 1977, Levels of prostaglandin F_2 alpha and E_1 and thromboxane B_1 in joint fluid in rheumatoid arthritis, *Scand. J. Rheum.* **6**:151.

Tsurufuji, S., Sato, H., Min, K. R., and Ohuchi, K., 1978, Difference in the anti-inflammatory effects of indomethacin between acute and chronic stages of carrageenin-induced inflammation, *J. Pharm. Dyn.* **1**:8.

Vane, J. R., 1976, Prostaglandin as mediators of inflammation in: *Advances in Prostaglandin and thromboxane Research* (B. Samuelson and R. Paoletti, ed.), *Raven Press, New York*, pp. 791–798.

Warren, K. S., Mahmoud, A. A. F., Boros, D. L., Rall, T. W., and Carpenter, C. C. J., 1974, *In vivo* suppression by cholera toxin of cell-mediated and foreign body inflammatory response. *J. Immunol.* **112**:996.

Weidemann, M. J., Peskar, B. A., Wrongemann, K., Reitschel, E. T., and Fischer, H., 1978, Prostaglandin and thromboxane synthesis in a pure macrophage population and the inhibition, by E-type prostaglandins, of chemiluminescence, *FEBS Lett.* **89**:136.

Zurier, R. B., Weissman, G., Hoffstein, S., Kammermann, S., and Tiu, M. H., 1974, Mechanisms of lysosomal enzyme release from human leukocytes. II. Effects of cAMP and cGMP, autonomic agonists and agents which affect microtubule function, *J. Clin. Invest.* **53**:297.

Zurier, R. B., Damjarrow, I., Miller, P. L., and Biewer, B. F., 1978, Prostaglandin E treatment prevents progression of nephritis in murine lupus erythematosus, *J. Clin. Lab. Immunol.* **1**:95.

15

Monocyte-Mediated Antibody-Dependent Cellular Cytotoxicity

DAVID G. POPLACK, DIANE E. COLE, and USHA SRINIVASAN

1. INTRODUCTION

During the past decade there has been increasing interest in the role of the mononuclear phagocyte in the immune response. It is now appreciated that these cells subserve a variety of important immunologic functions. In addition to their classical function of removing debris (such as senescent cells) from the circulation, mononuclear phagocytes are involved in antigen processing, antimicrobial resistance, antineoplastic activity, mediation of inflammation, control of granulopoiesis, and regulation of the immune response (Poplack and Blaese, 1980).

Considerable interest has been focused on the cytotoxic activity of monocytes and macrophages, a function which is believed to play a significant role in resistance to infection, tumor rejection, and certain "autoimmune" reactions. One mechanism by which mononuclear phagocytes are capable of invoking cytolysis is via antibody-dependent cellular cytotoxicity (ADCC). This process involves the destruction of a target cell by a nonimmune effector cell in the presence of an appropriate antitarget antibody. ADCC has been observed in a variety of *in vitro* human and animal systems which have employed a number of target cells including erythrocytes, lymphoid cells, tumors cells, and virally infected cultured cell lines. In addition, ADCC systems have been described for a number of different effector cells including promonocytes, monocytes/ macrophages, polymorphonuclear neutrophils, and lymphocytes. Although ADCC reactions have been extensively studied *in vitro,* to some extent their role *in vivo* remains speculative. However, there is increasing evidence that this process is a clinically significant one in man.

A common property of effector cells which are capable of mediating ADCC

DAVID G. POPLACK, DIANE E. COLE, and USHA SRINIVASAN • Pediatric Branch, National Cancer Institute, Bethesda, Maryland 20205.

is that they bear receptors for the Fc portion of IgG (MacDonald *et al.*, 1975; Shaw *et al.*, 1978). These receptors allow stable effector cell–target cell contact, a necessary prerequisite for target cell lysis (Milgrom and Shore, 1978). Another important feature of ADCC is that the type of target cell and the specific anti-target antibody appear to dictate the nature of the effector cell which mediates cytolysis (Milgrom and Shore, 1978; Nelson *et al.*, 1979; Shaw *et al.*, 1978; Klassen and Sagone, 1980; MacDonald *et al.*, 1975).

In this chapter we will discuss those ADCC reactions which are mediated by viable, functionally capable monocytes and/or macrophages (monocyte-mediated ADCC, MMADCC). The next section will attempt to describe the MMADCC phenomenon, what is known about the mechanism of the reaction as well as what factors may influence it; the last section will discuss the significance of MMADCC to *in vivo* monocyte function and clinically described disease processes.

2. MMADCC *IN VITRO*

In an early description of the interaction between monocytes and antibody-coated red blood cells (RBCs), LoBuglio *et al.* (1967) noted that type O Rh-positive cells coated with the IgG fraction of a hyperimmune anti-D antiserum bound firmly to human monocytes *in vitro*. This binding was followed by rapid morphological injury to the RBCs characterized by sphering, deformity, fragmentation, and profoundly increased osmotic fragility.

In 1972, Holm, expanding upon this observation, utilized a ^{51}Cr release method for *in vitro* quantitation of cell-mediated lysis of human RBCs and determined that human leukocytes or peritoneal macrophages, but not purified blood lymphocytes, could damage these RBCs in the presence of isologous or heterologous hyperimmune antisera. Subsequent studies by his group further confirmed the monocyte specificity of the killing of antibody-coated human erythrocytes. Purified monocytes and lymphocytes were tested for *in vitro* cytotoxicity against blood group A erythrocytes which had been treated with the IgG fraction of human hyperimmune anti-A serum. In the adherent purified monocyte preparation, the calculated killing of RBCs was 2–3 per monocyte; in contrast, the nonadherent population (lymphocytes) showed little or no lytic activity against the human erythrocyte targets. Since that time a number of different *in vitro* monocyte-mediated ADCC systems have been described (Table 1). What all of these systems have in common is that monocytes effect the killing of antibody-coated target cells.

As noted in Table 1, the majority of commonly used *in vitro* MMADCC systems utilize erythrocytes as targets. There are practical reasons for this. Both human RBCs and their specific anti-blood group antisera are easy to obtain in sufficient quantities. In addition, these systems have well-defined antigen–antibody interactions. Most importantly, it has been in this type of system that monocytes have been demonstrated to be the sole effector cell mediating lysis. This latter fact makes this type of MMADCC system most applicable for the study of monocyte effector function in man.

TABLE 1. ADCC SYSTEMS IN WHICH MONOCYTES FUNCTION AS EFFECTOR CELLS[a]

Target	Antibody	Reference
Human type A RBCs	Human hyperimmune anti-A	Holm (1972), Holm and Hammarstrom (1973), MacDonald *et al.* (1975), Fleer *et al.* (1978)
	Rabbit hyperimmune anti-A	Holm (1972)
Human type B RBCs	Human hyperimmune anti-B	Poplack *et al.* (1976), Nelson *et al.* (1979)
TNP-modified human type B RBCs	Goat anti-TNP, monkey anti-TNP	Nelson *et al.* (1979)
Human type 0 RBCs Rh positive	Anti-D	Kurlander *et al.* (1978), Fleer *et al.* (1978), Yust *et al.* (1980)
	Anti-CD	Shaw *et al.* (1978)
Sheep RBCs	Rat anti-SRBC	Hersey (1973)
Chicken RBCs	Rabbit hyperimmune anti-CRBC	MacDonald *et al.* (1975), Poplack *et al.* (1976), Nelson *et al.* (1979), Keaney *et al.* (1980)
β-Glutaraldehyde-treated chicken RBCs	Rat anti-CRBC	Gagnon and Joshua (1980)
Lymphoid cells	Sera from patients with SLE, transplantation rejections, multiparous women	Jonny *et al.* (1979)
Human T-lymphoblastoid cell line (CEM)	Rabbit hyperimmune anti-CEM	Klassen and Sagone (1980)
HSV-infected Chang liver cells	Human anti-HSV	Kohl *et al.* (1977)
TLx9 murine lymphoma of C57BL	Rabbit anti-TLx9	Mantovani *et al.* (1977)

[a]In some of these systems, lymphocytes may also mediate some ADCC activity.

One such MMADCC assay used in our laboratory is a "micro" modification of the system first described by Poplack *et al.* (1976). Target cells consist of human type B erythrocytes which are washed three times in isotonic buffered medium. RBCs (1×10^8) in 0.1 ml are radiolabeled during a 30-min 37°C incubation with 0.1 mCi $Na^{51}CrO_4$. The cells are then washed three times and adjusted to 4×10^6 cells/ml. Effector mononuclear cells are isolated from whole blood collected in preservative-free heparin. The peripheral blood mononuclear cell fraction (PBMC) is isolated by centrifugation over Ficoll–Hypaque (Boyum, 1968), washed three times, and adjusted to 2×10^6 cells/ml in RPMI-1640 supplemented with 10% fetal bovine serum. In a 96-well round-bottomed Linbro tissue culture plate, triplicate samples consisting of 100 μl PBMC, 50 μl ^{51}Cr-RBCs, and either 50 μl of hyperimmune anti-B serum ("test") or 50 μl medium ("control") are aliquoted. Following an 18-hr incubation at 37°C in a humidified 5% CO_2–95% air atmosphere, supernatants are harvested using a Titertek harvesting system and counts of ^{51}Cr released into the supernatant are quantitated:

$$\text{Percent RBCs lysed} = \%\ \text{specific release} = \frac{\begin{matrix}\text{average} \\ \text{counts in} \\ \text{"test"}\end{matrix} - \begin{matrix}\text{average} \\ \text{counts in} \\ \text{"control"}\end{matrix}}{\begin{matrix}\text{"total} \\ \text{releasable"} \\ \text{counts}\end{matrix} - \begin{matrix}\text{background} \\ \text{counts}\end{matrix}} \times 100$$

where "total releasable" counts are determined by incubating 50 μl ^{51}Cr RBCs with 150 μl of lysing buffer and "background" counts are derived from spontaneous lysis of RBCs in medium (50 μl ^{51}Cr RBCs + 150 μl medium). The percentage of monocytes in each preparation is determined by examination of nonspecific esterase-stained cytocentrifuge-prepared slides (Koski *et al.*, 1976) and the number of RBCs killed per monocyte is quantitated. PBMCs prepared in this way usually contain 20–30% esterase-positive cells (monocytes), resulting in an effector : target ratio of approximately 1 : 4. In this system a single normal monocyte is capable of mediating the lysis of 2–3 RBCs.

Depletion studies in which the monocytes were removed from the PBMC preparation demonstrated complete abrogation of cytotoxicity, confirming that in this particular system only the monocytes present in the mononuclear cell preparation are capable of mediating the ADCC reaction. As noted earlier, in any ADCC system the type of target cell and the specific antitarget antibody appear to dictate the nature of the effector cell which mediates cytolysis. Studies in systems similar to that described above have investigated (1) the contribution of the target cell and antibody to MMADCC, (2) the influence of various factors upon the *in vitro* MMADCC, and (3) the mechanism of target cell lysis.

2.1. NATURE OF THE TARGET CELL

It is now apparent that the nature of the target cell may profoundly influence the character of an MMADCC reaction. The influence of surface antigen orientation and its density on the target cell have been studied in depth. On human erythrocytes the number of antigenic sites present on type A or B RBCs (> 100,000 molecules/cell) is markedly different from that on type O Rh D-positive RBCs (15,000–30,000 D sites/cell). Kurlander *et al.* (1978) reported that optimal MMADCC of type O Rh-positive RBCs required the binding of only 1000–1500 molecules of purified anti-D per cell while specific lysis of type A (or type B) RBCs was less than 5% at 10,000 molecules of IgG anti-A (or IgG anti-B) per RBC. This suggests that the interaction between antibody-coated type A RBCs and monocytes requires a larger number of antigen–antibody binding sites than the interaction between monocytes and type O Rh-positive RBCs coated with anti-D serum.

The effect of enzymatic alteration of the erythrocyte membrane surface on MMADCC has also been studied in an attempt to evaluate the role of changes in membrane charge density and antigen configuration on the MMADCC reaction. Early investigators demonstrated that the use of trypsin-treated (Holm, 1972; Holm and Hammarstrom, 1973) or papain-treated (Urbaniak, 1976) human RBCs increased lysis in MMADCC. Milgrom and Shore (1977) confirmed that under normal conditions monocytes were the sole effector cells for human RBC lysis but noted that human RBCs treated with proteolytic enzymes (trypsin, papain) or neuraminidase were susceptible to lysis by lymphocytes as well as monocytes. These investigators hypothesized that this shift toward lymphocyte-mediated killing was due to a reduction in the surface charge density on the erythrocyte membrane as a consequence of the loss of sialic acid residues. In a more recent report, Yust *et al.* (1980a) confirmed that papain treatment of RBCs resulted in lysis by lymphocytes as well as monocytes; however, it did not appear to be the sole result of a reduction in surface charge. Using both transmission and scanning electron microscopy these investigators documented that enzyme treatment resulted in morphological changes in the RBCs which altered antigenic configuration and therefore antibody orientation.

Further evidence that the antigenic determinants on the cell surface influence the type of effector cell comes from experiments using TNP-modified erythrocyte targets (Nelson *et al.*, 1979). These studies demonstrated that while human type B RBCs coated with human hyperimmune anti-B serum were lysed only by monocytes, TNP-treated B RBCs could be lysed by either monocytes or lymphocytes.

2.2. NATURE OF THE ANTIBODY

In vitro red cells sensitized with non-complement-binding IgG antibodies adhere to mononuclear phagocytes as rosettes (LoBuglio *et al.*, 1967). This adherence of erythrocytes to monocytes leads to either cytolysis of the RBC outside the phagocyte or to phagocytosis with subsequent lysis (van der Meulen *et al.*, 1978). Studies fractionating the antierythrocyte antisera using a Sephadex G-200 column have demonstrated that RBC lysis is mediated only by the IgG fraction, not by IgM or IgA (Holm and Hammarstrom, 1973). Furthermore, it is known that human monocytes have receptors for the Fc portion of IgG, which preferentially bind IgG1 and IgG3. The work of Kurlander *et al.* (1978) supports the theory that MMADCC is mediated through these IgG subclasses by demonstrating that free IgG1 and IgG3 are 100 times more effective in inhibiting MMADCC of type O Rh^+ RBCs than either IgG2 or IgG4. Additionally, removal or alteration of the Fc fragment of the antibody by pepsin digestion or treatment with 2-mercaptoethanol (Lovchik and Hong, 1977) inhibits MMADCC.

2.3. OTHER FACTORS WHICH MAY INFLUENCE MMADCC

In addition to the three major factors which influence MMADCC (target, effector cell, and antibody) there have been a number of studies which have examined the role of a variety of other factors. Table 2 summarizes these studies. It is important to note that while a number of factors may inhibit the *in vitro* MMADCC reaction, none profoundly enhance it. Moreover, which of these factors are capable of effecting *in vivo* MMADCC is unclear.

TABLE 2. FACTORS WHICH INFLUENCE *IN VITRO* MMADCC

Factor	Effect upon MMADCC	Reference
Serum (fresh)	Increased	Kragballe *et al.* (1980), Kurlander *et al.* (1978)
Serum (heated)	Decreased	Kragballe *et al.* (1980)
Immune complexes	Decreased	Kragballe *et al.* (1980)
Platelets	Decreased	Kragballe *et al.* (1980)
Loading of monocytes with foreign particles:		
Carbonyl iron	Decreased	Holm and Hammarstrom (1973)
Heat-killed *Candida albicans*		
Latex		
Cell damage		
Silica	Decreased	O'Rourke *et al.* (1978)
Carrageenan		
Glucan	Decreased	Kohl *et al.* (1979)
Hypoxia (decreased O_2 pressure *in vitro*)	Decreased	Klassen and Sagone (1980), Borregaard and Kragballe (1980)
Radiation (3000–5000 rads)	No effect	Kovithavongs *et al.* (1975)
Antineoplastic agents		
Adriamycin	Decreased	Bolivar *et al.* (1980)
Cyclophosphamide		
Prednisone		
Procarbazine		
Vincristine		

2.4. MECHANISM OF LYSIS IN ADCC

The actual mechanism of lysis in MMADCC is incompletely understood. One necessary prerequisite for eventual target cell lysis is the stable adherence of the target to the effector cell. As alluded to above, van der Meulen *et al.* (1978) reported a strict correlation between adherence *in vitro* and the *in vivo* lysis of erythrocytes. In patients producing different subclasses of IgG autoantibodies, only those exhibiting IgG1 and IgG3 showed both adherence (rosetting) *in vitro* and overt signs of autoimmune hemolytic anemia. Those patients with IgG2 and IgG4 subclass antibodies demonstrated neither rosetting nor active *in vivo* hemolysis.

Erythrophagocytosis of antibody-coated cells by monocytes has been noted by many investigators. Although it has been demonstrated that this can be a mechanism of ^{51}Cr release from RBCs (Kurlander and Rosse, 1979), it is not believed to be the only mechanism (Hersey, 1973), since, in general, those chemicals which block phagocytosis do not inhibit ADCC. A variety of agents have been studied in this regard including the esterase inhibitors TLCK (tosyllysine chloromethyl ketone), PMSF (phenylmethane sulfonyl fluoride), and DFP (diisopropyl fluorophosphate); alkylating agents such as iodoacetic acid, NEM (*N*-ethylmaleimide), and PCMB (parachloromercuribenzoate); colchicine, a microtubule inhibitor (Spira, 1979; Katz *et al.*, 1980); and cytochalasin B (Spira,

1979). Interestingly, reactive oxygen species, which may participate in the lytic event (discussed below), are produced both on contact with target cells and as a consequence of phagocytosis (Fleer *et al.*, 1979).

In addition to stable effector–target contact, several other physical requirements necessary for target cell lysis have been studied. The ADCC reaction is known to be temperature dependent, proceeding well at 37°C but poorly at either 4 or 46°C. In contrast, cytolysis is neither dependent on the presence of divalent cations in the medium, nor is it inhibited by EDTA (Spira, 1979). In addition, MMADCC appears to be independent of nucleic acid replication or protein synthesis. Inhibitors of DNA synthesis (mitomycin C), RNA synthesis (actinomycin D), and protein synthesis (puromycin, cycloheximide and chloramphenicol) also fail to inhibit ADCC (Spira, 1979).

MMADCC is an energy-requiring event. Recently it has been demonstrated (by direct measurement of glycolytic energy metabolism and by inhibition of oxygen-dependent energy production) that MMADCC depends largely, if not exclusively, upon monocyte anaerobic glycolysis for the energy needs of effector function (Ladisch and Feig, 1982). Monocyte glycolysis is significantly augmented in association with MMADCC as evidenced by a nearly two-fold increase in lactate production. This increase occurs in the presence of sensitizing antierythrocyte antibody alone, other human sera, and purified IgG, but is not dependent on contact with a target cell. This suggests that IgG binding to the monocyte triggers an increase in monocyte glycolysis. These data support earlier studies in which it was found that inhibition of glycolysis by 2-deoxyglucose caused an inhibition of ADCC (Koller *et al.*, 1978). Alternatively, most reports confirm that MMADCC does not require oxygen-dependent energy metabolism. Inhibitors of oxidative phosphorylation including cyanide, 2,4-dinitrophenol, and sodium azide appear to exert no effect on MMADCC (Sharma and Piessens, 1979; Fleer *et al.*, 1979; LoBuglio *et al.*, 1979; Borregaard and Kragballe, 1980).

A great deal of controversy surrounds the delineation of the exact chemical reactions necessary for the lytic event of ADCC, in particular on the role of reactive oxygen species (ROS). Monocytes respond to phagocytosis of microorganisms with a series of metabolic changes termed the "respiratory burst." This is characterized by an increase in oxygen consumption, and hexose monophosphate shunt activity (HMPS), and the production of ROS such as superoxide (O_2^-), hydrogen peroxide (H_2O_2) (Klassen and Sagone, 1980), and hydroxyl radicals (OH^-) (Borregaard and Kragballe, 1980). As noted earlier, actual ingestion is not required for the generation of these latter three molecules; and it has been demonstrated that human monocytes treated with antimycin A (an inhibitor of phagocytosis) generate both O_2^- and H_2O_2 when incubated with opsonized zymosan (Reiss and Roos, 1978). Thus, it is possible that these ROS are involved in the mediation of extracellular target cell lysis. However, there are conflicting data regarding the role of ROS in MMADCC. Clark and Klebanoff (1977) and Katz *et al.* (1980) indirectly implicate ROS as a participant in the lytic event, by demonstrating that granulocyte-mediated ADCC and monocyte-mediated ADCC were significantly depressed in patients with chronic granulomatous disease (CGD). CGD is characterized by the inability of neutrophils and monocytes to produce reduced oxygen radicals in response to a phagocyte challenge. Fleer *et al.* (1979), however, found MMADCC in a similar system to be essentially normal. Moreover, scavengers of reactive oxygen species such as superoxide dismutase (O_2^-), catalase (H_2O_2), sodium benzoate (OH^-), sodium azide (O^-), histidine (O^-), and phenol (OH^-) have no effect on normal MMADCC against erythrocyte targets (Klassen and Sagone, 1980; Fleer *et al.*, 1979; Borregaard and Kragballe, 1980).

The single conclusion which can be garnered from these reports is that target lysis in MMADCC can occur as either an intracellular or an extracellular event and that reactive oxygen species may play a role.

3. MMADCC IN HUMAN DISEASE

There is now considerable evidence that *in vivo* MMADCC activity plays a role in a number of disease states in man. Perhaps the two most obvious conditions in which the destruction of sensitized erythrocytes by mononuclear phagocytes may be pathophysiologically significant are autoimmune hemolytic anemia (Frank *et al.*, 1975) and hemolytic disease of the newborn (Zawodnik *et al.*, 1976). However, there is an increasing body of information which suggests that MMADCC may play a role in a number of other disease states. This information has been obtained from *in vitro* assays which utilize either erythrocyte or nonerythrocyte target cells.

3.1. STUDIES UTILIZING ERYTHROCYTE TARGETS

We have studied MMADCC activity against ^{51}Cr-labeled antibody-coated human erythrocyte targets in a variety of clinical situations.

3.1.1. Aplastic Anemia

In initial studies we investigated (Poplack *et al.*, 1976) MMADCC activity in profoundly monocytopenic patients with aplastic anemia and noted that they demonstrated no *in vitro* RBC killing (Fig. 1). In contrast, these aplastic individuals did demonstrate significant ADCC activity against chicken erythrocytes, a predominantly lymphocyte-dependent cytolytic process. Furthermore, we observed that less monocytopenic aplastic anemia patients and normal individuals exhibit cytotoxic activity proportional to their monocyte numbers, confirming that this particular MMADCC assay is able to detect quantitative differences in monocyte number.

3.1.2. Wiskott–Aldrich Syndrome

Using the same assay system, we also investigated MMADCC (Poplack *et al.*, 1976) in patients with Wiskott–Aldrich syndrome, a sex-linked immunodefi-

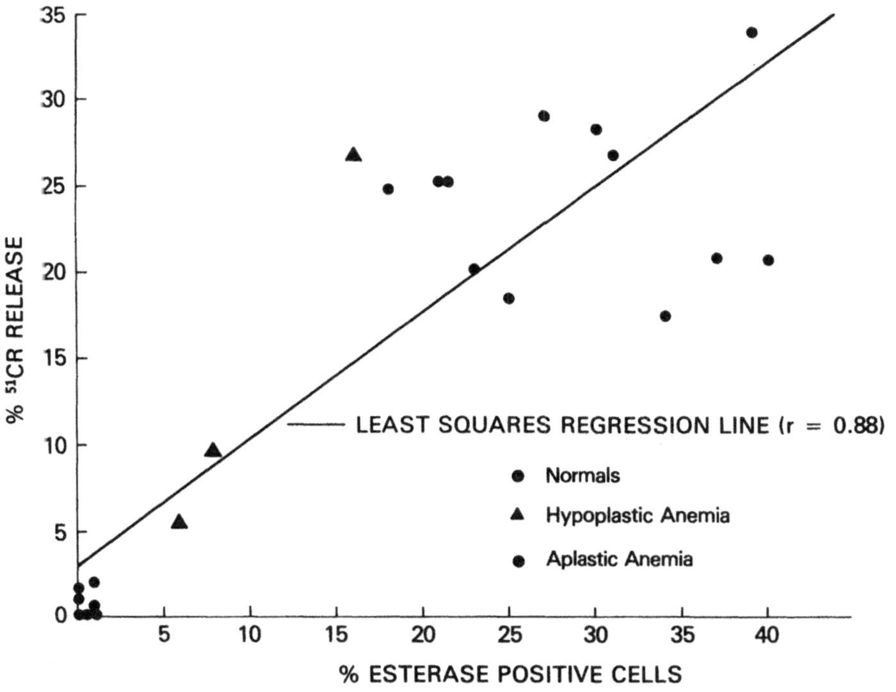

FIGURE 1. Correlation between monocyte number and cytotoxicity in normal, aplastic, and hypoplastic individuals. The correlation coefficient (r = 0.88) is highly significant ($p < 0.001$).

ciency disorder characterized by eczema, thrombocytopenia, and chronic infections. Despite the fact that these patients have normal numbers of circulating monocytes, we noted a profound defect in monocyte killer function (Fig. 2). This finding is of particular interest since there is other immunologic evidence to suggest that an abnormality in monocyte function may, in part, be responsible for the altered immune function observed in these patients (Altman *et al.*, 1974).

3.1.3. Familial Erythrophagocytic Lymphohistiocytosis

We also studied MMADCC (Ladisch *et al.*, 1978) in four patients with familial erythrophagocytic lymphohistiocytosis. This frequently fatal disorder is characterized by recurrent fever, hepatospenomegaly, leukopenia, anemia, thrombocytopenia, and diffuse tissue infiltration of cells of the macrophage series which demonstrate striking erythrophagocytosis. Although all four patients had a normal proportion of circulating monocytes, they had significantly depressed MMADCC (Fig. 3). The mechanism of this apparent defect is unclear. Studies of monocyte Fc receptors demonstrated identical affinity for antibody-coated erythrocytes as that found in normal individuals. The MMADCC defect in these patients appears to be part of a constellation of immune abnormalities observed in patients with this disorder (Ladisch *et al.*, 1978).

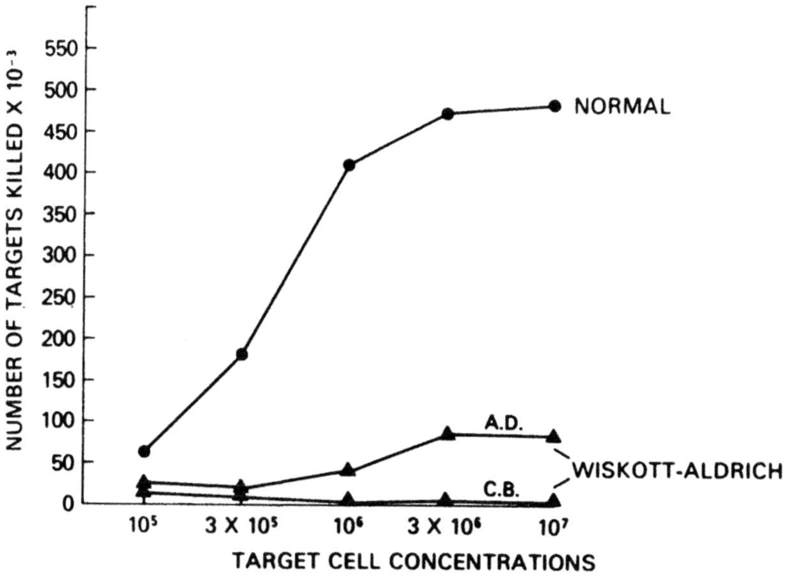

FIGURE 2. Defective monocyte cytotoxicity in patients with Wiskott–Aldrich syndrome. Graph shows cytotoxic activity of two patients at multiple target cell concentrations. These individuals manifest impaired cytotoxicity despite normal numbers of circulating monocytes.

3.1.4. MMADCC in Neonates

The neonatal period is a state of relative immunodeficiency during which newborns are more susceptible to many infections. Although the phagocytic and bactericidal ability of cord blood monocytes are equivalent to those of adult monocytes (Weston *et al.*, 1977), neonatal cord blood monocytes have been shown to be more susceptible to viral infection and replication than adult mono-

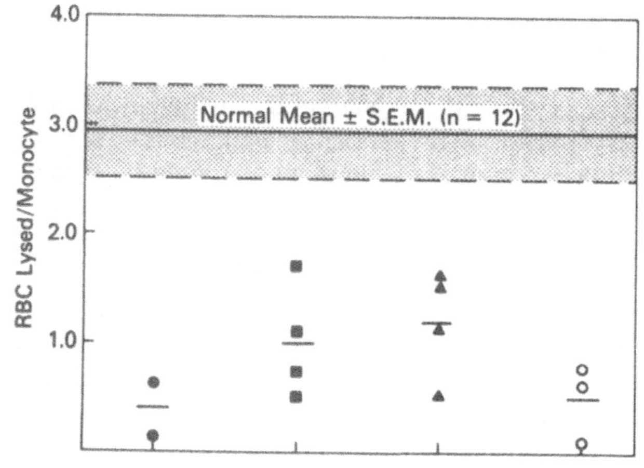

FIGURE 3. Lysis of antibody-coated erythrocytes by monocytes in four patients with familial erythrophagocytic lymphohistiocytosis. — = mean value.

cytes (Sullivan *et al.*, 1975). We have studied 20 cord blood samples and have demonstrated that MMADCC activity of human cord blood monocytes against antibody-coated human erythrocyte targets was equal to that of adult peripheral blood monocytes (Blaese *et al.*, 1979). Others obtained similar results from cord blood monocytes in MMADCC assays utilizing both erythrocyte (Milgrom and Shore, 1977) and HSV-1-infected Chang liver cell targets (Shore *et al.*, 1977; Kohl *et al.*, 1978a).

MMADCC activity in ABO and Rh fetal–maternal incompatibilities has been studied using antibody-sensitized human RBCs as target cells (Zawodnik *et al.*, 1976). In this study, cord RBCs from infants with Rh D fetal–maternal incompatibility were lysed by autologous or isologous monocytes in the absence of exogenous antiserum; in contrast, MMADCC activity was absent in five cases of ABO incompatibility. The authors speculated that MMADCC could be operative *in vivo* in hemolytic disease of the newborn.

3.1.5. MMADCC in Malignant Cells

The ability of malignant cells to express MMADCC activity has also been studied. Both the blast cells of a child with chronic myelomonocytic leukemia and those of a patient with acute monoblastic leukemia demonstrated MMADCC against antibody-coated erythrocytes (Thomas *et al.*, 1981, and our unpublished observations). Although this capacity is unlikely to play a role in the pathophysiology of these diseases, the ability of these cells to mediate monocyte-specific ADCC gives important information regarding the differentiation status of these cells.

3.1.6. Hodgkin's Disease

Pehamberger *et al.* (1980) studied MMADCC against antibody-coated human RBCs in 23 adult patients with advanced Hodgkin's disease and noted that although the lytic capacity of the individual monocytes was significantly higher in these patients, there was no correlation between MMADCC activity and disease status.

3.1.7. Rheumatoid Arthritis

MMADCC against antibody-coated chicken erythrocyte targets was studied in 10 adult patients with rheumatoid arthritis (Waytz and Douglas, 1979). The study demonstrated no difference in ADCC activity between the patients and normal controls, when mixed mononuclear (lymphocyte-predominant) and monocyte-depleted populations were compared; however, monocyte-enriched fractions from patients with rheumatoid arthritis mediated a significantly increased degree of cytotoxicity at lower effector : target ratios. The authors postulated that the enhanced effector function of the peripheral blood monocytes in this system may be an indication that mononuclear phagocytes are "activated" in patients with rheumatoid arthritis.

3.1.8. Atopic Dermatitis

Kragballe *et al.* (1980) investigated MMADCC against human erythrocytes from 23 adult patients with atopic dermatitis of varying severity. MMADCC was found to be significantly decreased in patients with widespread dermatitis compared to normals. In contrast, 8 patients with contact dermatitis and 13 control patients with extrinsic asthma or allergic rhinitis showed normal cytotoxicity. The investigators also noted that normal monocytes preincubated with patient serum did not show abnormal ADCC function, and the impairment of MMADCC activity in atopic dermatitis patients was not related to their serum IgE level.

3.1.9. Systemic Lupus Erythematosus and Systemic Sclerosis

Cooper *et al.* (1978) examined ADCC of peripheral blood monocytes against antibody-coated chicken erythrocytes in 18 patients with systemic lupus erythematosus and 13 patients with progressive systemic sclerosis and found it to be normal. Patients with systemic lupus erythematosus also demonstrate normal MMADCC activity with our assay system which employs antibody-coated human erythrocytes (unpublished data).

3.1.10. Hashimoto's Thyroiditis

Suzuki *et al.* (1980) studied 45 patients with Hashimoto's thyroiditis for their MMADCC activity in a system in which the anti-thyroglobulin-antibody-armed monocytes became cytotoxic against thyroglobulin-coated chicken erythrocytes. It was suggested that in these patients the monocytes might be armed by cytophilic antibodies *in vivo,* since monocytes of patients with Hashimoto's thyroiditis showed increased rosette formation with thyroglobulin-coated erythrocytes relative to monocytes from control subjects. This suggests a possible pathogenic role for monocytes in human autoimmune thyroiditis.

3.1.11. Asthma

Flaherty *et al.* (1978) noted a reduced MMADCC capacity of peripheral blood mononuclear cells against chicken erythrocytes in 15 patients with a history of asthma provoked by viral infections. It was speculated that the MMADCC mechanism contributes to containment and/or termination of respiratory viral infections in these patients.

3.2. STUDIES OF MMADCC UTILIZING NONERYTHROCYTIC TARGET CELLS

Patients with hematologic malignancies are prone to developing severe infections caused by the herpes virus group, including varicella zoster and herpes simplex (HSV). A method has been described which makes it possible to assess the ability of lymphocytes, monocyte–macrophages, and polymorphonuclear leukocytes to destroy HSV-infected target cells in the presence of antibody (Kohl *et al.*, 1977). *In vitro*, MMADCC appears to be one of the few mechanisms by which HSV-infected cells can be killed prior to the time of new viral production and cell-to-cell transfer of virus. It is not known if this applies *in vivo* in humans. Nevertheless, this system appears to be a useful *in vitro* method for assessing monocyte cytotoxicity. It has been studied in several situations including Hodgkin's disease (Kohl *et al.*, 1980) and the neonatal state (Shore *et al.*, 1977; Kohl *et al.*, 1978a).

One interesting study examined human colostral cell cytotoxicity (Kohl *et al.*, 1978). HSV-infected ^{51}Cr-labeled Chang liver cells were employed as the target cells, colostral cells from healthy women 2–6 days postpartum as effector cells, and pooled immune sera from individuals with past HSV infections as antibody. ADCC was found to be mediated exclusively by mononuclear adherent cells. ADCC was totally inhibited by preincubation of colostral cells with latex particles, confirming that a subpopulation of human colostral macrophages can mediate ADCC against virus-infected target cells. The authors speculated that either maternal colostral antibody or transplacentally acquired antibody together with colostral cells may help prevent the dissemination of HSV infection from the gastrointestinal tract in the neonate.

The above examples suggest that MMADCC may play a role in human disease processes. The evidence is obviously more compelling in some disorders than in others. A greater appreciation of the importance of MMADCC in the host immunologic defenses will require additional clinically related studies. Hopefully such studies will be performed simultaneously with other monocyte function studies (both of the effector and noneffector variety). Such information is necessary before the true contribution of MMADCC to man's host defense system can be ascertained.

REFERENCES

Altman, L. C., Snyderman, R., and Blaese, R. M., 1974, Abnormalities of chemotactic lymphokine synthesis and mononuclear leukocyte chemotaxis in Wiskott Aldrich syndrome, *J. Clin. Invest.* **54:**486.

Blaese, R. M., Poplack, D. G., and Muchmore, A. V., 1979, The mononuclear phagocyte system: Role in expression of immunocompetence in neonatal and adult life, *Pediatrics* **64**(Suppl.)**:**829.

Bolivar, R., Kohl, S., Pickering, L. K., and Walters, D. L., 1980, Effect of antineoplastic drugs on human leukocyte-mediated cytotoxicity against herpes simplex virus infected cells, *Cancer* **46:**1555.

Borregaard, N., and Kragballe, K., 1980, Role of oxygen in antibody-dependent cytotoxicity mediated by monocytes and neutrophils, *J. Clin. Invest.* **66:**676.

Boyum, A., 1968, Isolation of leukocytes from human blood, *Scand. J. Clin. Lab. Invest.* **21**(Suppl. 97)**:**77.

Clark, R. A., and Klebanoff, S. J., 1977, Studies on the mechanism of antibody-dependent polymorphonuclear leukocyte-mediated cytotoxicity, *J. Immunol.* **119:**1413.

Cooper, S. M., Harding, B., Mirick, G. R., Schneider, J., Quismorio, F. P., and Friou, G., 1978, Selective decrease in antibody-dependent cell-mediated cytotoxicity in systemic lupus erythematosus and progressive systemic sclerosis, *Clin. Exp. Immunol.* **34:**235.

Flaherty, D. K., Martin, J. M., Surfus, J. E., Koorstra, J. B., and Reed, C. E., 1978, Antibody-dependent cellular cytotoxicity of mononuclear cells from asthmatics tested in three *in vitro* assays, *J. Allergy Clin. Immunol.* **62**:156.

Fleer, A., van der Meulen, F. W., Linthout, E., von dem Borne, A. E. G. K., and Engelfriet, C. P., 1978, Destruction of IgG sensitized erythrocytes by human blood monocytes: Modulation of inhibition by IgG, *Br. J. Haematol.* **39**:425.

Fleer, A., Roos, D., von dem Borne, A. E. G. K., and Engelfriet, C. P., 1979, Cytotoxic activity of human monocytes towards sensitized red cells is not dependent on the generation of reactive oxygen species, *Blood* **54**:407.

Frank, M. M., Schreiber, A. D., and Atkinson, J. P., 1975, Studies of the interaction of antibody, complement and macrophages in the immune clearance of erythrocytes, in: *The Phagocytic Cell in Host Resistance* (J. A. Bellanti and D. H. Dayton, eds.), pp. 101–116, Raven Press, New York.

Gagnon, R. F., and Joshua, D. E., 1980, Antibody-dependent cell-mediated cytotoxicity (ADCC) assay for specific IgG antibody produced *in vitro*, *J. Immunol. Methods* **36**:243.

Hersey, P., 1973, Macrophage effector function: An *in vitro* system of assessment, *Transplantation* **15**:282.

Holm, G., 1972, Lysis of antibody treated human erythrocytes by human leukocytes and macrophages in tissue culture, *Int. Arch. Allergy Appl. Immunol.* **43**:671.

Holm, G., and Hammarstrom, S., 1973, Haemolytic activity of human blood monocytes: Lysis of human erythrocytes treated with anti-A serum, *Clin. Exp. Immunol.* **13**:29.

Jonny, M., Pazderka, F., Kovitharongs, T., Schlant, J., and Dossetor, J. B., 1979, Monocyte-specific antigens—Detection by the antibody-dependent cellular cytotoxicity (ADCC) method, *Transplant. Proc.* **XI**:1970.

Katz, P., Simone, C. B., Henkart, P. A., and Fauci, A. S., 1980, Mechanisms of antibody-dependent cellular cytotoxicity, *J. Clin. Invest.* **65**:55.

Keaney, M., McPhail, S., Jodouin, C.-A., and Richter, M., 1980, The antibody-dependent cell-mediated reaction. II. The effect of the concentration of anti-target cell antibodies of the identity of the human effector cell, *Immunology* **40**:205.

Klassen, D. K., and Sagone, A. L., Jr., 1980, Evidence for both oxygen and nonoxygen dependent mechanisms of antibody sensitized target cell lysis by human monocytes, *Blood* **56**:985.

Kohl, S., Starr, S. E., Oleske, J. M., Shore, S. L., Ashman, R. B., and Nahmias, A. J., 1977, Human monocyte-macrophage-mediated antibody-dependent cytotoxicity to herpes simplex virus-infected cells, *J. Immunol.* **118**:729.

Kohl, S., Sedat, S. S., Starr, S. E., Wood, P. A., and Nahmias, A. J., 1978a, Human neonatal and maternal monocyte-macrophage and lymphocyte-mediated antibody-dependent cytotoxicity to cells infected with herpes simplex, *J. Pediatr.* **93**:206.

Kohl, S., Malloy, M. M., Pickering, L. K., Morriss, F. H., Adcock, E. W., and Walters, D. L., 1978b, Human colostral cytotoxicity. 1. Antibody dependent cellular cytotoxicity against herpes simplex viral-infected cells mediated by colostral cells, *J. Clin. Lab. Immunol.* **1**:221.

Kohl, S., Pickering, L. K., and Diluzio, N. R., 1979, Inhibition of human monocyte-macrophage and lymphocyte cytotoxicity to herpes simplex-infected cells by glucan, *J. Immunol. Methods* **29**:361.

Kohl, S., Pickering, L. K., Sullivan, M. P., and Walters, D. L., 1980, Impaired monocyte-macrophage cytotoxicity in patients with Hodgkin's disease, *Clin. Immunol. Immunopathol.* **15**:577.

Koller, C. A., Laufman, H. B., and LoBuglio, A. F., 1978, Characterization of the monocyte antibody dependent cellular cytotoxicity (ADCC) against RBC targets, *Blood* **52**:152A.

Koski, I., Poplack, D. G., and Blaese, R. M., 1976, A non-specific esterase stain for the identification of monocytes and macrophages, in: *In Vitro Methods in Cell-Mediated and Tumor Immunity* (B. R. Bloom and J. R. David, eds.), pp. 359–362, Academic Press, New York.

Kovithavongs, T., Rice, G., Thong, K. T., and Dossetor, J. B., 1975, Effector cell activity in antibody mediated cell dependent immune lysis. II. Evidence for different populations of effector cells for different targets, *Cell. Immunol.* **18**:167.

Kragballe, K., Ellegaard, J., and Herlin, T., 1980a, Antibody dependent monocyte mediated cytotoxicity: The interference by platelets, immune complexes and normal serum, *Scand. J. Haematol.* **25**:67.

Kragballe, K., Herlin, T., and Jensen, J. R., 1980b, Impaired monocyte-mediated cytotoxicity in atopic dermatitis, *Arch. Dermatol. Res.* **269**:21.

Kurlander, R. J., and Rosse, W. F., 1979, Monocyte mediated destruction in the presence of serum of red cells coated with antibody, *Blood* **54**:1131.

Kurlander, R. J., Rosse, W. F., and Logue, G. L., 1978, Quantitative influence of antibody and complement coating of red cells on monocyte-mediated cell lysis, *J. Clin. Invest.* **61**:1309.

Ladisch, S., Holiman, B., Poplack, D. G., and Blaese, R. M., 1978, Immunodeficiency in familial erythrophagocytic lymphohistiocytosis, *Lancet* **1**:581.

Ladisch, S., Feig, S. A., 1982, Inhibition of monocyte-mediated antibody-dependent cellular cytoxicity by oubain: Relationship between cytoxic function, glycolysis and intracellular cation homeostasis, *J. Immunol.* **129**:282.

LoBuglio, A. F., Cotran, R. S., and Jandl, J. H., 1967, Red cells coated with immunoglobulin G: Binding and sphering by mononuclear cells in man, *Science* **158**:1582.

LoBuglio, A. F., Solvay, M. J., and Weiss, S. J., 1979, Characterization of human monocyte directed tumor cell cytotoxicity, *Blood* **54**:1031A.

Lovchik, J., and Hong, R., 1977, Antibody dependent cell mediated cytolysis (ADCC): Analyses and projections, *Prog. Allergy* **22**:1.

MacDonald, H. R., Bonnard, G. D., Sordat, B., and Zawodnik, S. A., 1975, Antibody-dependent cell-mediated cytotoxicity: Heterogeneity of effector cells in human peripheral blood, *Scand. J. Immunol.* **4**:487.

Mantovani, A., Caprioli, V., Gritti, P., and Spreafico, F., 1977, Human mature macrophages mediate antibody-dependent cellular cytotoxicity of tumor cells, *Transplantation* **24**:291.

Milgrom, H., and Shore, S. L., 1977, Assessment of monocyte function in the normal newborn infant by antibody-dependent cellular cytotoxicity, *J. Pediatr.* **91**:612.

Milgrom, H., and Shore, S. L., 1978, Lysis of antibody-coated human red cells by peripheral blood mononuclear cells: Altered effector cell profile after treatment of target cells with enzymes, *Cell. Immunol.* **39**:178.

Nelson, D. L., Poplack, D. G., Holiman, B. J., and Henkart, P. A., 1979, ADCC against human erythrocyte target cells: Role of the anti-target cell antibodies in determining lymphocyte killer activity, *Clin. Exp. Immunol.* **35**:447.

O'Rourke, E. J., Halstead, S. B., Allison, A. C., and Platts-Mills, T. A. E., 1978, Specific lethality of silica for human peripheral blood mononuclear phagocytes *in vitro*, *J. Immunol. Methods* **19**:137.

Pehamberger, H., Ludwig, H., Potzi, P., and Knapp, W., 1980, Increased monocyte-mediated antibody-dependent cellular cytotoxicity (ADCC) in Hodgkin's disease, *Br. J. Cancer* **4**:778.

Poplack, D. G., and Blaese, R. M., 1980, The mononuclear phagocytic system, in: *Immunological Disorders in Infants and Children* (E. R. Stiehm and V. A. Fulginite, eds.), pp. 109–126, Saunders, Philadelphia.

Poplack, D. G., Bonnard, G. D., Holiman, B. J., and Blaese, R. M., 1976, Monocyte-mediated antibody-dependent cellular cytotoxicity: A clinical test of monocyte function, *Blood* **48**:809.

Reiss, M., and Roos, D., 1978, Differences in oxygen metabolism of phagocytosing monocytes and neutrophils, *J. Clin. Invest.* **61**:480.

Sharma, S. D., and Piessens, W. F., 1979, Tumor cell killing by macrophages activated *in vitro* with lymphocyte mediators. IV. Role of energy metabolism, *Cell. Immunol.* **47**:106.

Shaw, G. M., Levy, P. C., and LoBuglio, A. F., 1978, Human lymphocyte, monocyte and neutrophil antibody-dependent cell-mediated cytotoxicity toward human erythrocytes, *Cell. Immunol.* **41**:122.

Shore, S. L., Milgrom, H., Wood, P. A., and Nahmias, A. J., 1977, Antibody-dependent cellular cytotoxicity to target cells infected with herpes simplex viruses: Functional adequacy in the neonate, *Pediatrics* **59**:22.

Spira, T. J., 1979, Mechanisms of monocyte-mediated antibody-dependent cellular cytotoxicity, Proceedings of the 13th International Leukocyte Culture Conference, Ottawa, Canada, p. 85.

Sullivan, J. L., Barry, D. W., Lucas, S. J., and Albrecht, P., 1975, Measles infection of human mononuclear cells, *J. Exp. Med.*, **142**:773.

Suzuki, S., Mitsunaga, M., Miyoshi, M., Hirakawa, S., Nakagawa, O., Miura, H., and Ofujui, T., 1980, Cytophilic antithyroglobulin antibody and antibody dependent monocyte-mediated cytotoxicity in Hashimoto's thyroiditis, *J. Clin. Endocrinol. Metab.* **51**:446.

Thomas, W. J., North, R. B., Poplack, D. G., Slease, R. B., and Duval-Arnould, B., 1981, Chronic myelomonocytic leukemia in childhood, *Am. J. Hematol.* **10:**181.

Urbaniak, S. J., 1976, Lymphoid cell dependent (K-cell) lysis of human erythrocytes sensitized with rhesus alloantibodies, *Br. J. Haematol.* **33:**409.

van der Meulen, F. W., van der Hart, M., Fleer, A., von dem Borne, A. E. G. K., Engelfriet, C. P., and van Loghem, J. J., 1978, The role of adherence to human mononuclear phagocytes in the destruction of red cells sensitized with non-complement binding IgG antibodies, *Br. J. Immunol.* **38:**541.

Waytz, P. H., and Douglas, S. D., 1979, Increased antibody dependent cell-mediated cytotoxicity by monocytes from patients with rheumatoid arthritis, *Arthritis Rheum.* **22:**590.

Weston, W. L., Carson, B. S., Barkin, R. M., Slater, A. D., Dustin, R. D., and Hecht, S. K., 1977, Monocyte-macrophage function in the newborn, *Am. J. Dis. Child.* **131:**1241.

Yust, I., Frisch, B., and Goldsher, N., 1980a, Antibody dependent cell mediated cytotoxicity against human red blood cells: Correlation of effector cell type with enzymatic alteration of the target cell surface, *Eur. J. Immunol.* **10:**127.

Yust, I., Goldsher, N., Greenfeld, R., and Rabinovitz, M., 1980b, Hemolysis due to human antibody-dependent cell-mediated cytotoxicity: Lysis of erythrocytes treated with anti-D serum, *Isr. J. Med. Sci.* **16:**174.

Zawodnik, S. A., Bonnard, A. D., and Gautier, E., 1976, Antibody dependent cell mediated destruction of human erythrocytes sensitized in ABO and rhesus fetal–maternal incompatibilities, *Pediatr. Res.* **10:**791.

16

Role of Macrophages in Immunopotentiation by Adjuvants

RICHARD M. SCHULTZ, JON R. SCHMIDTKE, and ARTHUR G. JOHNSON

1. INTRODUCTION

There is considerable evidence that macrophages can modulate the immune response *in vivo* (for reviews, see Unanue, 1972, 1980; Oppenheim and Seeger, 1976; Oehler *et al.*, 1978). Aside from their role as tumoricidal and microbicidal effector cells, evidence from *in vitro* studies indicates that macrophages are required for antigen- or mitogen-induced lymphocyte proliferation, antibody production, and the production of some lymphokines (Oppenheim and Rosenstreich, 1976). These responses are critically dependent on presenting antigen in association with macrophage surface membrane components of the major histocompatibility complex such as Ia and on growth and differentiation factors supplied by macrophages.

Adjuvants derived from bacterial preparations or components are frequently used to amplify the immune response. Understanding the mechanism(s) by which these adjuvants exert this augmentation becomes somewhat complex, since it is now appreciated that immune competency requires the interaction of several cell types and subsets, usually with regulatory and effector functions. Consequently, experiments with adjuvants have been conducted empirically, and the mechanism of action of a particular adjuvant remains presently a matter of conjecture. Over the past few years, evidence has accumulated that macrophages may be involved in the heightened immune response produced by

---

RICHARD M. SCHULTZ and JON R. SCHMIDTKE • Department of Immunology Research, Lilly Research Laboratories, Indianapolis, Indiana 46285. ARTHUR G. JOHNSON • Department of Microbiology and Immunology, The University of Minnesota, Duluth, Minnesota 55812.

these adjuvants. One common effect of adjuvants is their ability to stimulate macrophage secretory and effector function and thus possibly serve as a vector for their adjuvant properties (Nagao *et al.*, 1981; Oppenheim *et al.*, 1980b; Rosenstreich and Vogel, 1980; Wahl *et al.*, 1980).

The molecular basis for adjuvant action by macrophages is becoming more apparent. Recent studies have demonstrated that at least a part of the adjuvant action may be attributed to the release of soluble factors (monokines) from macrophages that affect other lymphoid cells and facilitate their responses (Diamantstein *et al.*, 1979). These include a mitogenic factor for lymphocytes termed lymphocyte-activating factor or IL-1 (Gery and Waksman, 1972; Oppenheim *et al.*, 1980a); a B-cell-activating factor (Wood and Gaul, 1974); and a thymocyte-differentiating factor (Beller and Unanue, 1977, 1980). Gillis and Mizel (1981) postulated that IL-1 mediates its effect on immune reactivity (enhancement of thymocyte mitogenesis and induction of antibody and cytotoxic T-cell responses) by maturation of a subset of immature T cells to the point where they are capable of T-cell growth factor (IL-2) production.

Adjuvants may also stimulate phagocytosis by macrophages *in vivo* and thereby remove and destroy extracellular antigen that has the potential for inducing negative responses in lymphocytes (Unanue, 1978). They may also act by enhancing the capacity of macrophages to process and present antigen to lymphocytes. For example, the immune response to bovine serum albumin bound to viable macrophages proved to be 1000- to 10,000-fold higher than that occurring when albumin was injected in soluble form (Spitznagel and Allison, 1970). Similarly, the injection of diphtheria toxoid at the skin site of a macrophage-rich delayed hypersensitivity reaction to tuberculin results in 2 to 4 times more antitoxin antibody production (Humphrey and Turk, 1963).

An alternative mechanism of adjuvant action is suggested by the ability of some adjuvants, including polyanions (Goren *et al.*, 1974) and dimethyldioctadecylammonium bromide (Van Der Meer *et al.*, 1979), to inhibit phagosome–lysosome fusion. The necessity to inject these adjuvants and antigen via the same route and preferentially in a mixture suggests that adjuvant may interfere with local antigen handling by macrophages. Similarly, i.v. injection of carrageenan, a frequently cited macrophage-toxic agent, with sheep red blood cells has been demonstrated to markedly reduce liver uptake and blood clearance of antigen, resulting in diversion of increased amounts of antigen to the spleen (Turner and Higginbotham, 1979). Enhanced hemagglutinating antibody (HA) titers and splenic plague-forming cell responses were noted in both antigen-primed and unprimed mice. The observed adjuvant effect of carrageenan appeared to reflect the influence of this polyanion on both antigen uptake and antigen disposal by the spleen. The local nature of the carrageenan effect is supported by the finding that the immune response to i.v. antigen is not affected by i.p. injection of carrageenan (Aschheim and Raffel, 1972; Bice *et al.*, 1971). In addition, adjuvants may indirectly inhibit antigen digestion by stimulating macrophage production of lysolecithin (Munder and Modelell, 1973; van Rooijen and van Nieuwmegen, 1979).

2. ASSOCIATION OF ADJUVANT ACTION WITH ENHANCED MACROPHAGE FUNCTION

In recent years several investigators (Arora and Crowle, 1978; Unanue, 1972; Wahl *et al.*, 1980) have suggested that macrophages might be involved in the heightened immune response produced by adjuvants. Indeed, one mechanism of adjuvant action may be through direct triggering of the macrophage, since synthetic and naturally occurring adjuvants have the common property of directly stimulating macrophage function (Table 1). Among the most commonly used adjuvants are heat-killed mycobacterial cells contained in Freund's adjuvant, bacterial peptidoglycans such as muramyl dipeptide (MDP), bacterial lipopolysaccharides (LPS), various viable bacterial preparations, glucans, and polynucleotides. For simplicity, we will restrict ourselves in this chapter to LPS, MDP, and polynucleotides. The relationship of chemical structure of adjuvant to macrophage activation will be presented along with evidence that macrophages are initial target cells for adjuvant action.

2.1. BACTERIAL LPS

Bacterial LPS has been known for over 20 years to be a potent immunologic adjuvant. Several investigators (Johnson *et al.*, 1956; McGhee *et al.*, 1979; Neter, 1969) have demonstrated that LPS enhances the antibody response *in vivo* to foreign erythrocytes or soluble proteins. LPS also prevents the induction of immunologic tolerance (Claman, 1963; Golub and Weigle, 1967) and bypasses

TABLE 1. ASSOCIATION OF ADJUVANT ACTIVITY WITH STIMULATION OF MACROPHAGE FUNCTION

Adjuvant	References
Alkyldiamine (CP20961)	Chang *et al.* (1980)
Amphotericin B	Lin *et al.* (1977), Stein *et al.* (1978)
Barium sulfate and beryllium salts	Blyden and Handschumacher (1977), Unanue *et al.* (1976)
2-Cyanaziridines (BM12.531)	Bicker (1978)
Dimethyldioctadecylammonium bromide	Gordon *et al.* (1980)
Evans blue dye	Arora and Crowle (1978)
β-(1→3)-Glucans	Chirigos *et al.* (1978), Cook *et al.* (1978)
LPS (lipid A)	McGhee *et al.* (1979), Rosenstreich and Vogel (1980), Wahl *et al.* (1980)
Lysolecithin analogs	Arnold *et al.* (1979), Tarnowski *et al.* (1978)
Muramyl dipeptide	Fevrier *et al.* (1978), Oppenheim *et al.* (1980a), Wahl *et al.* (1980)
Polynucleotides	Ahmed *et al.* (1974), Johnson and Johnson (1971)
Pyran copolymer (MVE)	Baird and Kaplan (1975), Chirigos *et al.* (1978), Meltzer and Oppenheim (1977)

the requirement for T-helper cells by facilitating immune responses in mice given haptenated, homologous erythrocytes (Hoffmann *et al.*, 1977; Schmidtke and Dixon, 1972) or a soluble protein antigen (Chiller and Weigle, 1973). However, the specific cell type by which LPS exerts its primary adjuvant effect has not been resolved.

LPS is a complex molecule comprising three main regions: the O-polysaccharide, the core polysaccharide, and the lipid A, linked to the latter by a trisaccharide (Luderitz *et al.*, 1971). It has now been clearly established that many of the biologic activities of LPS are attributable to the lipid A portion of the molecule. For example, several investigators have shown that macrophage activation by LPS results from a direct interaction between the lipid A activation signal and macrophages and appears to be entirely independent of lymphocytes (Alexander and Evans, 1971; Doe and Henson, 1979; Vogel *et al.*, 1979; Weinberg *et al.*, 1978). Using pure populations of cloned macrophages, Weinberg *et al.* (1978) demonstrated that LPS can act on macrophages in the complete absence of contaminating lymphocytes. The LPS effect on macrophages was reproduced by lipid A. Similarly, preparations of lipid A were mitogenic to B cells (Andersson *et al.*, 1973; Chiller *et al.*, 1973) and induced polyclonal antibody synthesis and secretion (Andersson *et al.*, 1973) to a similar extent as the intact LPS molecule.

2.1.1. Effects of LPS on Macrophage Activities

Several macrophage activities have been shown to be directly enhanced by LPS treatment without lymphocyte participation. Bacterial LPS stimulates macrophages to increase phagocytosis of colloidal gold (Bennett and Cohn, 1966), and synthesis and release of collagenase (Wahl *et al.*, 1977), plasminogen activator (Gordon *et al.*, 1974; Wahl *et al.*, 1980), lysosomal acid and neutral hydrolases (Bennett and Cohn, 1966; Allison *et al.*, 1973), and prostaglandins (Ellner and Spagnuolo, 1979; Kurland and Bockman, 1978; Schultz *et al.*, 1979). Furthermore, several cytokines are elaborated by LPS-treated macrophages or monocytes, including interferons (Borecky *et al.*, 1974; Maehara and Ho, 1977), B-cell-activating factor (Wood, 1979a,b), LAF (Meltzer and Oppenheim, 1977), colony-stimulating factor (CSF) (Apte *et al.*, 1980), and a factor that induces fibroblast proliferation (Wahl *et al.*, 1980). Moreover, macrophages are directly rendered nonspecifically tumoricidal by LPS treatment *in vitro* or *in vivo* (Alexander and Evans, 1971; Schultz *et al.*, 1978). Stadler and De Weck (1980) demonstrated with flow-cytometric analysis that mouse peritoneal macrophages exposed to LPS had elevated cellular RNA content which paralleled improved adherence of plated macrophages in culture. Due to the ability of macrophages to make all the major mediators of endotoxin action, Rosenstreich and Vogel (1980) suggested a central role of macrophages in the host response to endotoxin. Using several different parameters of macrophage function, Wahl *et al.* (1980) demonstrated that the macrophage-activating potential of LPS and mycobacteria-derived water-soluble adjuvant was retained in the adjuvant-active subcomponents of these molecules.

2.1.2. Use of the C3H/HeJ Model

The C3H/HeJ mouse strain, which is resistant to essentially all effects of lipid A (Chedid *et al.*, 1976; Rosenstreich and Glode, 1975; Skidmore *et al.*, 1975; Watson and Riblet, 1974, 1975), has proven to be a useful model for evaluating the mechanisms underlying the biologic effects of LPS. Michalek *et al.* (1980) used adoptive transfer of bone marrow cells from LPS-sensitive mice (strain C3H/HeN) to evaluate the contribution of lymphoreticular cells to five effects of endotoxin on the host: immunogenicity, adjuvanticity, lethality, interferon induction, and induction of CSF. Adjuvanticity was determined by measuring the ability of LPS to induce mice to respond to trinitrophenyl-conjugated homologous mouse erythrocytes. C3H/HeJ mice became sensitive to each of the five effects after adoptive transfer of C3H/HeN bone marrow cells. The defect of C3H/HeJ mice is controlled by a single gene identical or closely linked to the LPS gene on chromosome 4 (Ruco *et al.*, 1978). C3H/HeJ spleen cells are unable to generate proliferative responses (Coutinho, 1976; Rosenstreich and Glode, 1975), to respond to the adjuvant activity of LPS, or to develop thymus-independent immune responses to LPS (Coutinho *et al.*, 1974).

Work from several laboratories has demonstrated that C3H/HeJ macrophages respond poorly to LPS (reviewed in Vogel *et al.*, 1981). These macrophages are defective in tumoricidal capacity (Ruco *et al.*, 1978; Schultz and Chirigos, 1980) and respond poorly to the lymphokine migration inhibitory factor (Tagliabue *et al.*, 1978). Doe and Henson (1979) showed that C3H/HeJ macrophages exhibit a highly selective defect characterized by unresponsiveness to the lipid A activation signal of protein-free LPS and resistance to the toxic effects of high concentrations of LPS. The observations of Rosenstreich and Vogel (1980) support the hypothesis that some of the LPS unresponsiveness of C3H/HeJ mice is related to the activation defect that macrophages of this strain possess. They clearly showed that BCG infection reverses the LPS unresponsiveness of C3H/HeJ mice *in vivo,* and similarly, *in vitro* lymphokine supernatants enable C3H/HeJ macrophages to produce IL-1 in response to LPS. From these studies, Rosenstreich and Vogel (1980) speculated that a certain differentiation or activation state may be prerequisite for LPS sensitivity.

2.1.3. Role of Macrophages in LPS-Induced Adjuvant Action

Other studies have indicated that enhancement of macrophage activity by LPS could account for adjuvanticity. The administration of antigen with macrophage and LPS greatly enhances immune responses (Unanue *et al.*, 1969; Spitznagel and Allison, 1970). Subsequent studies have shown that LPS induces the release of IL-1 from macrophages (Meltzer and Oppenheim, 1977; Oppenheim *et al.*, 1980a; Rosenstreich and Mizel, 1978) and that highly purified IL-1 enhances antibody response (Farrar and Koopman, 1979; Koopman *et al.*, 1977). McGhee *et al.* (1979) demonstrated that both T lymphocytes and macrophages must be derived from LPS-responsive mice to obtain an LPS-induced enhancement of the immune responses to particulate antigens.

2.2. MDP

Attempts to isolate the active fraction from mycobacteria responsible for this organism's extraordinary modulation of the immune response culminated recently in the synthesis and characterization of a muramyl dipeptide (*N*-acetylmuramyl-L-alanyl-D-isoglutamine, MDP) as the minimal active unit (Lederer *et al.*, 1975). The successful molecular definition of this compound, subsequent synthesis of its multiple derivatives and recognition of their diverse actions on the immune system was a major factor in launching the new field of immunopharmacology. Although MDP affects several cells involved in immune expression, the ensuing discussion will be restricted to the profound effects this chemically defined adjuvant, with a molecular weight of less than 500, and its derivatives have on the monocyte-macrophage system. Two extensive reviews on the wide range of other effects of MDP have been published recently (Parant, 1980; Chedid *et al.*, 1978).

2.2.1. Effects of MDP on Macrophage Movements and Proliferation

MDP at the low levels of 0.1–1 μg/ml has been found in three investigations to inhibit the migration of guinea pig and rat peritoneal exudate cells without evidence of cytotoxicity (Nagao *et al.*, 1979; Yamamoto *et al.*, 1978; Adam *et al.*, 1978). A direct action on the macrophages was postulated, and data have been presented that this effect may not be explainable on the basis of release of macrophage-inhibiting factor (MIF) from contaminating lymphocytes (Nagao *et al.*, 1979; Yamamoto *et al.*, 1978). Reduction of nonadherent cells to 0.1% did not change the capacity of MDP to inhibit migration (Nagao *et al.*, 1979). A relationship between this latter ability and the ability to increase antibody formation was found by all three groups. For example, Adam *et al.* (1978) found three structural analogs of MDP, which were incapable of elevating antibody, also to be unable to inhibit macrophage migration; whereas three adjuvant-active analogs inhibited migration. Since a stereospecific structure was shown to be required for both activities, it raises the intriguing question as to whether or not a specific receptor for MDP exists on macrophages which may initiate multiple functions of this cell (e.g., secretion of monokines, activation to cytotoxicity, increased adherence, etc.). However, no evidence for such a receptor has been found as yet.

Tanaka *et al.* (1980) reported a two- to threefold increase in the number of macrophages attaching to glass or plastic surfaces when 10 μg/ml of MDP was added for 1–3 days. A 30% increase in the number of macrophages which exhibited spreading also was noted. The results were influenced strongly by the kind of serum used in culture. Concentrations of MDP as low as 0.01 μg were effective under optimal conditions. Cummings *et al.* (1980) also reported enhanced spreading of macrophages from MDP-treated mice during 2 hr of adherence. This was associated with an increase in protein, lactate dehydrogenase, and a β-glucosaminidase.

Hadden (1978), Hadden and Englard (1979), and Hadden *et al.* (1979) studied the effects on macrophage and lymphocyte proliferation of MDP, isoprinosine, levamisole, and SM 1213, a synthetic, substituted monosaccharide with a structural relationship to MDP. In contrast to levamisole and isoprinosine, only a minimal inhibition (10%) of lymphocyte proliferation in the presence of phytohemagglutinin was exhibited by MDP. SM 1213 had no effect. With respect to guinea pig macrophage proliferation induced by macrophage mitogenic factor (MMF), however, MDP exerted strong inhibitory properties (90%), presumably through elevation of cAMP levels, with an ID_{50} of 0.01 μg/ml. No cytotoxic effect was exhibited by MDP in the absence of MMF.

2.2.2. Activation of Macrophage Tumoricidal Capacity by MDP

Nonspecific enhancement of resistance to tumors is a property of various mycobacteria. Retention of this activity was tested following synthesis of MDP. Although the latter represents the minimal adjuvant active unit of the *Mycobacterium*, Juy and Chedid (1975) found that a correlation did not exist between the antibody-enhancing capacity of MDP and the *in vivo* activation of macrophage tumoricidal ability. Thus, MDP was unable to induce cytotoxic properties in macrophages *in vivo* in contrast to two other more crude fractions (WSA and IPM). Nevertheless, MDP was capable of *in vitro* activation of murine peritoneal macrophages to a state cytotoxic for the target mastocytoma cells. Muramyl L-alanine, a nonadjuvant derivative of MDP, was incapable of either *in vivo* or *in vitro* activation of macrophages. Activation of macrophages by MDP has been associated by Hadden and Englard (1979) with elevation of cGMP levels. Matter (1979) confirmed the *in vitro* activation of macrophages by MDP and correlated it with several *in vivo* systems.

In addition, Galelli *et al.* (1980) documented that the inactive adjuvant derivative of MDP, *N*-acetyl-muramyl-D-alanyl-D-isoglutamine, (MDP)DD, also failed to activate peritoneal macrophages *in vitro* to inhibit the growth of mastocytoma cells. However, when (MDP)DD was coupled to an inert carrier, poly(DL-alanyl)-poly(L-lysine), activity equal to MDP surprisingly was demonstrable. Since (MDP)DD-A-L, like (MDP)DD, continued to be devoid of adjuvant action on antibody formation, the lack of correlation between the *in vitro* inducement of macrophage cytotoxicity for tumor cells and adjuvant action was confirmed.

In the aforementioned cytotoxicity experiments, it was not certain that MDP exerted a direct action on macrophages. By demonstrating that MDP could activate cloned macrophage cell lines, however, Taniyama and Holden (1979) were able essentially to eliminate the possibility that MDP might have acted through contaminating lymphocytes to activate macrophages.

Tenu *et al.* (1980) also found that MDP caused an increase in the cytostatic activity of murine macrophages for mastocytoma cells in culture. Thus, MDP incubated for 48 hr *in vitro* with either thioglycollate- or trehalose dimycollate-induced macrophages to which the target cells were added, inhibited the uptake of tritiated thymidine almost completely when 5% fetal calf serum was in the culture medium.

Recently, Sone and Fidler (1980, 1981) have described a striking synergism between MDP and lymphokines in activation of the tumoricidal capacity of rat alveolar macrophages. When the macrophages were incubated first with subthreshold amounts of MAF for as short a time as 15 min, the addition of subliminal amounts of MDP rendered the cells cytotoxic for syngeneic, allogeneic, and xenogeneic tumor cells. Furthermore, the incorporation of either MDP or MAF, or both, within liposomes did not negate the synergism.

2.2.3. Effect on Phagocytosis and Bactericidal Capacity

An increase in the phagocytic index in animals injected with MDP was reported by Tanaka *et al.* (1977). As in most other effects of MDP, stereospecificity was demonstrable with this property also, inasmuch as *N*-acetylmuramyl-L-alanyl-L-isoglutamine was not active. A later study by this same group (Tanaka *et al.*, 1979) extended these findings to show that essentially no strain differences in carbon clearance existed among seven different strains of mice; however, females exhibited greater reactivity than males at low dosage levels. Again, only adjuvant-active structures exhibited RES stimulation.

The injection of MDP, but not (MDP)DD, 1 day before challenge with *Klebsiella pneumoniae* was found by Chedid *et al.* (1978) to protect mice against this microorganism. Such nonspecific protection is thought to be due to stimulation of macrophage activity. Parant *et al.* (1978a) reported the capacity of MDP given s.c. to enhance carbon clearance in the adult mouse and increase survival of 8- and 2-day-old mice against *K. pneumoniae*. Of interest was the fact that the profound increase in nonspecific resistance usually conferred by the LPS of gram-negative bacteria in adult mice was not functional in mice of this early age. Of considerable practical importance was the finding by this group that a derivative of MDP, MDP-(γ-L-lysine), protected 7-day-old mice dramatically against *Klebsiella* when given orally, 1 day before challenge. In addition, a cross-linked oligomer of MDP of approximately 6000 daltons exhibited marked ability in protecting mice against this organism (Parant *et al.*, 1978). Galland *et al.* (1982) extended this study of the capacity of MDP to increase resistance to *K. pneumoniae* by using a local bacterial challenge in starved mice. Significant bacterial containment and a reduction in mortality were seen with MDP treatment.

A new class of derivatives devoid of the muramyl moiety was tested by Parant *et al.* (1981). The peptidolipid 1-O-(L-Ala-D-isoGln-L-Ala)-glycerol-3-mycolate demonstrated strong stimulation of nonspecific resistance against bacterial infections. An extensive characterization of the ability of MDP and multiple derivatives to enhance carbon clearance in mice, rats, and guinea pigs was published by Waters and Ferraresi (1980). A single i.p. or s.c. injection of MDP at dosages of 20–2000 μg into CF-1 mice resulted in increased carbon clearance. When either serine or valine was substituted for alanine, equal or greater clearance resulted. However, the LL and DL stereoisomers were inactive, as were the dipeptide alone and threonine, leucine, proline, and glycine substitutions for alanine. MDP exerted a greater effect in female than male mice or rats. On the other hand, no stimulatory effect was seen in guinea pigs, a species in which MDP is a good adjuvant with respect to antibody formation.

An increase in *in vitro* phagocytosis and killing of microorganisms following treatment with MDP and derivatives has been demonstrated by several investigators. Thus, Hadden *et al.* (1979) found that MDP at concentrations ranging from 0.12 to 12 μg/ml increased both the number of macrophages which ingested *Listeria* and the number of bacteria ingested per cell. Against *Candida,* Nozawa *et al.* (1980) demonstrated that MDP, 100 μg/ml, stimulated candidicidal activity of normal mouse macrophages by fourfold. LPS proved to be much more active, however. Similarly, Cummings *et al.* (1980) found that injection of MDP rapidly activated macrophages. Fifty micrograms of this synthetic adjuvant given s.c. 18 hr before *Candida* challenge, was responsible for a 60% survival of mice receiving a 100% lethal dose of the yeast. Survival was also prolonged if MDP was given 1 min or 1 day after challenge. Simultaneous experiments adding MDP to cultured macrophages showed that a slightly higher percent exhibited phagocytosis and ingestion of *Candida* 1 day after initiation of culture. In addition, macrophages from MDP-treated mice killed twice as many *Candida* as control cells at 1, 2, and 3 hr. MDP(DD) was inactive.

2.2.4. Increased Production of Superoxide

Following phagocytosis of opsonized particles, macrophages generate two metabolites of oxygen, superoxide anion (O_2^-) and hydrogen peroxide (H_2O_2), which are responsible, in the main, for the killing of phagocytosed microorganisms. Pabst and Johnston (1980) have reported that 1 μM MDP-primed cultures of peritoneal macrophages to a twofold increase in amounts of O_2^- following stimulation of these cells to membrane activation by phorbol myristic acid or opsonized zymosan. This effect was less than that seen with 1 μg LPS, however, which elicited a sevenfold increase. A lipophilic derivative of MDP, 6-O(2-tetradecylhexadecanonyl)-MDP, was found to be twice as active as MDP in a later study (Pabst *et al.*, 1980).

Profound changes in morphology of resident mouse peritoneal macrophages were effected by 0.5 μg MDP, including enhanced pseudopod formation after 4 hr. An increased O_2^--generating capacity by these cells correlated with the enhanced spreading in that again, stereoisomers of MDP, which were not adjuvant active, also did not induce more O_2^-. A direct action of MDP on macrophages was predicted inasmuch as (1) the addition of lymphocytes to the macrophage cultures did not alter the response, (2) nude mice without mature T lymphocytes reacted positively to MDP, and (3) the cultured macrophage-like cell line J744.1 responded to MDP after 4 hr with increased O_2^- (Pabst and Johnston, 1980).

In a second investigation, Cummings *et al.* (1980) related the above *in vitro* observations to action in the intact animal by demonstrating that s.c. administration of 25–100 μg MDP to mice 18 hr before harvesting, primed peritoneal macrophages to produce up to five times more O_2^-. Near-peak levels were reached at 3 hr and they persisted for longer than 48 hr.

An increase in glucosamine incorporation by MDP (Takada *et al.*, 1979) as well as glucose 1-C oxidation (Imai *et al.*, 1980) has been reported.

2.2.5. Release of Monokines by MDP

MDP, as might be expected, also has been found to induce the secretion of monokines from cells of the monocyte-macrophage system. In an early paper, Staber *et al.* (1978) recorded the ability of MDP to elevate the colony-stimulating activity of supernatant fluids from cultures of C57BL/6 adherent peritoneal exudate cells. Wood and Staruch (1980) found a factor expressed by human monocytes which enhanced murine IgM PFC when incubated with as little as 10 ng/ml MDP. MDP at 100 and 10 μg was reported by Oppenheim *et al.* (1980b) to stimulate unfractionated and adherent, but not nonadherent, human mononuclear cells to secrete a monokine which was mitogenic for murine thymocytes. It resembled murine LAF (IL-1) in its molecular weight. The derivative 6-O-stearoyl MDP was also active, but MDP(DD) only minimally so. Adherent mouse peritoneal exudate cells were stimulated by MDP to produce IL-1, as was the macrophage cell line P388D1. The latter required a longer incubation period of 4 days, however, in contrast to 1–3 days for peritoneal cells.

Akagawa and Tokunaga (1980) have reported that MDP when added at 50, 100, and 200 μg to a clone of ML cells could not induce these immature cells to differentiate into macrophages. However, when 50 μg MDP was incubated with the J774.1 line, a factor was secreted which when added to ML cells stimulated them to acquire Fc receptors and phagocytize. In addition, if this concentration of MDP was added to mature ML cells, a like factor was produced which induced premature ML cells to differentiate. Thus, in this instance MDP per se did not trigger differentiation. Rather, it induced secretion of differentiating factors from cells capable of synthesizing this monokine.

Further evidence of the release of monokines by MDP emerged from the finding by Parant *et al.* (1980) that while indomethacin blocked the febrile response induced by MDP, circulating pyrogens were still demonstrable following transfer of serum from treated rabbits to normal animals. In *in vitro* experiments using rabbit peritoneal macrophages, endogenous pyrogen was elicited by MDP, a condition which was not inhibited by a dose of indomethacin which blocked the synthesis of prostaglandins. On the other hand, no endogenous pyrogens were produced when such cells were incubated with both cycloheximide and MDP.

The release by 10 μg MDP of a pyrogen from rabbit mononuclear cells as well as blood leukocytes has been documented by Dinarello (1982). The derivatives *N*-acetyl-muramyl-L-alanyl-D-glutamic acid (MDPA) and dimethyl MDPA were inactive. Of interest was the finding that MDP at 100 and 1000 μg/ml stimulated the release of pyrogen from human mononuclear cells. Since MDPA and dimethyl MDPA are effective adjuvants to antibody synthesis, their reduced pyrogenicity indicated that inducement of these two properties can be separated, and appropriate analogs without pyrogenicity could be useful as adjuvants in vaccines for human usage.

MDP also has been shown to release helper factors stimulating *in vitro* antibody formation when incubated with murine adherent cells (Fevrier *et al.*, 1978). Deletion of macrophages by an antimacrophage antiserum negated the production of this activity. This supernatant factor was active across histocompatibility barriers.

MDP enhanced antibody formation *in vitro* in cultures of Peyers' patches derived from normal or orally primed LPS-responsive C3H/HeN mice. It also mimicked LPS in failing to induce antibody synthesis in Peyers' patch cultures from C3H/HeJ mice (Kiyono *et al.*, 1981). An effect on macrophages was suggested in experiments showing MDP promoted a good immune response in C3H/HeJ cultures when macrophages from C3H/HeN mice were added. Since macrophages from LPS-nonresponsive C3H/HeJ mice did not permit a like effect, the suggestion was made that macrophages from LPS-nonresponsive C3H/HeJ mice are defective in promoting MDP adjuvancy (Kiyono *et al.*, 1981). However, no data on whether or not this effect of MDP was mediated by a monokine are available as yet.

The secretion of plasminogen activator by thioglycollate- or streptococci-elicited macrophages was reported to be inhibited partially by MDP, whereas muramyl pentapeptide (*N*-acetyl-muramyl-L-Ala-D-Glu-meso-A_2pm-D-Ala-D-Ala) was a potent inhibitor (Drapier *et al.*, 1980).

Elevation of macrophage secretory activity was reported by Wahl *et al.* (1979) with regard to a variety of products. Thus, collagenase activity was increased markedly 48 hr after guinea pig macrophages had been incubated with 100 μg MDP or WSA. MDP(DD) was inactive. Prostaglandin E_2 and, in turn, cAMP levels were increased also by both compounds. In addition, both evoked from macrophages the release of a mediator causing fibroblast proliferation. Again MDP(DD) was inactive.

2.3. POLYRIBONUCLEOTIDES

2.3.1. Structure–Activity Relationship

Synthetic double-stranded polyribonucleotide complexes, which are formed by polymerization of mononucleotide-diphosphates by *streptomyces lysodeikticus* polynucleotide phosphorylase and subsequent mixing of complementary single-stranded polynucleotide strands, exert marked stimulatory effects on the immune response (reviewed in Johnson, 1979). Both complexes of polyadenylic and polyuridylic acid (poly A : U) and of polyinosinic and polycytidylic acid (poly I : C) appear to be equally effective as adjuvants. There appears to be a requirement for the double helix in adjuvant action, since the single strands show little, if any, activity (Schmidtke and Johnson, 1971). A complex composed of two complementary high-molecular-weight polynucleotides has also been found to be required for macrophage activation (Schultz, 1980; Schultz and Chirigos, 1980). It is intriguing that interferon induction by macrophage cultures has a similar structure requirement (Schultz, 1980), and Neumann (1979) has suggested that induction of macrophage interferon might be correlated with adjuvant activity of immunopotentiators. It is not presently known if the inertness of the single strands is due to their rapid destruction *in vivo* by serum nucleases or whether specific cell receptors exist for a structural conformation peculiar to the double-stranded complex.

Both poly A : U and poly I : C stimulate the production of antibodies to a variety of antigens (Braun and Nakano, 1965; Johnson, 1976; Johnson and Johnson, 1971). Moreover, doses of protein as low as 1 ng were rendered antigenic by polynucleotide treatment (Schmidtke and Johnson, 1971). Johnson (1976) demonstrated that the polynucleotides are effective as adjuvants by multiple routes and need not be given together with antigen. Subsequently, Morris and Johnson (1978) observed enhanced antibody responses when poly A : U was given together with the immunizing antigen, while suppressor cells were activated by poly A : U treatment prior to antigenic stimulation.

2.3.2. Role of Macrophages in Polynucleotide-Induced Adjuvant Action

Johnson and Johnson (1971) demonstrated that poly A : U and poly I : C further increased the already potent enhancing action of macrophage-associated antigen on antibody synthesis. In these experiments, thioglycollate-elicited peritoneal macrophages were incubated *in vitro* with antigens ± polynucleotide, and washed four times prior to their reinjection into syngeneic mice. Due to the resultant boost in antibody when incubated with polynucleotide, the authors suggested a direct action of the adjuvant on macrophages. They also observed that the inhibition of macrophage adjuvant action by actinomycin D was overcome in the presence of poly A : U. Similarly, Ahmed *et al.* (1974) found that murine B cells could be stimulated to undergo blastogenic transformation by poly I : C and LPS, and that the addition of normal peritoneal exudate cells augmented this response.

A role for the monocyte-macrophage in adjuvant action by synthetic polynucleotides was further suggested by several other studies. Winchurch and Braun (1969) found that the anergic, immunologic status of newborn mice could be negated by the injection of either poly A : U or adult syngeneic macrophages. From these studies, it was suggested that poly A : U might hasten the immunological maturation of macrophages in the newborn. Daughaday *et al.* (1977) observed that incubation of rabbit pulmonary alveolar macrophages with poly I : C results in enhanced IgG receptor activity in comparison to untreated cells. In addition, several investigators have demonstrated that poly A : U and poly I : C directly render macrophages nonspecifically tumoricidal *in vitro* and *in vivo* (Alexander and Evans, 1971; Schultz *et al.*, 1977). Interferon appeared to be involved in poly I : C-induced macrophage cytotoxicity, since highly purified anti-interferon globulin blocked macrophage activation (Schultz and Chirigos, 1979).

3. CONCLUDING REMARKS

It is becoming increasingly clear that a number of synthetic and biologic adjuvants can have time- and dose-dependent regulatory properties causing either enhancement or inhibition of various immune responses (for reviews, see Dukor *et al.*, 1979; Renoux, 1980). Due to the potential usefulness of these agents in treating and possibly preventing infectious diseases, immunodeficiencies, autoimmune diseases, and neoplasia, there has been a dramatic proliferation of recent papers on immunopharmacology and on agents which modulate various parameters of the immune response. This chapter has focused on three chemically well-defined adjuvants which have been subjected to intense study. The more complex bacterial vaccines and crude microbial preparations are well beyond the scope of this chapter.

Many of the presently available adjuvants appear to directly affect multiple target cells and differ in their activity depending on the mode and schedule of their application. In this chapter, we have discussed some of the evidence for macrophage involvement in immunopotentiation by adjuvants. The central role of the macrophage in the immune response comes as a result of various interrelated functions: (1) the capacity of the macrophage to remove and degrade extracellular antigen; (2) their capacity to hold a few immunogenic moieties at the cell surface and thus initiate the immune inductive process; and (3) their capacity to secrete molecules that regulate lymphocyte proliferation and differentiation. Calderon and Unanue (1975) suggested that the key role of the macrophage in immune induction stems from the way in which immunity developed during phylogeny. In their view, specific immunity developed as a function necessary to complement and make more efficient the essential phagocyte function of antigen uptake and elimination, at the same time ensuring the lack of immunity to self. The provocative correlation between the adjuvant effect and the ability of a compound to directly influence macrophage functional activity suggests the hypothesis that macrophages may contribute to the nonspecific immunoenhancing effects of adjuvants. The judicial use of conditions, or appropriate derivatives of adjuvants, provides hope for man's selective regulation of the variety of endogenous functions exerted by macrophages in the retention of health and well-being.

ACKNOWLEDGMENTS. We thank Dr. Claude Leclerc, Institut Pasteur, Paris, for assistance in compiling the bibliography on MDP.

REFERENCES

Adam, A., Souvannavong, V., and Lederer, E., 1978, Nonspecific MIF-like activity induced by the synthetic immunoadjuvant: *N*-acetylmuramyl-L-alanyl-D-isoglutamine (MDP), *Biochem. Biophys. Res. Commun.* **85**:684.

Ahmed, A., Strong, D. M., and Scher, I., 1974, Blastogenic transformation of murine B cells by polynucleotides and carbohydrate polymers: The influence of macrophages, *Fed. Proc.* **33**:645.

Akagawa, S., and Tokunaga, T., 1980, Effect of synthetic muramyl dipeptide (MDP) on differentiation of myeloid leukemic cells, *Microbiol. Immunol.* **24**:1005.

Alexander, P., and Evans, R., 1971, Endotoxin and double stranded RNA render macrophages cytotoxic, *Nature New Biol.* **232**:76.

Allison, A. C., Davies, P., and Page, R. C., 1973, Effects of endotoxin on macrophages and other lymphoreticular cells, *J. Infect. Dis.* **128**(Suppl.):212.

Andersson, J., Melchers, F., Galanos, G., and Luderitz, O., 1973, The mitogenic effect of lipopolysaccharide on bone-marrow-derived mouse lymphocytes: Lipid A as the mitogenic part of the molecule, *J. Exp. Med.* **137**:943.

Apte, R. N., Hertogs, C. H. F., and Pluznik, D. H., 1980, Regulation of lipopolysaccharide-induced granulopoiesis and macrophage formation by spleen cells, *J. Immunol.* **124**:1223.

Arnold, B., Staber, F. G., and Miller, J. F. A. P., 1979, Lysolecithin analogs as adjuvants in delayed-type hypersensitivity in mice. II. Studies on the mode of action, *Eur. J. Immunol.* **9**:367.

Arora, M. P., and Crowle, A. J., 1978, Adjuvanticity of Evans blue dye: Preliminary characterization of its mechanisms and mode of application in mice, *J. Reticuloendothelial Soc.* **24**:271.

Aschheim, L., and Raffel, S., 1972, The immunodepressant effect of carrageenan, *J. Reticuloendothelial Soc.* **11**:253.

Baird, L. G., and Kaplan, A. M., 1975, Immunoadjuvant activity of pyran copolymer, *Cell. Immunol.* **20**:167.

Beller, D. I., and Unanue, E. R., 1977, Thymic maturation *in vitro* by a secretory product from macrophages, *J. Immunol.* **121**:1861.

Beller, D. I., and Unanue, E. R., 1980, Role of macrophages in the regulation of thymocyte proliferation and differentiation, in: *Macrophage Regulation of Immunity* (E. R. Unanue and A. S. Rosenthal, eds.), pp. 361–378, Academic Press, New York.

Bennett, W. E., and Cohn, Z. A., 1966, The isolation and selected properties of blood monocytes, *J. Exp. Med.* **123**:145.

Bice, D. E., Schwartz, H. J., Lake, W. W., and Salvaggio, J. E., 1971, The effect of carrageenan on the establishment of delayed hypersensitivity, *Int. Arch. Allergy Appl. Immunol.* **41**:628.

Bicker, U., 1978, Immunomodulating effects of BM12.531 in animals and tolerance in man, *Cancer Treat. Rep.* **62**:1987.

Blyden, G., and Handschumacher, R. E., 1977, Purification and properties of human lymphocyte activating factor (LAF), *J. Immunol.* **118**:1631.

Borecky, L., Lackovic, V., Fuchsberger, N., and Hajnicka, V., 1974, Stimulation of interferon production in macrophages, in: *Activation of Macrophages. Proc. Second Workshop Conference Hoechst* (W.-H. Wagner and H. Hahn, eds.), pp. 111–122, American Elsevier Publishing Co., New York.

Braun, W., and Nakano, M., 1965, Antibody formation: Stimulation by polyadenylic acids, *Science* **157**:819.

Calderon, J., and Unanue, E. R., 1975, An evaluation of the role of macrophages in immune induction, *Fed. Proc.* **34**:1737.

Chang, Y., Pearson, C. M., and Abe, C., 1980, Adjuvant polyarthritis. IV. Induction by a synthetic adjuvant: Immunologic, histopathologic, and other studies, *Arthritis Rheum.* **23**:62.

Chedid, L., Parant, M., Damais, C., Parant, F., Juy, D., and Galleli, A., 1976, Failure of endotoxin to increase nonspecific resistance to infection of lipopolysaccharide low responder mice, *Infect. Immun.* **13**:722.

Chedid, L., Audibert, F., and Johnson, A. G., 1978, Biological activities of muramyl dipeptide, a synthetic glycopeptide analogous to bacterial immunoregulating agents, in: *Progress in Allergy*, Vol. 25 (P. Kallos, B. H. Waksman, and A. L. deWick, eds.), pp. 63–105, Karger, Basel.

Chiller, J. M., and Weigle, W. O., 1973, Termination of tolerance to human gamma globulin in mice by antigen and bacterial lipopolysaccharide (endotoxin), *J. Exp. Med.* **137**:740.

Chiller, J. M., Skidmore, B. J., Morrison, D. C., and Weigle, W. O., 1973, Relationship of the structure of bacterial lipopolysaccharides to its function in mitogenesis and adjuvanticity, *Proc. Natl. Acad. Sci. USA* **70**:2129.

Chirigos, M. A., Stylos, W. A., Schultz, R. M., and Fullen, J. R., 1978, Chemical and biological adjuvants capable of potentiating tumor cell vaccine, *Cancer Res.* **38**:1085.

Claman, H. N., 1963, Tolerance to a protein antigen in adult mice and the effect of non-specific factors, *J. Immunol.* **91**:833.

Cook, J. A., Taylor, D., Cohen, C., Rodrigue, J., Malshet, V., and DiLuzio, N. R., 1978, Comparative evaluation of the role of macrophages and lymphocytes in mediating the antitumor action of glucan, in: *Immune Modulation and Control of Neoplasia by Adjuvant Therapy* (M. A. Chirigos, ed.), pp. 183–200, Raven Press, New York.

Coutinho, A., 1976, Genetic control of B-cell responses. II. Identification of the spleen B-cell defect in C3H/HeJ mice, *Scand. J. Immunol.* **5**:129.

Coutinho, A., Gronowicz, E., Bullock, W., and Moller, G., 1974, Mechanism of thymus-independent immunocyte triggering: Mitogenic activation of B-cells results in specific immune responses, *J. Exp. Med.* **139**:74.

Cummings, N. P., Pabst, M. J., and Johnston, R. B., Jr., 1980, Activation of macrophages for enhanced release of superoxide anion and greater killing of *Candida albicans* by injection of muramyl dipeptide, *J. Exp. Med.* **152**:1659.

Daughaday, C. C., Schmidt, M. E., and Douglas, S. D., 1977, Effects of polynucleotides and levamisole on alveolar macrophage morphology and receptor activity, *Infect. Immun.* **17**:161.

Diamantstein, T., Oppenheim, J. J., Unanue, E. R., Wood, D. D., Handschumacher, R. E., Rosenstreich, D. L., and Waksman, B. H., 1979, Nonspecific "lymphocyte activating" factors produced by macrophages, *Cell Immunol.* **46**:422.

Dinarello, C. A., 1982, Leukocytic pyrogen, in: *Lymphokines, Vol. 7* (E. Pick, ed.), pp. 23–74, Academic Press, New York.

Doe, W. F., and Henson, P. M., 1979, Macrophage stimulation by bacterial lipopolysaccharides. III. Selective unresponsiveness of C3H/HeJ macrophages to the lipid A differentiation signal, *J. Immunol.* **123**:2304.

Drapier, J. C., Bouchahda, A., Lemaire, G., and Petit, J. F., 1980, Plasminogen activator of elicited mouse peritoneal macrophages: Control of the secretion and of the intracellular activity by peptidoglycan derived immunomodulators, *Int. J. Immunopharmacol.* **2**:211.

Dukor, P., Tarcsay, L., and Baschang, G., 1979, Immunostimulants, in: *Annual Reports in Medicinal Chemistry—14* (J. Weisbach, ed.), pp. 146–167, Academic Press, New York.

Ellner, J. J., and Spagnuolo, P. J., 1979, Suppression of antigen and mitogen induced human T lymphocyte DNA synthesis by bacterial lipopolysaccharide: Mediation by monocyte activation and production of prostaglandins, *J. Immunol.* **123**:2689.

Farrar, J. J., and Koopman, W. J., 1979, Characterization of macrophage and lymphocyte derived mitogenic factors and their effect on the antibody response *in vitro*, in: *Biology of the Lymphokines* (S. Cohen, E. Pick, M. Landy, and J. J. Oppenheim, eds.), pp. 325–346, Academic Press, New York

Fevrier, M., Birrien, J. L., LeClerc, C., Chedid, L., and Liacopoulos, P., 1978, The macrophage, target cell of the synthetic adjuvant muramyl dipeptide (MDP), *Eur. J. Immunol.* **8**:558.

Galelli, A., Le Garrec, Y., Chedid, L., Lefrancher, P., Derrien, M., and Level, M., 1980, Macrophage stimulation *in vitro* by an inactive muramyl dipeptide derivative after conjugation to a multi-poly(DL-alanyl)-poly(L-lysine) carrier, *Infect. Immun.* **28**:1.

Galland, R. B., Trachtenberg, L. S., Rynerson, N., and Polk, H. C., Jr., 1982, Non-specific enhancement of resistance to local bacterial infection in starved mice, *Arch. Surg. (Chicago)* **117**:161.

Gery, I., and Waksman, B., 1972, Potentiation of the T-lymphocyte response to mitogens. II. The cellular source of potentiating mediator(s), *J. Exp. Med.* **136**:143.

Gillis, S., and Mizel, S. B., 1981, T-cell lymphoma model for the analysis of interleukin l-mediated T-cell activation, *Proc. Natl. Acad. Sci. USA* **78**:1133.

Golub, E. S., and Weigle, W. O., 1967, Studies on the induction of immunologic unresponsiveness. I. Effects of endotoxin and phytohemagglutinin, *J. Immunol.* **98**:1241.

Gordon, S., Unkeless, J. C., and Cohn, Z. A., 1974, Induction of macrophage plasminogen activator by endotoxin stimulation and phagocytosis, *J. Exp. Med.* **140**:995.

Gordon, W. C., Prager, M. D., and Carroll, M. C., 1980, The enhancement of humoral and cellular immune responses by dimethyldioctadecylammonium bromide, *Cell. Immunol.* **49**:329.

Goren, M. B., Brokl, O., and Schaefer, W. B., 1974, Lipids of putative relevance to virulence in *Mycobacterium tuberculosis:* Correlation of virulence with elaboration of sulfatides and strongly acidic lipids, *Infect. Immun.* **9**:142.

Hadden, J. W., 1978, Effects of isoprinosine, levamisole, muramyl dipeptide and SM 1213 on lymphocyte and macrophage function *in vitro*, *Cancer Treat. Rep.* **62**:1981.

Hadden, J., and Englard, A., 1979, Molecular aspects of macrophage activation and proliferation, in: *Pharmacology of Immunoregulation* (G. Werner, ed.), p. 273, Academic Press, New York.

Hadden, J. W., Englard, A., Sadlik, J. R., and Hadden, E. M., 1979, The comparative effects of isoprinosine, levamisole, muramyl dipeptide and SM 1213 on lymphocyte and macrophage proliferation and activation *in vitro*, *Int. J. Immunopharmacol.* **1**:17.

Hoffmann, M. K., Galanos, C., Koenig, S., and Oettgen, H. F., 1977, B-cell activation by lipopolysaccharide: Distinct pathways for induction of mitosis and antibody production, *J. Exp. Med.* **146**:1640.

Humphrey, J. H., and Turk, J. L., 1963, The effect of an unrelated delayed-type hypersensitivity reaction on the antibody response to diphtheria toxoid, *Immunology* **6**:119.

Imai, K., Tomioka, M., Nagao, S., Kushima, K., and Tanaka, A., 1980, Biochemical evidence for activation of guinea pig macrophages by muramyl dipeptide, *Biomed. Res.* **1**:300.

Johnson, A. G., 1976, The adjuvant action of synthetic polynucleotides on the immune response, in: *Immune RNA* (E. P. Cohen, ed.), p. 17, CRC Press, Cleveland.

Johnson, A. G., 1979, Modulation of the immune system by synthetic polynucleotides, *Springer Semin. Immunopathol.* **2**:149.

Johnson, A. G., Gaines, S., and Landy, M., 1956, Studies on the O antigen of *Salmonella typhosa*. V. Enhancement of antibody response to protein antigen by the purified lipopolysaccharide, *J. Exp. Med.* **103**:225.

Johnson, H. G., and Johnson, A. G., 1971, Regulation of the immune system by synthetic polynucleotides, *J. Exp. Med.* **133**:649.

Juy, D., and Chedid, L., 1975, Comparison between macrophage activation and enhancement of nonspecific resistance to tumors by mycobacterial immunoadjuvants, *Proc. Natl. Acad. Sci. USA* **72**:4105.

Kiyono, H., McGhee, J. R., Kearney, J. F., and Michalek, S. M., 1981, Enhancement of *in vitro* immune responses of murine Peyer's patch cultures by concanavalin A, muramyl dipeptide and lipopolysaccharide, *Scand. J. Immunol.* **15**:329.

Koopman, W. J., Farrar, J. J., Oppenheim, J. J., Fullar-Bonar, J., and Dougherty, S., 1977, Association of a low molecular weight helper factor(s) with thymocyte proliferative activity, *J. Immunol.* **119**:55.

Kurland, J. I., and Bockman, R. S., 1978, Prostaglandin E production by human blood monocytes and mouse peritoneal macrophages, *J. Exp. Med.* **147**:952.

Lederer, E., Adam, A., Ciorbaru, R., Petit, J. F., and Wietzerbin, J., 1975, Cell walls of *Mycobacteria* and related organisms: Chemistry and immunostimulant properties, *Mol. Cell. Biochem.* **7**:87.

Lin, H., Medoff, G., and Kobayashi, G. S., 1977, Effects of amphotericin B on macrophages and their precursor cells, *Antimicrob. Agents Chemother.* **11**:154.

Luderitz, O., Westphal, O., Staub, A. M., and Nikaido, H., 1971, Isolation and chemical and immunological characterization of bacterial lipopolysaccharides, in: *Microbial Toxins, Vol. IV* (G. Weinbaum, S. Kadis, and S. J. Ajl, eds.), pp. 145–233, Academic Press, New York.

McGhee, J. R., Farrar, J. J., Michalek, S. M., Mergenhagen, S. E., and Rosenstreich, D. L., 1979, Cellular requirements for lipopolysaccharide adjuvanticity, *J. Exp. Med.* **149**:793.

Maehara, N., and Ho, M., 1977, Cellular origin of interferon induced by bacterial lipopolysaccharide, *Infect. Immun.* **15**:78.

Matter, A., 1979, The effects of muramyl dipeptide (MDP) in cell-mediated immunity: A comparison between *in vitro* and *in vivo* systems, *Cancer Immunol. Immunother.* **6**:201.

Meltzer, M. S., and Oppenheim, J. J., 1977, Biodirectional amplification of macrophage–lymphocyte interactions: Enhanced lymphocyte activation factor production by activated adherent mouse peritoneal cells, *J. Immunol.* **118**:77.

Michalek, S. M., Moore, R. N., McGhee, J. R., Rosenstreich, D. L., and Mergenhagen, S. E., 1980, The primary role of lymphoreticular cells in the mediation of host responses to bacterial endotoxin, *J. Infect. Dis.* **141**:55.

Morris, C. K., and Johnson, A. G., 1978, Regulation of the immune system by synthetic polynucleotides. VII. Suppression induced by pretreatment with poly A : U, *Cell. Immunol.* **39**:345.

Munder, P. G., and Modelell, M., 1973, Adjuvant induced formation of lysophosphatides and their role in the immune response, *Int. Arch. Allergy Appl. Immunol.* **45**:133.

Nagao, S., Tanaka, A., Yamamoto, Y., Koga, T., Onoue, K., Shiba, T., Kusumoto, K., and Kotani, S., 1979, Inhibition of macrophage migration by muramyl peptides, *Infect. Immun.* **24**:308.

Nagao, S., Miki, T., and Tanaka, A., 1981, Macrophage activation by muramyl dipeptide (MDP) without lymphocyte participation, *Microbiol. Immunol.* **25**:41.

Neter, E., 1969, Endotoxin and the immune response, *Curr. Top. Microbiol. Immunol.* **47**:82.

Neumann, C., 1979, Is the induction of macrophage-interferon a parameter for adjuvant activity?, *J. Invest. Dermatol.* **72**:273.

Nozawa, R. T., Sekiguchi, R., and Yokota, T., 1980, Stimulation by conditioned medium of L 929 fibroblasts, *E. coli* lipopolysaccharide and muramyl dipeptide of candidocidal activity of mouse macrophages, *Cell. Immunol.* **53**:116.

Oehler, J. R., Herberman, R. B., and Holden, H. T., 1978, Modulation of immunity by macrophages, *Pharmacol. Ther. A* **2**:551.

Oppenheim, J. J., and Rosenstreich, D. L., 1976, Signals regulating *in vitro* activation of lymphocytes, *Prog. Allergy* **20**:65.

Oppenheim, J. J., and Seeger, R. C., 1976, The role of macrophages in the induction of cell-mediated immunity *in vitro*, in: *Immunobiology of the Macrophage* (D. S. Nelson, ed.), pp. 111–130, Academic Press, New York.

Oppenheim, J. J., Moore, R., Gmelig-Meyling, F., Togawa, A., Wahl, S., Mathieson, B. J., Dougherty, S., and Carter, C., 1980a, Role of cytokine- and endotoxin-induced monokines in lymphocyte proliferation, differentiation, and immunoglobulin production, in: *Macrophage Regulation of Immunity* (E. R. Unanue and A. S. Rosenthal, eds.), pp. 379–398, Academic Press, New York.

Oppenheim, J. J., Togawa, A., Chedid, L., and Mizel, S., 1980b, Components of mycobacteria and muramyl dipeptide with adjuvant activity induce lymphocyte activating factor, *Cell. Immunol.* **50**:71.

Pabst, M. J., and Johnston, R. B., 1980, Increased production of superoxide anion by macrophages exposed *in vitro* to muramyl dipeptides or lipopolysaccharide, *J. Exp. Med.* **151**:101.

Pabst, M. J., Cummings, N. P., Shiba, T., Kusumoto, S., and Kotani, S., 1980, Lipophilic derivative of muramyl dipeptide is more active than muramyl dipeptide in priming macrophages to release superoxide anion, *Infect. Immun.* **29**:617.

Parant, M., 1980, Biological properties of a new synthetic adjuvant, muramyl di-peptide (MDP), in: *Immunostimulation* (L. Chedid, P.-A. Miescher and H. J. Mueller-Eberhard, eds.), pp. 111–128, Springer-Verlag, Berlin.

Parant, M., Parant, F., and Chedid, L., 1978a, Enhancement of the neonate's nonspecific immunity to *Klebsiella* infection by muramyl dipeptide, a synthetic immunoadjuvant, *Proc. Natl. Acad. Sci. USA* **75**:3395.

Parant, M., Damais, C., Audibert, F., Parant, F., Chedid, L., Sache, E., Lefrancier, P., Choay, J., and Lederer, E., 1978b, *In vivo* and *in vitro* stimulation of nonspecific immunity by the β-D-*p*-aminophenyl glycoside of *N*-acetylmuramyl-L-alanyl-D-isoglutamine and an oligomer prepared by cross-linking with glutaraldehyde, *J. Infect. Dis.* **138**:378.

Parant, M., Riveau, G., and Chedid, L., 1980, Influence of indomethacin on various immunopharmacological effects of muramyl dipeptide (MDP), *Agents Actions [Suppl]* **7**:33.

Parant, M. A., Audibert, F. M., Chedid, L., Level, M. R., Lefrancier, P. L., Choay, J. P., and Lederer, E., 1981, Immunostimulant activities of a lipophilic muramyl dipeptide derivative, and of des-muramyl peptidolipid analogs, *Infect. Immun.* **27**:826.

Renoux, G., 1980, Trends in immunopotentiation, *Int. J. Immunopharmacol.* **2**:1.

Rosenstreich, D., and Glode, L., 1975, Difference in B-cell mitogen responsiveness between closely related strains of mice, *J. Immunol.* **115**:777.

Rosenstreich, D. L., and Mizel, S. B., 1978, The participation of macrophages and macrophage cell lines in the activation of T lymphocytes by mitogens, *Immunol. Rev.* **40**:102.

Rosenstreich, D. L., and Vogel, S. N., 1980, Central role of macrophages in the host response to endotoxin, in: *Microbiology 1980* (D. Schlessinger, ed.), pp. 11–15, Am. Soc. Microbiology, Washington, D.C.

Ruco, L. P., Meltzer, M. S., and Rosenstreich, D. L., 1978, Macrophage activation for tumor cytotoxicity: Control of macrophage tumoricidal capacity by the LPS gene, *J. Immunol.* **121**:543.

Schmidtke, J. R., and Dixon, F. J., 1972, Immune response to a hapten coupled to a nonimmunogenic carrier: Influence of lipopolysaccharide, J. Exp. Med. **136**:392.

Schmidtke, J. R., and Johnson, A. G., 1971, Regulation of the immune system by synthetic polynucleotides. I. Characterization of adjuvant action on antibody synthesis, *J. Immunol.* **106**:1191.

Schultz, R. M., 1980, Macrophage activation by interferons, in: *Lymphokine Reports*, Vol. 1 (E. Pick, ed.), pp. 63–97, Academic Press, New York.

Schultz, R. M., and Chirigos, M. A., 1979, Selective neutralization by anti-interferon globulin of macrophage activation of L-cell interferon, *Brucella abortus* ether extract, *Salmonella typhimurium* lipopolysaccharide, and polyanions, *Cell Immunol.* **48**:52.

Schultz, R. M., and Chirigos, M. A., 1980, Macrophage activation for nonspecific tumor cytotoxicity, in: *Advances in Pharmacology and Chemotherapy*, Vol. 17 (R. J. Schnitzer, ed.), pp. 157–193, Academic Press, New York.

Schultz, R. M., Papamatheakis, J. D., and Chirigos, M. A., 1977, Interferon: An inducer of macrophage activation by polyanions, *Science* **197**:674.

Schultz, R. M., Pavlidis, N. A., and Chirigos, M. A., 1978, Macrophage involvement in the antitumor activity of *Brucella abortus* ether extract (Bru-Pel) against experimental lung carcinoma metastases, *Cancer Res.* **38**:3427.

Schultz, R. M., Stoychkov, J. N., Pavlidis, N., Chirigos, M. A., and Olkowski, Z. L., 1979, Role of E-type prostaglandins in the regulation of interferon-treated macrophage cytotoxic activity, *J. Reticuloendothelial Soc.* **26**:93.

Skidmore, B. J., Chiller, J. M., Morrison, D. C., and Weigle, W. O., 1975, Immunologic properties of bacterial lipopolysaccharides (LPS): Correlation between mitogenic, adjuvant and immunogenic activities, *J. Immunol.* **114**:770.

Sone, S., and Fidler, I. J., 1980, Synergistic activation by lymphokines and muramyl dipeptide of tumoricidal properties in rat alveolar macrophages, *J. Immunol.* **125**:2454.

Sone, S., and Fidler, I. J., 1981, *In vitro* activation of tumoricidal properties in rat alveolar macrophages by synthetic muramyl dipeptide encapsulated in liposomes, *Cell Immunol.* **57**:42.

Spitznagel, J. K., and Allison, A. C., 1970, Mode of action of adjuvants: Effects of antibody responses to macrophage-associated bovine serum albumin, *J. Immunol.* **104**:128.

Staber, F. G., Gisler, R. H., Schumann, G., Tarcsay, L., Schlafli, E., and Dukor, P., 1978, Modulation of myelopoiesis by different bacterial cell-wall components: Induction of colony-stimulating activity (by pure preparations, low-molecular-weight, degradation products and a synthetic low-molecular analog of bacterial cell-wall components) *in vitro*, *Cell. Immunol.* **37**:174.

Stadler, B. M., and De Weck, A. L., 1980, Flow-cytometric analysis of mouse peritoneal macrophages, *Cell. Immunol.* **54**:36.

Stein, S. H., Plut, E. J., Shine, T. E., and Little, J. R., 1978, The importance of different murine cell types in the immunopotentiation produced by amphotericin methyl ester, *Cell. Immunol.* **40**:211.

Tagliabue, A., McCoy, J. L., and Herberman, R., 1978, Refractoriness to migration inhibitory factor of macrophages of LPS nonresponder mouse strains, *J. Immunol.* **121**:1223.

Takada, H., Tsujimoto, M., Kato, K., Kotani, S., Kusumoto, S., Inage, M., Shiba, T., Yano, I., Kawata, S., and Yokogawa, K., 1979, Macrophage activation by bacterial cell walls and related synthetic compounds, *Infect. Immun.* **25**:48.

Tanaka, A., Nagao, S., Saito, R., Kotani, S., Kusumoto, S., and Shiba, T., 1977, Correlation of stereochemically specific structure in muramyl dipeptide between macrophage activation and adjuvant activity, *Biochem. Biophys. Res. Commun.* **77**:621.

Tanaka, A., Nagao, S., Nagao, R., Kotani, S., Shiba, T., and Kusumoto, S., 1979, Stimulation of the reticuloendothelial system of mice by muramyl dipeptide, *Infect. Immun.* **24**:302.

Tanaka, A., Nagao, S., Imai, K., and Mori, R., 1980, Macrophage activation by muramyl dipeptide as measured by macrophage spreading and attachment, *Microbiol. Immunol.* **24**:547.

Taniyama, T., and Holden, H. T., 1979, Direct augmentation of cytolytic activity of tumor-derived macrophages and macrophage cell lines by muramyl dipeptide, *Cell. Immunol.* **48**:369.

Tarnowski, G. S., Mountain, I. M., Stock, C. C., Munder, P. G., Weltzein, H. U., and Westphal, O., 1978, Effect of lysolecithin and analogs on mouse ascites tumors, *Cancer Res.* **38**:339.

Tenu, J. P., Lederer, E., and Petit, J. F., 1980, Stimulation of thymocyte mitogenic protein secretion and of cytostatic activity of mouse peritoneal macrophages by trehalose dimycolate and muramyl dipeptide, *Eur. J. Immunol.* **10**:647.

Turner, E. V., and Higginbotham, R. D., 1979, Effects of intravenous carrageenan on immune responses and on the reticuloendothelial system, *J. Reticuloendothelial Soc.* **26:**763.

Unanue, E. R., 1972, The regulatory role of macrophages in antigenic stimulation, *Adv. Immunol.* **15:**95.

Unanue, E. R., 1978, The regulation of lymphocyte functions by the macrophage, *Immunol. Rev.* **40:**227.

Unanue, E. R., 1980, Cooperation between mononuclear phagocytes and lymphocytes in immunity, *N. Engl. J. Med.* **303:**997.

Unanue, E. R., Askonas, B. A., and Allison, A. C., 1969, A role of macrophages in the stimulation of immune responses by adjuvants, *J. Immunol.* **103:**71.

Unanue, E. R., Keily, J. M., and Calderon, J., 1976, The modulation of lymphocyte functions by molecules secreted by macrophages, *J. Exp. Med.* **144:**155.

Van Der Meer, C., Hofhuis, F. M. A., and Willers, J. M. N., 1979, Delayed-type hypersensitivity and acquired cellular resistance in mice immunized with killed *Listeria monocytogenes* and adjuvants, *Immunology* **37:**77.

van Rooijen, N., and van Nieuwmegen, R., 1979, Liposomes in immunology: Impairment of the adjuvant effect of liposomes by incorporation of the adjuvant lysolecithin and the role of macrophages, *Immunol. Commun.* **8**(4):381.

Vogel, S. N., Marshall, S. T., and Rosenstreich, D. L., 1979, Analysis of the effects of lipopolysaccharide on macrophages: Differential phagocytic responses of C3H/HeN and C3H/HeJ macrophages *in vitro*, *Infect. Immun.* **25:**328.

Vogel, S. N., Weinblatt, A. C., and Rosenstreich, D. L., 1981, Inherent macrophage defects in mice, in: *Immunologic Defects in Laboratory Animals, Volume 1* (M. E. Gershwin and B. Merchant, eds.), pp. 327–357, Plenum Press, New York.

Wahl, L. M., Olsen, C. E., Sandberg, A. L., and Mergenhagen, S. E., 1977, Prostaglandin regulation of macrophage collagenase production, *Proc. Natl. Acad. Sci. USA* **74:**4955.

Wahl, L. M., Wahl, S. M., and McCarthy, J. B., 1980, Adjuvant activation of macrophage functions, in: *Macrophage Regulation of Immunity* (E. R. Unanue and A. S. Rosenthal, eds.), pp. 491–504, Academic Press, New York.

Wahl, S. M., Wahl, L. M., McCarthy, J. B., Chedid, L., and Mergenhagen, S., 1979, Macrophage activation by mycobacterial water-soluble components and synthetic muramyl dipeptide, *J. Immunol.* **122:**2226.

Waters, R. V., and Ferraresi, R. W., 1980, Muramyl dipeptide stimulation of particle clearance in several animal species, *J. Reticuloendothelial Soc.* **28:**457.

Watson, J., and Riblet, R., 1974, Genetic control of responses to bacterial lipopolysaccharides in mice. I. Evidence for a single gene that influences mitogenic responses to lipopolysaccharides, *J. Exp. Med.* **140:**1147.

Watson, J., and Riblet, R., 1975, Genetic control of responses to bacterial lipopolysaccharides in mice. II. A gene that influences a membrane component involved in the activation of bone marrow derived lymphocytes by lipopolysaccharides, *J. Immunol.* **114:**1462.

Weinberg, J. B., Chapman, H. A., and Hibbs, J. B., 1978, Characterization of the effects of endotoxin on macrophage tumor cell killing, *J. Immunol.* **121:**72.

Winchurch, R., and Braun, W., 1969, Antibody formation: Premature initiation by endotoxin or synthetic polynucleotides in newborn mice, *Nature (London)* **223:**843.

Wood, D. D., 1979a, Purification and properties of human B cell-activating factor, *J. Immunol.* **123:**2395.

Wood, D. D., 1979b, Mechanism of action of human B cell-activating factor, *J. Immunol.* **123:**2400.

Wood, D. D., and Gaul, S. L., 1974, Enhancement of the humoral response of T cell-depleted murine spleens by a factor derived from human monocytes *in vitro*, *J. Immunol.* **113:**925.

Wood, D. D., and Staruch, M. J., 1980, Biochemical properties and cellular requirements of BAF, in: *Biochemical Characterization of Lymphokines* (A. L. de Weck, F. Kristensen, and M. Landy, eds.), pp. 423–425, Academic Press, New York.

Yamamoto, Y., Nagao, S., Tanaka, T., Koga, T., and Inoue, K., 1978, Inhibition of macrophage migration by synthetic muramyl dipeptide, *Biochem. Biophys. Res. Commun.* **80:**923.

Index

GPSR Compliance

The European Union's (EU) General Product Safety Regulation (GPSR) is a set of rules that requires consumer products to be safe and our obligations to ensure this.

If you have any concerns about our products, you can contact us on ProductSafety@springernature.com

In case Publisher is established outside the EU, the EU authorized representative is:

Springer Nature Customer Service Center GmbH
Europaplatz 3
69115 Heidelberg, Germany

Batch number: 10838290

Printed by Printforce, the Netherlands